Metaverse Applications for Intelligent Healthcare

Loveleen Gaur
University of South Pacific, Fiji & Taylor's University, Malaysia

Noor Zaman Jhanjhi
Taylor's University, Malaysia

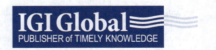

A volume in the Advances in Medical Technologies and Clinical Practice (AMTCP) Book Series

Published in the United States of America by
IGI Global
Medical Information Science Reference (an imprint of IGI Global)
701 E. Chocolate Avenue
Hershey PA, USA 17033
Tel: 717-533-8845
Fax: 717-533-8661
E-mail: cust@igi-global.com
Web site: http://www.igi-global.com

Copyright © 2024 by IGI Global. All rights reserved. No part of this publication may be reproduced, stored or distributed in any form or by any means, electronic or mechanical, including photocopying, without written permission from the publisher.
Product or company names used in this set are for identification purposes only. Inclusion of the names of the products or companies does not indicate a claim of ownership by IGI Global of the trademark or registered trademark.

Library of Congress Cataloging-in-Publication Data

Names: Gaur, Loveleen, editor. | Zaman, Noor, 1972- editor.
Title: Metaverse applications for intelligent healthcare / edited by
   Loveleen Gaur, and Noor Zaman Jhanjhi.
Description: Hershey, PA : Medical Information Science Reference, [2023] |
   Includes bibliographical references and index. | Summary: "This book
   introduces various applications of the metaverse in healthcare,
   including virtual consultations, remote patient monitoring, and virtual
   rehabilitation. The book discusses how the metaverse can be used to
   provide immersive experiences that empower patients and providers, while
   also offering unique learning opportunities. The book is ideal for
   researchers, practitioners, healthcare professionals, scholars, and
   students who are interested in exploring the cutting-edge technology of
   AI and the metaverse in healthcare. It offers insights into the future
   of healthcare, and how these technologies can be used to provide better
   care to patients. By combining the latest research in AI and the
   metaverse, this book provides a comprehensive overview of the potential
   applications of these technologies in healthcare"-- Provided by
   publisher.
Identifiers: LCCN 2023025174 (print) | LCCN 2023025175 (ebook) | ISBN
   9781668498231 (hardcover) | ISBN 9781668498248 (ebook)
Subjects: MESH: Artificial Intelligence | Virtual Reality |
   Telerehabilitation | Hospital Information Systems
Classification: LCC R859 (print) | LCC R859 (ebook) | NLM W 26.55.A7 |
   DDC 362.10285--dc23/eng/20230630
LC record available at https://lccn.loc.gov/2023025174
LC ebook record available at https://lccn.loc.gov/2023025175

This book is published in the IGI Global book series Advances in Medical Technologies and Clinical Practice (AMTCP) (ISSN: 2327-9354; eISSN: 2327-9370)

British Cataloguing in Publication Data
A Cataloguing in Publication record for this book is available from the British Library.

All work contributed to this book is new, previously-unpublished material.
The views expressed in this book are those of the authors, but not necessarily of the publisher.

For electronic access to this publication, please contact: eresources@igi-global.com.

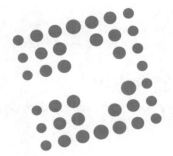

Advances in Medical Technologies and Clinical Practice (AMTCP) Book Series

ISSN:2327-9354
EISSN:2327-9370

Editor-in-Chief: Srikanta Patnaik, SOA University, India

MISSION

Medical technological innovation continues to provide avenues of research for faster and safer diagnosis and treatments for patients. Practitioners must stay up to date with these latest advancements to provide the best care for nursing and clinical practices.

The **Advances in Medical Technologies and Clinical Practice (AMTCP) Book Series** brings together the most recent research on the latest technology used in areas of nursing informatics, clinical technology, biomedicine, diagnostic technologies, and more. Researchers, students, and practitioners in this field will benefit from this fundamental coverage on the use of technology in clinical practices.

COVERAGE

- Nutrition
- Nursing Informatics
- Patient-Centered Care
- E-Health
- Telemedicine
- Clinical Studies
- Neural Engineering
- Clinical Nutrition
- Medical Imaging
- Biomechanics

IGI Global is currently accepting manuscripts for publication within this series. To submit a proposal for a volume in this series, please contact our Acquisition Editors at Acquisitions@igi-global.com or visit: http://www.igi-global.com/publish/.

The Advances in Medical Technologies and Clinical Practice (AMTCP) Book Series (ISSN 2327-9354) is published by IGI Global, 701 E. Chocolate Avenue, Hershey, PA 17033-1240, USA, www.igi-global.com. This series is composed of titles available for purchase individually; each title is edited to be contextually exclusive from any other title within the series. For pricing and ordering information please visit http://www.igi-global.com/book-series/advances-medical-technologies-clinical-practice/73682. Postmaster: Send all address changes to above address. Copyright © 2024 IGI Global. All rights, including translation in other languages reserved by the publisher. No part of this series may be reproduced or used in any form or by any means – graphics, electronic, or mechanical, including photocopying, recording, taping, or information and retrieval systems – without written permission from the publisher, except for non commercial, educational use, including classroom teaching purposes. The views expressed in this series are those of the authors, but not necessarily of IGI Global.

Titles in this Series

For a list of additional titles in this series, please visit:
http://www.igi-global.com/book-series/advances-medical-technologies-clinical-practice/73682

AI-Based Digital Health Communication for Securing Assistive Systems
Vijeyananthan Thayananthan (University of South Wales, UK)
Medical Information Science Reference • © 2023 • 299pp • H/C (ISBN: 9781668489383) • US $325.00

AI and IoT-Based Technologies for Precision Medicine
Alex Khang (Global Research Institute of Technology and Engineering, USA)
Engineering Science Reference • © 2023 • 562pp • H/C (ISBN: 9798369308769) • US $360.00

Wearable and Implantable Electrocardiography for Early Detection of Cardiovascular Diseases
Shaik Asif Hussain (Middle East College, Oman) J. Chinna Babu Jyothi (Annamacharya Institute of Technology and Sciences, India) and Nizar Albassam (Middle East College, Oman)
Medical Information Science Reference • © 2023 • 158pp • H/C (ISBN: 9781668448755) • US $315.00

Advancements in Bio-Medical Image Processing and Authentication in Telemedicine
Rijwan Khan (ABES Institute of Technology, India) and Indrajeet Kumar (Graphic Era Hill University, Dehradun, India)
Medical Information Science Reference • © 2023 • 380pp • H/C (ISBN: 9781668469576) • US $325.00

Recent Advancements in Smart Remote Patient Monitoring, Wearable Devices, and Diagnostics Systems
Furkh Zeshan (COMSATS University Islamabad, Lahore, Pakistan) and Adnan Ahmad (COMSATS University Islamabad, Lahore, Pakistan)
Medical Information Science Reference • © 2023 • 274pp • H/C (ISBN: 9781668464342) • US $345.00

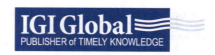

701 East Chocolate Avenue, Hershey, PA 17033, USA
Tel: 717-533-8845 x100 • Fax: 717-533-8661
E-Mail: cust@igi-global.com • www.igi-global.com

Table of Contents

Preface xiv

Chapter 1
Demystifying Metaverse Applications for Intelligent Healthcare 1
    Loveleen Gaur, Taylor's University, Malaysia
    Devanshi Gaur, Florida International University, USA
    Anam Afaq, Amity University, Noida, India

Chapter 2
Metaverse: Virtual Gyms and Sports 24
    Siva Raja Sindiramutty, Taylor's University, Malaysia
    Noor Zaman Jhanjhi, Taylor's University, Malaysia
    Sayan Kumar Ray, Taylor's University, Malaysia
    Husin Jazri, Taylor's University, Malaysia
    Navid Ali Khan, Taylor's University, Malaysia
    Loveleen Gaur, University of the South Pacific, Fiji
    Abdalla Gharib, Zanzibar University, Tanzania
    Amaranadha Reddy Manchuri, Kyungpook National University, South Korea

Chapter 3
Metaverse: Virtual Meditation 93
    Siva Raja Sindiramutty, Taylor's University, Malaysia
    Noor Zaman Jhanjhi, Taylor's University, Malaysia
    Sayan Kumar Ray, Taylor's University, Malaysia
    Husin Jazri, Taylor's University, Malaysia
    Navid Ali Khan, Taylor's University, Malaysia
    Loveleen Gaur, University of the South Pacific, Fiji

Chapter 4
A Combined Survey on Machine Learning for Cognitive Radio Deployed on
Secure WBAN Environments 159
    M. V. Karthikeyan, St. Joseph's Institute of Technology, India
    Tephillah Sophia, St. Joseph's Institute of Technology, India
    M. Senthil Murugan, St. Joseph's Institute of Technology, India
    D. Suresh, St. Joseph's Institute of Technology, India
    M. Samayaraj Murali Kishanlal, St. Joseph's Institute of Technology, India
    T. Siva, St. Joseph's Institute of Technology, India

Chapter 5
A Metaverse-Based Approach to Rehabilitation Healthcare 182
    V. Vivekitha, Sri Ramakrishna Engineering College, India
    S. Caroline Vinnetia, Bannari Amman Institute of Technology, India
    R. Sri Roshini, Dr. N.G.P. Institute of Technology, India

Chapter 6
Deep Learning Perspectives for Prediction of Diabetic Foot Ulcers 203
    Aman Sharma, Jaypee University of Information Technology, India
    Archit Kaushal, Jaypee University of Information Technology, India
    Kartik Dogra, Jaypee University of Information Technology, India
    Rajni Mohana, Jaypee University of Information Technology, India

Chapter 7
Metaverse System for Patients` Safety 229
    Calin Ciufudean, Stefan cel Mare University, Romania
    Corneliu Buzduga, Ştefan cel Mare University, Romania

Chapter 8
Ethical Considerations in the Use of the Metaverse for Healthcare 248
    Loveleen Gaur, Taylor's University, Malaysia
    Devanshi Gaur, Florida International University, USA
    Anam Afaq, Amity University, Noida, India

Chapter 9
Metaverse for Healthcare: Possible Potential Applications (Virtual Reality
Technologies), Opportunities, Challenges, and Future Directions 274
    Hafiz Asif, Islamia University of Bahawalpur, Pakistan
    Rabia Zahid, Islamia University of Bahawalpur, Pakistan
    Uzma Bashir, Islamia University of Bahawalpur, Pakistan
    Waseem Afzal, Islamia University of Bahawalpur, Pakistan

Misbah Firdous, Islamia University of Bahawalpur, Pakistan
Ahsan Zahid, Islamia University of Bahawalpur, Pakistan
Muhammad Hasnain, Islamia University of Bahawalpur, Pakistan

Chapter 10
The Future of Telemedicine: Emerging Technologies, Challenges, and
Opportunities 306
    Robertas Damaševičius, Vytautas Magnus University, Lithuania
    Olusola O. Abayomi-Alli, Kaunas University of Technology, Lithuania

Compilation of References 339

About the Contributors 400

Index 404

Detailed Table of Contents

Preface xiv

Chapter 1
Demystifying Metaverse Applications for Intelligent Healthcare 1
    Loveleen Gaur, Taylor's University, Malaysia
    Devanshi Gaur, Florida International University, USA
    Anam Afaq, Amity University, Noida, India

The metaverse is a virtual, interlinked digital world where users can connect, socialise, and participate in numerous activities using virtual, augmented, and other innovative technologies. It is a phrase borrowed from science fiction recently gaining popularity in the information and technology sector. It's a sizable, shared, 3D virtual environment that illustrates a collective, shared online space that stretches beyond traditional internet experiences. The chapter explores and investigates how immersive technologies, such as virtual reality, augmented reality, and others, might improve several facets of healthcare and make it more intelligent, effective, and patient-centred.

Chapter 2
Metaverse: Virtual Gyms and Sports 24
    Siva Raja Sindiramutty, Taylor's University, Malaysia
    Noor Zaman Jhanjhi, Taylor's University, Malaysia
    Sayan Kumar Ray, Taylor's University, Malaysia
    Husin Jazri, Taylor's University, Malaysia
    Navid Ali Khan, Taylor's University, Malaysia
    Loveleen Gaur, University of the South Pacific, Fiji
    Abdalla Gharib, Zanzibar University, Tanzania
    Amaranadha Reddy Manchuri, Kyungpook National University, South Korea

In recent years, the concept of the metaverse has garnered substantial attention as an emerging digital realm that combines virtual reality, augmented reality, and various interactive technologies to create immersive and interconnected digital spaces. As traditional fitness routines and sports activities transform due to technological advancements, virtual gyms and sports have emerged as innovative solutions to engage individuals in physical activities within the metaverse. Dive into the dynamic realm of the metaverse with this chapter on virtual gyms and sports. The metaverse's business models, user experience design, and scaling strategies are explored, as are its applications in healthcare, therapy, and sports training. As the curtain falls, the authors delve into virtual fan engagement, community building, and future trends. The dynamic landscape of the metaverse awaits your exploration within these pages. Join the researchers in navigating the boundless possibilities of virtual gyms and sports, unraveling their impact on society, industry, and beyond.

Chapter 3
Metaverse: Virtual Meditation 93
    Siva Raja Sindiramutty, Taylor's University, Malaysia
    Noor Zaman Jhanjhi, Taylor's University, Malaysia
    Sayan Kumar Ray, Taylor's University, Malaysia
    Husin Jazri, Taylor's University, Malaysia
    Navid Ali Khan, Taylor's University, Malaysia
    Loveleen Gaur, University of the South Pacific, Fiji

The rise of the metaverse as a digital domain for diverse activities has birthed an innovative application known as 'metaverse virtual meditation.' This concept seamlessly merges technology and mindfulness, employing virtual reality (VR) and augmented reality (AR) to craft serene digital landscapes. These immersive settings, ranging from natural vistas to abstract spaces, enable users to overcome physical constraints and distractions, facilitating mindfulness, stress reduction, and emotional resilience. The chapter navigates the fusion of technology and contemplative practices, from traditional meditation to modern VR and AR experiences. Stress reduction, heightened focus, and inclusivity are among the advantages highlighted. The convergence of visuals, biofeedback, brain-computer interfaces (BCIs), and AI-driven personalization is explored for tailored meditation. Design principles, interactive elements, and natural components play a crucial role in shaping tranquil virtual environments.

Chapter 4
A Combined Survey on Machine Learning for Cognitive Radio Deployed on
Secure WBAN Environments 159
    M. V. Karthikeyan, St. Joseph's Institute of Technology, India
    Tephillah Sophia, St. Joseph's Institute of Technology, India
    M. Senthil Murugan, St. Joseph's Institute of Technology, India
    D. Suresh, St. Joseph's Institute of Technology, India
    M. Samayaraj Murali Kishanlal, St. Joseph's Institute of Technology, India
    T. Siva, St. Joseph's Institute of Technology, India

Wireless body area network (WBAN) security and cognitive radio networks (CRNs) are two separate topics in the field of wireless communication, but they can be related in some ways. WBANs are wireless networks that are designed to operate on or around the human body, typically for medical or healthcare applications. These networks often involve small, low-power devices that can monitor vital signs, track movement, or even deliver medication. Security is a critical concern in WBANs, as they often deal with sensitive personal information and may be vulnerable to various types of attacks. Some of the security challenges in WBANs include confidentiality, integrity, availability, privacy, and authentication. CRNs are wireless networks that allow devices to dynamically adapt to their environment by changing their transmission and reception parameters. This technology can improve the efficiency and reliability of wireless communication, but it also introduces security challenges, an attacker may try to manipulate the cognitive radio's sensing mechanism or jam the spectrum to disrupt the network. potential connections between WBAN security and CRNs. For instance, cognitive radios can be used to enhance the security of WBANs by providing more secure communication channels or detecting and mitigating attacks. Some of the security mechanisms developed for WBANs, such as secure authentication and encryption protocols, can be applied to CRNs to improve their security posture. WBAN security and CRNs are distinct topics, there is potential for these technologies to complement each other and enhance the overall security of wireless networks. the relationship between WBAN and CRN's is the specific objective is the primarily centered around spectrum management, interference mitigation, and secure spectrum sharing. By intelligently adapting to the wireless environment and optimizing spectrum usage, CR can enhance the security and reliability of WBAN communication in healthcare and other contexts where WBANs are deployed.

Chapter 5
A Metaverse-Based Approach to Rehabilitation Healthcare 182
    V. Vivekitha, Sri Ramakrishna Engineering College, India
    S. Caroline Vinnetia, Bannari Amman Institute of Technology, India
    R. Sri Roshini, Dr. N.G.P. Institute of Technology, India

Rehabilitative healthcare is focused on restoring physical and cognitive abilities in individuals following injuries or diseases and has largely relied on traditional methods such as physical therapy and medical interventions over time. However, the metaverse, a collaborative virtual environment, has opened new possibilities for the field of rehabilitation. In comparison to traditional rehabilitation, this technology provides increased accessibility and convenience by allowing individuals to participate in therapy from the comfort of their own homes. The immersive and engaging nature of virtual reality (VR) and augmented reality (AR) technologies increases patient motivation and compliance with therapy regimens. Through the integration of telemedicine, wearable technologies, and artificial intelligence, rehabilitation can become more sophisticated and personalized. The use of these technologies can enable the acquisition, analysis, and tracking of patient data, as well as providing real-time feedback for the improvement of treatment regimens and outcomes.

Chapter 6
Deep Learning Perspectives for Prediction of Diabetic Foot Ulcers 203
    Aman Sharma, Jaypee University of Information Technology, India
    Archit Kaushal, Jaypee University of Information Technology, India
    Kartik Dogra, Jaypee University of Information Technology, India
    Rajni Mohana, Jaypee University of Information Technology, India

A significant complication of diabetes mellitus, diabetic foot ulcers (DFUs), can have devastating repercussions if they are not identified and treated right away. Machine learning algorithms have gained more attention recently for their potential to anticipate DFUs before they manifest, enabling early management and preventing consequences. In this chapter, the authors examine how convolutional neural networks (CNNs) can be used to forecast DFUs. The performance of DenseNet, EfficientNet, and a regular CNN are specifically compared. With labels identifying the presence or absence of a DFU, the authors use a dataset of medical photographs of diabetic feet to train each model. The objective is to assess the effectiveness of these models and look at how each layer affects the precision of the predictions. The authors also hope to provide some light on how the algorithms are able to pinpoint foot regions that are most likely to get DFUs. They also look into how each CNN model's different layers affect prediction accuracy.

Chapter 7
Metaverse System for Patients` Safety 229
    Calin Ciufudean, Stefan cel Mare University, Romania
    Corneliu Buzduga, Ştefan cel Mare University, Romania

For the hospital environment information technology (IT) is essential, as it determines the quality of hospitalization of patients, and creates patterns that help organize medical activity conceptually, therefore it determines the quality of medical care, and ultimately it determines the security of patients and hospital personnel, both from the point of view of monitoring in real-time gas concentration (oxygen, CO, CO2) in hospital rooms, air humidity, air temperature, and pressure. The system the authors designed and developed is an application of Telemedicine with the main purpose to streamline the patients' and medical personnel's security in case of fire or an over-limit concentration of harmful gases. Data gathered by sensors are processed by a microcontroller and it is sent every quarter of an hour to medical personnel smartphones in a user-friendly graphical display.

Chapter 8
Ethical Considerations in the Use of the Metaverse for Healthcare 248
    Loveleen Gaur, Taylor's University, Malaysia
    Devanshi Gaur, Florida International University, USA
    Anam Afaq, Amity University, Noida, India

The promotion of augmenting and enhancing healthcare in the ethical metaverse setting should be guided by the fundamental bioethical principles of beneficence, nonmaleficence, autonomy, and justice, focusing on minimising risks and adverse outcomes. Implementing a patient-centred strategy and establishing responsible regulatory measures are essential for harnessing the advantages of metaverse technology in the healthcare sector while effectively tackling the associated problems. The chapter explores the ethical considerations surrounding using metaverse technology within the healthcare sector.

Chapter 9
Metaverse for Healthcare: Possible Potential Applications (Virtual Reality Technologies), Opportunities, Challenges, and Future Directions 274
    Hafiz Asif, Islamia University of Bahawalpur, Pakistan
    Rabia Zahid, Islamia University of Bahawalpur, Pakistan
    Uzma Bashir, Islamia University of Bahawalpur, Pakistan
    Waseem Afzal, Islamia University of Bahawalpur, Pakistan
    Misbah Firdous, Islamia University of Bahawalpur, Pakistan
    Ahsan Zahid, Islamia University of Bahawalpur, Pakistan
    Muhammad Hasnain, Islamia University of Bahawalpur, Pakistan

2021 is known as the first Year of the Metaverse, and around the world, internet giants are eager to devote themselves to it. Metaverse is the augmented virtual world formed by convergence of virtual and physical space. Users interact within this created world, meeting each other virtually, immersing themselves in performing virtual activities, which subsequently could lead to real experiences. Conventionally, the healthcare "industry" is conservative in deploying future ready technology. Demonstrating significant improvement in healthcare outcomes using the metaverse will be difficult to prove. This overview discusses the untapped potential of metaverse applications in healthcare, and also points out the advantages, disadvantages, limitations, and challenges in actual deployment of the metaverse in clinical practice in the real world. This alone will ultimately lead to the development of a business model, insurance reimbursement, and behavioral modification necessary for accepting and using a hitherto unused method in patient care.

Chapter 10
The Future of Telemedicine: Emerging Technologies, Challenges, and
Opportunities 306
    Robertas Damaševičius, Vytautas Magnus University, Lithuania
    Olusola O. Abayomi-Alli, Kaunas University of Technology, Lithuania

Telemedicine, or the delivery of healthcare services via distant communication technology, has grown in importance in recent years. Telemedicine has the ability to alter healthcare delivery and enhance access to treatment for patients in rural and underserved locations. However, there are significant barriers to mainstream telemedicine adoption and implementation, including data privacy and security, funding, and the need for standardization. The authors review telemedicine's current situation and future potential by discussing new technologies that will shape the future of telemedicine, such as 5G networks, augmented and virtual reality, and wearable gadgets. Then the chapter discusses the growing use of telemedicine and its role in improving access to healthcare in rural and underserved areas. In addition to discussing the benefits for telemedicine, the chapter delves into the problems and limits that must be solved before it may achieve its full potential. Finally, it analyzes the future of telemedicine, including prospective uses and interaction with traditional healthcare systems.

Compilation of References 339

About the Contributors 400

Index 404

Preface

In a rapidly evolving world, the intersection of healthcare, artificial intelligence, and the metaverse is ushering in a new era of possibilities. We are delighted to introduce *Metaverse Applications for Intelligent Healthcare*, a reference book that delves deep into the synergistic potential of AI and the metaverse to transform healthcare as we know it.

The age of artificial intelligence in healthcare has dawned, offering innovative solutions that extend far beyond traditional practices. AI is now an indispensable ally, aiding in diagnosis, treatment, and management of diverse medical conditions. From the analysis of medical images to drug discovery and patient care, it has opened up new frontiers in healthcare. As healthcare professionals, we recognize the profound impact AI has on our daily practices, and this book aims to provide a comprehensive guide to its applications in our field.

Simultaneously, the metaverse, a realm where real and virtual converge, has transcended the boundaries of gaming and entertainment to enter the domain of healthcare. In this virtual universe, healthcare professionals can interact with patients, conduct remote consultations, monitor health, and even facilitate rehabilitation. The metaverse is not just a space for recreation; it is an innovative tool for learning, empowerment, and delivering exceptional experiences to both patients and providers.

The amalgamation of AI and the metaverse in healthcare is a promising trend that holds the potential to revolutionize the industry. The book brings together insights from leading experts in the field to showcase how these technologies can make healthcare more accessible, efficient, and personalized. As technology continues to evolve, we anticipate a proliferation of AI and metaverse applications in healthcare, forever changing the way we deliver and receive medical care.

This reference book is aimed at a wide range of healthcare professionals, practitioners, and researchers seeking to harness the power of AI and the metaverse. From virtual reality in medical training to augmented reality in surgical procedures, from gamification in healthcare to telemedicine and mental health treatment using virtual platforms, this book covers a diverse array of topics that are of great relevance

Preface

in the modern healthcare landscape. We have also included discussions on wearable technology, the metaverse in radiology, and much more.

Chapter Overview

Chapter 1 takes an in-depth look at the metaverse, a virtual interconnected digital world where innovative technologies such as virtual reality and augmented reality converge. Explore how these immersive technologies can transform various aspects of healthcare, making it more intelligent, effective, and patient-centered.

Chapter 2 dives into the dynamic realm of the metaverse with a focus on virtual gyms and sports. Discover how the metaverse is reshaping traditional fitness routines and sports activities, offering innovative solutions for engaging individuals in physical activities. Explore its applications in healthcare, therapy, and sports training, and uncover the future trends and possibilities within this dynamic landscape.

Chapter 3 explores the innovative concept of "Metaverse Virtual Meditation." Learn how technology seamlessly merges with mindfulness, using virtual reality and augmented reality to create serene digital landscapes. Discover the advantages of this fusion, including stress reduction, heightened focus, and personalized meditation experiences. Explore the design principles and elements that shape tranquil virtual environments.

In chapter 4, we delve into the realms of Wireless Body Area Networks (WBANs) and Cognitive Radio Networks (CRNs) in this chapter. While they are distinct topics in wireless communication, find out how they can be related and explore the critical security concerns in WBANs. Discover the potential of CRNs to enhance wireless communication efficiency and reliability while addressing new security challenges.

Discover how the metaverse is transforming rehabilitative healthcare in Chapter 5. Explore the possibilities of virtual reality and augmented reality technologies for rehabilitation, offering increased accessibility and convenience for patients. Dive into the immersive and engaging nature of these technologies and how they enhance patient motivation and compliance. Learn how telemedicine, wearable technologies, and AI are advancing rehabilitation practices.

Explore the use of convolutional neural networks (CNNs) to predict diabetic foot ulcers (DFUs) in Chapter 6. Compare the performance of different CNN models and examine how they can identify foot regions susceptible to DFUs. Gain insights into the potential of machine learning to enable early management and prevention of DFUs.

Chapter 7 looks into the importance of information technology in hospital environments and its impact on patient safety. Explore a telemedicine application designed to enhance security by monitoring gas concentrations and environmental parameters. Learn how data from sensors are processed and transmitted to medical personnel's smartphones, ensuring patient safety in real-time.

Chapter 8 navigates the ethical considerations surrounding the use of the metaverse in healthcare. Explore how the principles of beneficence, nonmaleficence, autonomy, and justice guide the promotion of ethical metaverse healthcare. Learn how responsible regulatory measures and a patient-centered strategy are essential for leveraging metaverse technology while minimizing risks.

2021 marked the "Year of the Metaverse," and Chapter 9 discusses the potential of metaverse applications in healthcare. Explore the advantages, disadvantages, limitations, and challenges in deploying the metaverse in clinical practice. Understand how this technology can lead to the development of new business models, insurance reimbursement, and behavioral modifications in patient care.

Telemedicine's growth and potential are the focus of Chapter 10. Explore new technologies such as 5G networks, augmented and virtual reality, and wearable gadgets that will shape the future of telemedicine. Understand how telemedicine can improve healthcare access in rural and underserved areas while addressing challenges such as data privacy and security. Dive into the future of telemedicine and its interaction with traditional healthcare systems.

Our hope is that *Metaverse Applications for Intelligent Healthcare* serves as a valuable resource for our readers, guiding them through the evolving landscape of healthcare technologies. As healthcare transforms, let us embrace this revolution together, adapting, innovating, and delivering a brighter, healthier future for all.

With sincere dedication to the advancement of healthcare,

Loveleen Gaur
University of South Pacific, Fiji & Taylor's University, Malaysia

Noor Zaman Jhanjhi
Taylor's University, Malaysia

Chapter 1
Demystifying Metaverse Applications for Intelligent Healthcare

Loveleen Gaur
https://orcid.org/0000-0002-0885-1550
Taylor's University, Malaysia

Devanshi Gaur
Florida International University, USA

Anam Afaq
Amity University, Noida, India

ABSTRACT

The metaverse is a virtual, interlinked digital world where users can connect, socialise, and participate in numerous activities using virtual, augmented, and other innovative technologies. It is a phrase borrowed from science fiction recently gaining popularity in the information and technology sector. It's a sizable, shared, 3D virtual environment that illustrates a collective, shared online space that stretches beyond traditional internet experiences. The chapter explores and investigates how immersive technologies, such as virtual reality, augmented reality, and others, might improve several facets of healthcare and make it more intelligent, effective, and patient-centred.

DOI: 10.4018/978-1-6684-9823-1.ch001

1. INTRODUCTION

In our rapidly evolving world, technological advancements are mounting across every field, giving us a plentitude of opportunities for growth (Bhandari et al., 2022; Chaudhary et al., 2022a; Mathur and Gaur, 2021). The field of healthcare solutions is no exception, as it too moves forward in employing innovation to improve our well-being (Bhandari et al., 2022; Gaur, Afaq, Singh, et al., 2021). The idea of the metaverse has developed as one of these innovations that might completely alter the playing field. Users can explore virtual settings and engage with virtual objects and representations in immersive digital worlds called the metaverse. Through innovative and user-friendly applications, emerging metaverse technologies like virtual reality (VR), augmented reality (AR), and mixed reality (MR) are poised to revolutionise healthcare and medicine (Afaq et al., 2021; Rana et al., 2022). Healthcare workers can practise skills and procedures in lifelike 3D virtual environments by adopting metaverse-based simulations in medical education and training. Before high-risk surgeries, surgeons might practise complex systems (Santosh et al., 2021). Medical students can work together in the metaverse to visualise and interact with virtual patients, human anatomy, and simulated clinical scenarios.

Telehealth powered by the metaverse will enable doctors to interact with patients electronically and in real-time using 3D avatars for diagnosis and treatment (Ahmed, Biswas, et al., 2022; Gaur et al., 2023). Doctors may view virtual symptoms on a lifelike avatar body and graphically show treatments. When a doctor is performing an examination, AR glasses can instantly overlay patient information and data in their field of vision (Gaur and Garg, 2023).

Customised exposure therapy and immersive distraction techniques can be employed in VR metaverse environments to treat phobias, anxiety, PTSD, and chronic pain in mental healthcare. Patients might experience simulated stressors in safe environments. After neurological damage and musculoskeletal injury, mixed reality mirrors and motion capture can help patients restore their motor function during therapy. Physical, occupational, and cognitive therapy are more attractive in gamified VR environments. The metaverse also provides benefits for preventative health and well-being through mindfulness exercises in virtual nature, fitness apps with virtual trainers, and social interactions that reduce isolation. As metaverse platforms develop, healthcare is positioned to advance by becoming more intuitive, immersive, and intelligent.

Consequently, metaverse-enabled VR and AR technologies bring revolutionary applications to medical education, diagnosis, treatment, mental health, rehabilitation, and well-being (Gaur, Afaq, Solanki, et al., 2021). As healthcare finally joins the digital age, the metaverse promises more readily available, high-quality care and better health outcome(Gaur, Singh, et al., 2022; Sharma et al., 2022). Integrating virtual reality, augmented reality, artificial intelligence, and other cutting-edge technology, metaverse applications present fascinating potential for intelligent healthcare (Chaudhary et al., 2022b; Sahu et al., 2023). By increasing patient experiences, advancing medical education, providing remote monitoring, and facilitating individualised care, these technologies have the potential to revolutionise healthcare (Afaq et al., 2022). Some technological benefits of metaverse in healthcare are depicted in the below mentioned figure 1.

Figure 1. Relevance of metaverse in healthcare

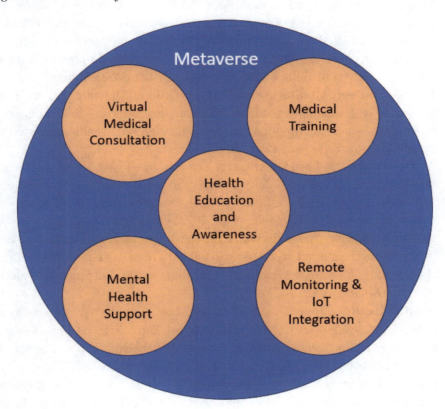

2. NEED OF STUDYING METAVERSE APPLICATIONS IN HEALTHCARE

Many advantages can be derived by analysing Metaverse applications in the healthcare context.

- **Innovation in Healthcare Delivery:** The utilisation of metaverse applications has the potential to transform healthcare service delivery significantly. This encompasses various advancements, including virtual consultations, telemedicine, remote patient monitoring, and personalised care (Santosh and Gaur, 2021).
- **Enhancing Patient Experiences:** Immersive virtual environments have the potential to improve patient experiences by rendering consultations and treatments more pleasant, accessible, and engaging (Gaur, Bhatia, Jhanjhi, et al., 2021; Protic et al., 2022).
- **Medical Training and Simulation:** Metaverse technologies have the potential to be employed in medical training, enabling healthcare workers to engage in simulated practice sessions. This utilisation offers the opportunity to refine procedural techniques, strengthen clinical decision-making abilities, and augment overall skills within a secure and hazard-free setting.
- **Remote Patient Monitoring and Intervention:** The integration of the Metaverse with wearables and IoT devices facilitates the real-time monitoring of patients, hence enabling the timely identification of health concerns and proactive action (Afaq and Gaur, 2021).
- **AI-Driven Personalized Healthcare:** Artificial intelligence inside Metaverse systems is employed to deliver individualised healthcare advice and assistance, enhancing the efficacy of treatment programmes and improving patient outcomes (Gaur, Jhanjhi, et al., 2022; Ghose et al., 2023).
- **Health Education and Behavior Change:** It can be useful to explore how interactive and gamified experiences in the Metaverse can educate individuals about health-related topics, motivate behaviour change, and promote healthier lifestyles(Solanki et al., 2022).
- **Mental Health Support and Therapy:** Using interactive and gamified experiences inside the Metaverse can impart knowledge on health-related subjects, encourage individuals to modify their behaviours, and foster the adoption of better lifestyles (Afaq et al., 2023a; Ghose et al., 2022).
- **Clinical Research and Drug Development:** The utilisation of metaverse applications has the potential to optimise the procedures involved in clinical research, hence resulting in enhanced efficiency of trials and accelerated medication development (Ahmed, Shaharier, et al., 2022; Biswas et al., 2023).
- **Data Privacy and Security:** Understanding the significance of data privacy and security in Metaverse healthcare apps is crucial to getting valuable insights and comprehending the measures required to protect sensitive patient information (Gaur and Sahoo, 2022).

- **Addressing Challenges and Ethical Considerations:** It is imperative to comprehend the ethical ramifications of implementing Metaverse applications in the healthcare sector and devise conscientious approaches to mitigate them.

By attaining these goals, individuals can make valuable contributions to the progress and conscientious integration of Metaverse applications within the healthcare sector. This, in turn, can result in enhanced patient care, superior outcomes, and heightened efficiency within the healthcare system.

3. TRANSFORMATION OF HEALTHCARE LANDSCAPE BY METAVERSE

3.1. Telemedicine and Virtual Consultations

Metaverse systems facilitate the provision of virtual consultations and telemedicine services by healthcare practitioners. Patients can engage with medical professionals, including doctors, specialists, and therapists, via avatars within immersive virtual environments. This technology improves accessibility, particularly for patients who live in remote or underdeveloped areas, while decreasing the necessity for in-person appointments (Naved et al., 2023). Virtual consultations have the potential to enhance patient experiences by providing a more comfortable and tailored environment, hence facilitating the development of stronger doctor-patient connections. These practices are improved in terms of immersion, engagement, and efficiency. The utilisation of the metaverse contributes significantly to the evolution of telemedicine and virtual consultation.

- **Full Disclosure:** Giving patients Immersive Virtual Environments: Metaverse platforms offer a means for patients and healthcare professionals to convene within virtual worlds, characterised by their immersive and interactive nature, whereby they assume the shape of avatars. The immersion in virtual consultations contributes to an enhanced overall experience, resulting in increased personalisation and naturalness (Maurya et al., 2023).
- **Avatar Customization and Identity Protection:** Patients can personalise their avatars to depict themselves in a manner that aligns with their preferences, enabling them to uphold a certain degree of anonymity if they so want. This can be particularly advantageous for individuals seeking mental health assistance or engaging in conversations about delicate health matters.
- **Enhanced Communication:** Metaverse applications provide functionalities such as gesture recognition, facial expressions analysis, and body language

simulation, thereby improving the quality of communication between healthcare personnel and patients.
- **Collaborative Healthcare:** Metaverse systems facilitate collaborative healthcare by allowing several providers, specialists, or family members to engage in virtual consultations concurrently. The adoption of a multidisciplinary approach has the potential to enhance the comprehensiveness of care planning.
- **Medical Visualisation:** The metaverse incorporates virtual reality (VR) technology to facilitate the display of medical data in three-dimensional formats. This technology enables healthcare professionals to effectively visualise and comprehend medical pictures, including magnetic resonance imaging (MRI) and computed tomography (CT) scans, in a more intuitive manner, resulting in enhanced accuracy of diagnoses and improved efficacy of treatment plans.
- **Remote Patient Monitoring Integration:** Integrating the metaverse with remote patient monitoring devices and wearables enables patients to exchange real-time health data while engaging in virtual consultations effectively. This functionality empowers medical professionals to make evidence-based decisions and closely track their patients' progress.
- **Tele-surgery and Remote Procedures:** In prospective scenarios, it is plausible that advanced metaverse applications may facilitate tele-surgery, thereby granting surgeons the ability to conduct treatments remotely using robotic assistance. This development has the potential to enhance the availability of specialised medical care.
- **Continuity of Care:** Metaverse applications have the potential to provide continuous connections between patients and healthcare practitioners, hence promoting the maintenance of care beyond individual virtual consultations. Virtual follow-up meetings can facilitate the monitoring of patient progress and the modification of treatment programmes as necessary.
- **Global Access to Specialised Care:** The metaverse facilitates the transcending of geographical limitations, thereby granting patients the ability to avail themselves of specialist healthcare services provided by professionals throughout the globe, eliminating the necessity for extensive travel.

3.2. Medical Training and Simulation

Virtual simulations provide a valuable means for medical students, clinicians, and surgeons to practice intricate procedures, mitigating the inherent risks connected with actual patients. Simulated situations can be modified to present learners with challenges that cater to their diverse ability levels, offering a very beneficial and enriching learning encounter. This methodology can boost clinical decision-making, mitigate medical errors, and augment the overall proficiency of healthcare professionals. By optimising the educational experience for healthcare professionals and students alike. The metaverse offers several advantages in the realm of medical teaching and simulation:

- **Realistic Simulations:** Metaverse systems can generate medical simulations that exhibit realism, accurately reproducing intricate medical scenarios and procedures. The realism achieved in this simulation enables healthcare professionals and students to engage in a secure and devoid-of-risk setting for practice.
- **Hands-on Experience:** Medical simulations conducted in metaverse environments offer a practical learning opportunity that enhances traditional classroom instruction. Learners can participate in medical operations actively, enhancing their technical proficiency and self-assurance.
- **Access to Specialised Training:** The metaverse facilitates overcoming geographical limitations, granting individuals the opportunity to acquire specialised medical training irrespective of their physical location. Healthcare workers can gain knowledge from global specialists without physical travel.
- **Interdisciplinary Training:** Metaverse apps facilitate interdisciplinary training, providing medical teams with the opportunity to interact and engage in coordinated reactions during emergencies.
- **Adjustable Scenarios:** The ability levels of learners can be readily accommodated by adjusting simulated circumstances within the metaverse. The provision of flexibility in training programmes guarantees that the content and structure of the training can be customised to meet each participant's specific requirements and advancements.
- **Feedback and Assessment:** Metaverse simulations frequently have integrated evaluation tools that offer learners immediate feedback. The aforementioned feedback loop identifies areas that require improvement and monitors learners' progress over time.
- **Team Training and Communication:** Using metaverse simulations fosters collaboration and enhances communication proficiency within the healthcare community. Participants can engage in decision-making, coordination, and communication exercises in a simulated clinical environment.
- **Enhanced Medical Training and Education:** The metaverse is poised to revolutionise medical training and education in several impactful ways. Firstly, it offers enhanced learning opportunities by enabling remote medical training, eliminating the need for physical training centres, and accommodating the busy schedules of healthcare professionals. Learners can

also simulate complex medical procedures and rare cases, gaining invaluable experience handling challenging scenarios not often encountered in real-life practice. Moreover, the metaverse fosters a culture of learning from mistakes, allowing healthcare professionals to practice error management and adverse event handling without patient risk. Additionally, it serves as a platform for Continuing Medical Education (CME) through virtual conferences, workshops, and webinars, ensuring that medical professionals remain up-to-date with the latest advancements and best practices.

- **Transformation of Healthcare Education:** Into a broader framework, the metaverse can revolutionise healthcare education. The training programme provides a complete methodology integrating immersive experiences, error control techniques, and remote accessibility features. Healthcare organisations have the potential to utilise metaverse platforms as a means to enhance the allocation of resources, decrease expenses, and ensure fair and equal availability of top-notch education. The importance of the metaverse in healthcare education extends beyond conventional limits, facilitating the development of a more effective and comprehensive healthcare workforce, ultimately yielding advantages for patients and healthcare systems.

3.3. Remote Patient Monitoring

Integrating the metaverse with wearable devices and IoT sensors facilitates the continuous real-time monitoring of patients' vital signs and health indicators. The collected data can be represented within a virtual environment, enabling healthcare practitioners to enhance their ability to monitor and manage patients' health more efficiently. Rapidly identifying irregularities can result in prompt interventions and proactive management of care, ultimately improving patient outcomes and mitigating the need for hospitalisations. Incorporating the metaverse can greatly enhance remote patient monitoring (RPM) by offering immersive and interactive approaches for gathering, processing, and visualising patient data. The utilisation of the metaverse presents numerous advantages within remote patient monitoring:

- **Data Analysis and AI Insights:** The integration of the metaverse with artificial intelligence (AI) algorithms enables the analysis of extensive datasets and the identification of patterns and deviations. AI-driven insights can support healthcare providers in making data-driven decisions for patient care.
- **Personalised Patient Care:** Using the metaverse facilitates the implementation of customised care plans tailored to particular patients' data.

Healthcare providers can customise treatment regimens and interventions to accommodate the unique demands of individual patients.
- **Patient Education and Empowerment:** Through the metaverse, patients can access educational resources, interactive tutorials, and self-management tools. This empowers patients to take an active role in their healthcare journey.
- **Secure Data Sharing:** Protecting sensitive patient information should be a primary concern for metaverse applications. The implementation of effective encryption and access controls is vital to maintaining the confidentiality of patient data. Through the utilisation of the metaverse, healthcare practitioners can engage in remote patient monitoring. This approach enables the delivery of care centred around the patient, driven by data, and ultimately contributes to enhanced patient outcomes, diminished hospital readmissions, and overall improvement in healthcare management. The ongoing advancement of technology is anticipated to result in an expanded role for the metaverse in remote patient monitoring, thereby bringing about significant transformations in the delivery and experience of healthcare.

3.4. Health Education and Behavior Change

Applications in the metaverse have the potential to significantly contribute to health education and facilitate the adoption of behaviour modification (Afaq et al., 2023b). The utilisation of interactive and gamified experiences has the potential to effectively engage users and facilitate the communication of health information about illness prevention, medication adherence, and lifestyle adjustments. Virtual environments can replicate and mimic harmful habits' potential outcomes and ramifications, motivating individuals to embrace and adopt healthier lifestyles. Through immersive and interactive technology, the metaverse can effectively include users in a captivating and tailored manner to their needs. This has the potential to enhance the effectiveness of health education and facilitate the attainment of behaviour change goals. The metaverse plays a significant role in facilitating health education and promoting behaviour change:

- **Interactive Learning Experiences:** The utilisation of metaverse applications facilitates the provision of health education that is both interactive and personalised. These applications employ gamified simulations and situations, engaging users in interesting learning experiences. These immersive experiences facilitate and encourage active engagement in health-related activities, augmenting knowledge retention. Furthermore, the metaverse possesses the capacity to gather user data and preferences, hence enabling

the provision of tailored health education information. This ensures that educational resources are pertinent and applicable to each user.
- **Virtual Health Classes and Workshops:** The metaverse provides an optimal platform for facilitating virtual health classes and workshops encompassing various subjects, such as nutrition, physical activity, stress mitigation, and psychological well-being. Remote participation enables individuals to engage in health education from a distance, enhancing accessibility to a broader and more heterogeneous demographic. The democratising health education facilitates the cultivation of individuals with a higher level of knowledge and understanding, ultimately leading to healthier communities.
- **Practical Skill Building:** The utilisation of metaverse applications allows individuals to engage in the development of practical health-related skills inside a secure and regulated virtual setting. The metaverse offers a platform for training various skills, ranging from first aid administration to cultivating mindfulness practises. Additionally, the platform provides behaviour modification programmes designed to assist individuals in adopting healthier habits. These programmes utilise gamification techniques and rewards as motivational tools to encourage long-term dedication to achieving their goals.
- **Virtual Health Coaching and Empathy Development:** Within the metaverse, individuals can utilise virtual health coaches or AI-driven virtual assistants that provide tailored direction and assistance in attaining health-related goals. Moreover, immersive experiences can replicate the experience of living with particular health conditions, promoting empathy and comprehension among users. The heightened level of empathy has the potential to exert a beneficial influence on attitudes and behaviours about health, hence fostering a healthcare community that is more helpful and knowledgeable.
- **Community Engagement and Support:** Community engagement and progress monitoring are facilitated by utilising virtual support groups and health communities within the metaverse, fostering inclusivity and providing individuals with emotional support. Individuals can exchange their experiences, confrontations, and achievements, establishing a network that encourages support and motivation in pursuing health-related goals. In addition, the metaverse monitors users' health-related actions and progress towards behaviour modification objectives, enabling them to observe their accomplishments and strengthen beneficial habits, thus fostering ongoing dedication.

3.5. Personalised Healthcare and AI Assistants

Integrating artificial intelligence (AI) with metaverse technology enables the analysis of extensive patient data, facilitating the provision of customised healthcare advice. AI-powered virtual health assistants can provide personalised guidance, medication intake reminders, and lifestyle modification recommendations, all derived from individual health profiles. A higher degree of personalisation can result in enhanced treatment outcomes and increased patient involvement in managing their health. The convergence of the metaverse and AI assistants facilitates the provision of tailored healthcare services:

- **Data Integration and Analysis:** Integrating the metaverse with healthcare systems, wearables, and IoT devices enables the gathering a wide range of patient data. As mentioned, artificial intelligence (AI) assistants can analyse the data to generate valuable insights about a patient's health condition, risk factors, and possible health issues.
- **Virtual Health Consultations:** Virtual health consultations involve the application of predictive analytics and continuous learning in the healthcare sector, allowing artificial intelligence (AI) to anticipate potential health problems and consequences through the analysis of patient data. Implementing this proactive method enables healthcare providers to intervene and mitigate unfavourable outcomes rapidly. AI assistants engage in an ongoing process of learning through the analysis of patient interactions, thereby augmenting their knowledge repository and enabling them to offer healthcare advice that is more accurate and relevant.
- **Remote Patient Monitoring:** The integration of the metaverse with artificial intelligence (AI) has the potential for remote patient monitoring, enabling timely treatments for patients with chronic illnesses and improving disease management protocols. AI assistants also offer customised health education resources designed to target specific health issues and bridge informational deficiencies, empowering patients in their pursuit of healthcare. Moreover, in the metaverse, adaptable user interfaces are developed to cater to the distinct preferences and accessibility needs of each user, hence enhancing the overall calibre of the user experience. The integration of artificial intelligence (AI) assistants inside the metaverse facilitates enhanced accessibility, efficiency, and patient-centricity in the realm of personalised healthcare. Patients are provided with individualised assistance and guidance along their healthcare trajectory, resulting in improved health outcomes and a more gratifying patient encounter. Additionally, AI-driven insights can help healthcare

providers make well-informed decisions and deliver proactive care, ultimately contributing to better population health.

3.6. Therapeutic Interventions and Mental Health Support

The utilisation of metaverse apps has the potential to yield positive outcomes in providing therapeutic interventions and mental health assistance. Virtual reality (VR)-based exposure therapy has demonstrated potential in treating phobias, post-traumatic stress disorder (PTSD), and anxiety disorders. Furthermore, virtual support groups and mental health counselling sessions can facilitate patient engagement with peers and foster emotional support within a secure and confidential setting. The metaverse plays a significant role in promoting treatments and providing support for mental health:

- **Virtual Reality-Based Exposure Therapy:** The metaverse's virtual reality settings provide exposure therapy for people with phobias, anxiety disorders, and PTSD. The utilisation of controlled virtual environments allows patients to address their concerns systematically, hence facilitating the process of desensitisation and promoting therapeutic advancement.
- **Mindfulness and Stress Reduction:** Within the metaverse, individuals can access guided mindfulness and relaxation experiences designed to assist in managing stress and anxiety. Virtual meditation and deep breathing exercises have been found to establish tranquil and immersive settings that promote emotional well-being.
- **Virtual Support Community**: In the realm of the metaverse, virtual support groups serve as a platform for persons with comparable mental health difficulties, fostering a sense of community and providing emotional support. Furthermore, the utilisation of virtual consultations with mental health specialists enhances the accessibility of therapy, hence providing advantages to individuals residing in remote geographical locations or facing limitations in physical mobility.
- **Therapist-Patient Interaction:** The use of the metaverse provides opportunities for those grappling with mood disorders, emotional dysregulation, attention impairments, and impulse control disorders to engage in interactive experiences aimed at teaching emotional regulation skills and cognitive training activities.

While the metaverse shows great promise in enhancing therapeutic interventions and mental health support, it is essential to consider ethical and privacy considerations and supplement virtual support with in-person care when necessary. Integrating the metaverse into mental health services can improve mental health outcomes, reduce stigma, and make mental health support more inclusive and accessible for diverse populations.

3.7. Clinical Research and Drug Development

The utilisation of metaverse apps has the potential to enhance and streamline clinical research and medication development procedures. Utilising virtual trials and simulations can improve the efficiency and cost-effectiveness of clinical trials by facilitating streamlined data collection, recruitment, and monitoring processes. This has the potential to expedite the process of discovering and obtaining approval for novel therapies, hence yielding benefits for patients on a global scale. The utilisation of the metaverse in clinical research and medication development offers significant advantages:

- **Virtual Clinical Trials:** Virtual clinical trials have been significantly transformed by the advent of the metaverse since it allows for distant participation via immersive virtual settings. This eliminates the necessity for physical study sites and enhances patient involvement through immersive experiences.
- **Realistic Simulations:** In the metaverse, scholars can generate authentic simulations of medical disorders and drug interactions, thereby enabling the virtual evaluation of prospective treatments before their implementation in real-world trials. This practice enhances the design and safety of clinical trials.
- **Data Collection and Analysis:** Integrating the metaverse with wearable devices and Internet of Things (IoT) sensors facilitates real-time data collection during clinical trials. As mentioned earlier, artificial intelligence algorithms are utilised to analyse the data, facilitating pattern detection and trend identification. Additionally, implementing remote monitoring systems guarantees the prompt reporting of undesirable events.
- **Collaboration and Data Sharing**: In the metaverse, researchers collaborate seamlessly across many geographical areas, facilitating effective data sharing and exchanging knowledge. Metaverse technology additionally facilitates decentralised clinical trials, thereby mitigating the necessity for frequent in-person visits and enabling participants to contribute data from their residences remotely.
- **Virtual FDA Meetings and Regulatory Approval:** The metaverse enables virtual engagement with regulatory bodies, enhancing the efficiency of research presentation and the process of obtaining regulatory approval.

Moreover, it has the potential to serve as a means of disseminating information to the general public regarding current clinical research endeavours, thereby fostering engagement and enhancing knowledge.
- **Efficient Data Management:** The immersive nature of the metaverse facilitates a patient-centric approach, emphasising patient feedback and experience significantly throughout the study process. In addition, this technology optimises data management, guaranteeing secure storage and facilitating the retrieval of research data. Consequently, it enhances the overall efficiency of clinical trials.

While the metaverse holds significant potential for clinical research and drug development, addressing data privacy and security concerns is crucial, adhering to regulatory guidelines and ensuring that virtual findings are validated in real-world settings. By leveraging the capabilities of the metaverse, researchers can accelerate the drug development process, make clinical trials more accessible to diverse populations, and ultimately advance medical discoveries for the benefit of patients worldwide.

3.8. Data Privacy and Security

Incorporating the metaverse into the healthcare sector necessitates a heightened emphasis on safeguarding data privacy and security. Developers and healthcare providers must implement strong encryption and data protection protocols to ensure the safety of sensitive patient information within the digital domain. Maintaining data privacy and security is crucial in utilising the metaverse across many fields, such as healthcare, education, and other sectors. The metaverse offers potential solutions to the challenges around data privacy and security:

- **Data Security and Encryption:** Data security and encryption are vital concerns for metaverse systems, as they prioritise protecting sensitive information during virtual interactions. This is achieved through the implementation of robust encryption methods. The implementation of secure communication protocols guarantees the preservation of data confidentiality.
- **User Authentication and Access Controls:** Effective user authentication techniques validate participants' identities, while access controls restrict data access only to authorised users. These methods mitigate the risk of unauthorised access or manipulation of sensitive data.
- **Privacy Measures:** Within certain situations, the metaverse facilitates user anonymity or pseudonymity, providing enhanced privacy safeguards. This holds significance in sensitive domains such as mental health assistance because individuals may opt to withhold their identities.

- **Data Management and Consent:** Metaverse systems adhere to the principle of data minimisation, wherein they just gather essential information in order to mitigate the potential for data breaches. The incorporation of strong consent processes is a key feature, as it guarantees that users explicitly provide permission for the collection and utilisation of their data. Additionally, these methods provide clear and comprehensive information regarding how data will be used, allowing users to withdraw their approval if desired.
- **Infrastructure and Compliance:** Metaverse providers utilise robust cloud infrastructure and data centres that prioritise security measures. They also conduct periodic security assessments to ensure the integrity of their systems. Additionally, these providers strictly adhere to data protection rules, such as the General Data Protection Regulation (GDPR). Implementing compliance measures, in conjunction with regular security audits and updates, protects user data from physical and cyber dangers.
- **Enhanced Security Measures:** Metaverse applications incorporate end-to-end encryption, establish explicit policies for data deletion and retention, foster cybersecurity awareness and training, and may even implement bug bounty programmes to promptly identify and resolve potential vulnerabilities, thereby ensuring a robust level of security for users.

Through robust data privacy and security protocols, the metaverse has the potential to establish a secure and reliable setting for users, fostering a sense of trust in the ethical utilisation of technology and facilitating widespread acceptance across diverse sectors such as healthcare, education, entertainment, and beyond.

3.9. Virtual Support Groups

Peer assistance is frequently advantageous for those with chronic illnesses and mental health disorders. Support groups based in the metaverse offer a platform for individuals to engage with others confronting comparable difficulties, cultivating camaraderie and psychological assistance. Virtual support groups can overcome geographical constraints, enabling improved connectedness and the exchange of experiences among individuals undergoing similar health challenges. The metaverse presents numerous advantages for virtual support groups, as it furnishes a conducive setting for interpersonal engagements, emotional assistance, and a collective feeling of affiliation among folks confronting comparable difficulties. The metaverse plays a significant role in enabling virtual support groups.

- **Global Reach and Accessibility:** The metaverse facilitates the enhancement of global connectivity and inclusion by transcending geographical limitations,

so enabling individuals from diverse locations to participate in virtual support groups. This promotes the growth of support networks and encourages interpersonal connections among persons who may otherwise face limited chances to interact with local support groups.
- **Anonymity and Privacy:** The utilisation of metaverse platforms allows individuals to maintain anonymity or employ pseudonyms, so creating a secure environment for the exchange of experiences and emotions while protecting their genuine identities. This attribute promotes a heightened sense of comfort and cultivates an inclusive atmosphere among the individuals engaged.
- **Immersive and Interactive Experience:** Metaverse systems offer a comprehensive and engaging platform that facilitates immersive and interactive experiences, hence augmenting user engagement, personalisation, and the depth of discourse. Users are able to assume the form of virtual avatars and engage in interactions within virtual settings. This surpasses the conventional video conferencing encounter.
- **Facilitated Sharing and Expression:** Virtual support groups within the metaverse serve as a conducive platform for individuals to effectively share and articulate their emotions and experiences. This is achieved through the utilisation of gesture-based interactions and the utilisation of virtual body language, facilitating users in successfully expressing their emotions. The employment of metaverse platforms enables individuals to maintain anonymity or employ pseudonyms, so creating a secure environment for the exchange of experiences and emotions while protecting genuine identities. This attribute enables an enhanced state of comfort and nurtures a welcoming atmosphere among the parties concerned.
- **Diverse Support Topics:** The metaverse provides a diverse range of support group themes encompassing mental health, chronic illness, addiction rehabilitation, and other relevant subject matters. Moreover, it facilitates active participation through the utilisation of periodic meetings, gatherings, therapeutic interventions, and educational programmes.
- **Regular Meetings and Events:** Participants involved in virtual support groups have the ability to form relationships with other individuals at any given time, thereby facilitating ongoing social support and alleviating feelings of isolation. Moreover, the metaverse enables cross-language connections and caters to specific communities, accommodating persons with diverse linguistic backgrounds and addressing their unique needs and concerns.

3.10. AI-Driven Personalized Healthcare

The integration of metaverse technology and artificial intelligence (AI) facilitates the implementation of healthcare therapies tailored to individual needs and characterised by high accuracy. Artificial intelligence (AI) algorithms can evaluate extensive patient data to discern patterns, ascertain risk factors, and propose potential therapy courses. Artificial intelligence (AI)--enabled virtual health assistants can aid patients in navigating their healthcare experiences by offering personalised suggestions and timely reminders. The utilisation of the metaverse in the context of AI-driven customised healthcare yields several benefits:

- **Data-Driven Healthcare Insights:** Integrating the metaverse with healthcare devices, wearables, and IoT sensors, along with using AI analytics, facilitates the collection of real-time patient data and offers significant insights into individual health state and medical history. The concept of proactive health risk assessment refers to the practice of identifying and evaluating potential health risks before they manifest into actual health problems.
- **Personalised Treatment and Predictive Care:** Artificial intelligence (AI), in conjunction with the metaverse, facilitates the creation of individualised treatment regimens for patients by leveraging their distinct health profiles. Moreover, artificial intelligence (AI) can forecast impending health difficulties. The utilisation of real-time monitoring and virtual consultations has become increasingly prevalent in various fields. Using AI-powered monitoring systems in the metaverse facilitates the real-time tracking of patient health data, hence offering prompt feedback and alarms in response to noteworthy alterations. AI assistants play a crucial role in facilitating virtual health consultations by providing pertinent medical information and responding to common patient inquiries.
- **Remote Patient Monitoring:** Using artificial intelligence in conjunction with the metaverse facilitates remote monitoring of patients with chronic ailments while assisting in adaptive user interfaces. Moreover, the utilisation of AI-powered simulations inside the metaverse contributes to the drug discovery process by facilitating the prediction of therapeutic effectiveness and potential adverse reactions in targeted groups of patients.

Through the utilisation of artificial intelligence (AI) capabilities inside the metaverse, the provision of personalised healthcare is enhanced, resulting in increased accessibility, efficiency, and a greater focus on the needs of individual patients. Patients are provided with personalised assistance and guidance along their healthcare trajectory, resulting in enhanced health results and a more gratifying patient encounter. Furthermore, the utilisation of AI-driven insights has the potential to assist healthcare practitioners in making educated decisions and providing proactive care, thereby making a significant contribution to improving public health.

4. KEY CHALLENGES

The integration and responsible utilisation of the metaverse in the healthcare industry necessitate resolving various problems, notwithstanding its promising opportunities for intelligent healthcare. Several significant issues arise in this context:

- **Data Privacy, Security, and Compliance:** The preservation of privacy and security for sensitive health data within the metaverse, adhering to healthcare standards, is paramount in mitigating the risks of data breaches and unauthorised access.
- **Ethical Considerations:** The task of striking a balance between the advantageous immersive aspects of the metaverse and the ethical concerns about permission, autonomy, and user experience design presents a formidable challenge. Developing interfaces that prioritise user-friendliness while upholding individual rights and preferences is imperative. The preservation of reliability and precision in AI algorithms and virtual simulations within the metaverse holds significant importance in healthcare applications. The ethical utilisation of artificial intelligence (AI), which focuses on mitigating prejudice, promoting explainability, and fostering transparency, is of utmost importance to facilitate equitable and responsible decision-making.
- **Equity and Accessibility:** The prioritisation of equity, accessibility, and training is crucial in efforts to bridge the digital divide and ensure fair access to metaverse technologies, especially for persons who have limited resources or technological proficiency. The imperative of providing education and preparing healthcare personnel for integrating metaverse technology cannot be denied.
- **Regulatory Compliance:** Obtaining regulatory approval for virtual clinical trials and effectively navigating the intricate healthcare regulatory environment pose a significant obstacle. In addition, healthcare providers have financial and logistical challenges when managing the cost and infrastructure requirements associated with metaverse platforms and AI-driven healthcare apps.

5. CONCLUSION

Incorporating the metaverse into intelligent healthcare systems exhibits significant potential for revolutionising healthcare delivery, experience, and personalisation. When integrated with artificial intelligence, the metaverse's immersive and interactive characteristics bring about significant transformations in multiple healthcare domains, encompassing telemedicine, virtual consultations, medical training, remote patient monitoring, and mental health assistance.

Through the metaverse, healthcare practitioners can surmount geographical limitations, enhance the availability of specialised medical services, and foster patient involvement through more captivating and individualised means. Virtual settings inside the metaverse serve as platforms that enable the creation of realistic simulations. These simulations can enhance the safety and effectiveness of medical training, as well as promote research and drug discovery through the utilisation of virtual clinical trials.

Furthermore, the metaverse provides patients with enhanced capabilities through immersive health education, individualised treatment strategies, and ongoing monitoring, resulting in enhanced health outcomes and more effective management of chronic ailments. Moreover, establishing virtual support groups within the metaverse engenders a communal atmosphere, cultivating emotional assistance and mitigating sentiments of seclusion among individuals confronted with comparable obstacles.

Nevertheless, with the increasing prevalence of metaverse applications in the healthcare sector, it is imperative to preserve data privacy, security, and ethical issues. Achieving an optimal equilibrium between technical advancement and protecting confidential patient data will be binding in establishing confidence and promoting the ethical use of metaverse technologies within the healthcare sector.

The future of intelligent healthcare appears hopeful due to the continuous improvements in metaverse technology and artificial intelligence. By acknowledging and using the potential of the metaverse, the healthcare sector can persistently advance, providing tailored and patient-focused healthcare, expanding medical education and research, and eventually augmenting the general welfare of humans worldwide. The collaboration of stakeholders in addressing difficulties and capitalising on possibilities will inevitably result in the metaverse assuming a crucial role in positively defining the future of healthcare.

REFERENCES

Afaq, A., & Gaur, L. (2021). The Rise of Robots to Help Combat Covid-19. *2021 International Conference on Technological Advancements and Innovations (ICTAI)*, (pp. 69–74). IEEE. 10.1109/ICTAI53825.2021.9673256

Afaq, A., Gaur, L., & Singh, G. (2022). A Latent Dirichlet allocation Technique for Opinion Mining of Online Reviews of Global Chain Hotels. *2022 3rd International Conference on Intelligent Engineering and Management (ICIEM)*, (pp. 201–206). IEEE. 10.1109/ICIEM54221.2022.9853114

Afaq, A., Gaur, L., & Singh, G. (2023a). Social CRM: Linking the dots of customer service and customer loyalty during COVID-19 in the hotel industry. *International Journal of Contemporary Hospitality Management, Emerald Publishing Limited*, *35*(3), 992–1009. doi:10.1108/IJCHM-04-2022-0428

Afaq, A., Gaur, L., & Singh, G. (2023b). A trip down memory lane to travellers' food experiences. *British Food Journal, Emerald Publishing Limited*, *125*(4), 1390–1403. doi:10.1108/BFJ-01-2022-0063

Afaq, A., Gaur, L., Singh, G., & Dhir, A. (2021). *COVID-19: transforming air passengers' behaviour and reshaping their expectations towards the airline industry. Tourism Recreation Research*. Routledge. doi:10.1080/02508281.2021.2008211

Ahmed, S., Biswas, M., Hasanuzzaman, M., Mahi, M. J. N., Islam, M. A., Chaki, S., & Gaur, L. (2022). A Secured Peer-to-Peer Messaging System Based on Blockchain. *2022 3rd International Conference on Intelligent Engineering and Management (ICIEM)*, (pp. 332–337). IEEE. 10.1109/ICIEM54221.2022.9853040

Ahmed, S., Shaharier, M. M., Roy, S., Lima, A. A., Biswas, M., Mahi, M. J. N., & Chaki, S. (2022), "An Intelligent and Multi-Functional Stick for Blind People Using IoT. *2022 3rd International Conference on Intelligent Engineering and Management (ICIEM)*, (pp. 326–331). IEEE. 10.1109/ICIEM54221.2022.9853012

Bhandari, M., Parajuli, P., Chapagain, P., & Gaur, L. (2022). Evaluating Performance of Adam Optimization by Proposing Energy Index. In K. C. Santosh, R. Hegadi, & U. Pal (Eds.), *Recent Trends in Image Processing and Pattern Recognition* (pp. 156–168). Springer International Publishing. doi:10.1007/978-3-031-07005-1_15

Biswas, M., Chaki, S., Mallik, S., Gaur, L., & Ray, K. (2023). Light Convolutional Neural Network to Detect Eye Diseases from Retinal Images: Diabetic Retinopathy and Glaucoma. in M.S. Kaiser, S. Waheed, A. Bandyopadhyay, M. Mahmud, & K. Ray (Eds.), *Proceedings of the Fourth International Conference on Trends in Computational and Cognitive Engineering*. Springer Nature Singapore, Singapore. 10.1007/978-981-19-9483-8_7

Chaudhary, M., Gaur, L., & Chakrabarti, A. (2022a). Comparative Analysis of Entropy Weight Method and C5 Classifier for Predicting Employee Churn. *2022 3rd International Conference on Intelligent Engineering and Management (ICIEM)*, (pp. 232–236). IEEE. 10.1109/ICIEM54221.2022.9853181

Chaudhary, M., Gaur, L., & Chakrabarti, A. (2022b). Detecting the Employee Satisfaction in Retail: A Latent Dirichlet allocation and Machine Learning approach. *2022 3rd International Conference on Computation, Automation and Knowledge Management (ICCAKM)*, (pp. 1–6). IEEE. 10.1109/ICCAKM54721.2022.9990186

Gaur, L., Afaq, A., Arora, G. K., & Khan, N. (2023). Artificial intelligence for carbon emissions using system of systems theory. *Ecological Informatics*, *76*, 102165. doi:10.1016/j.ecoinf.2023.102165

Gaur, L., Afaq, A., Singh, G., & Dwivedi, Y. K. (2021). Role of artificial intelligence and robotics to foster the touchless travel during a pandemic: A review and research agenda. *International Journal of Contemporary Hospitality Management, Emerald Publishing Limited*, *33*(11), 4079–4098. doi:10.1108/IJCHM-11-2020-1246

Gaur, L., Afaq, A., Solanki, A., Singh, G., Sharma, S., Jhanjhi, N. Z., My, H. T., & Le, D.-N. (2021). Capitalizing on big data and revolutionary 5G technology: Extracting and visualizing ratings and reviews of global chain hotels. *Computers & Electrical Engineering*, *95*, 107374. doi:10.1016/j.compeleceng.2021.107374

Gaur, L., Bhatia, U., Jhanjhi, N. Z., Muhammad, G., & Masud, M. (2021). Medical image-based detection of COVID-19 using Deep Convolution Neural Networks. *Multimedia Systems*. doi:10.100700530-021-00794-6 PMID:33935377

Gaur, L., & Garg, P. K. (2023). *Emerging Trends, Techniques, and Applications in Geospatial Data Science*. IGI Global. doi:10.4018/978-1-6684-7319-1

Gaur, L., Jhanjhi, N. Z., Bakshi, S., & Gupta, P. (2022). Analyzing Consequences of Artificial Intelligence on Jobs using Topic Modeling and Keyword Extraction. *2022 2nd International Conference on Innovative Practices in Technology and Management (ICIPTM)*, (pp. 435–440). IEEE. 10.1109/ICIPTM54933.2022.9754064

Gaur, L., & Sahoo, B. M. (2022). Explainable AI in ITS: Ethical Concerns. In *Explainable Artificial Intelligence for Intelligent Transportation Systems: Ethics and Applications* (pp. 79–90). Springer. doi:10.1007/978-3-031-09644-0_5

Gaur, L., Singh, G., Hinchey, M., Singh, G., & Jain, V. (2022). Applications of computational intelligence techniques to software engineering problems. *Innovations in Systems and Software Engineering*, *18*(2), 231–232. doi:10.100711334-021-00394-7

Ghose, P., Biswas, M., & Gaur, L. (2023). BrainSegNeT: A Lightweight Brain Tumor Segmentation Model Based on U-Net and Progressive Neuron Expansion. In F. Liu, Y. Zhang, H. Kuai, E. P. Stephen, & H. Wang (Eds.), *Brain Informatics* (pp. 249–260). Springer Nature Switzerland. doi:10.1007/978-3-031-43075-6_22

Ghose, P., Sharmin, S., Gaur, L., & Zhao, Z. (2022). Grid-Search Integrated Optimized Support Vector Machine Model for Breast Cancer Detection. *2022 IEEE International Conference on Bioinformatics and Biomedicine (BIBM)*, (pp. 2846–2852). IEEE. 10.1109/BIBM55620.2022.9995703

Mathur, S., & Gaur, L. (2021). Predictability, Power and Procedures of Citation Analysis. In D. Goyal, A.K. Gupta, V. Piuri, M. Ganzha, & M. Paprzycki (Eds.), *Proceedings of the Second International Conference on Information Management and Machine Intelligence*. Springer Singapore, Singapore. 10.1007/978-981-15-9689-6_6

Maurya, A., Munoz, J. M., Gaur, L., & Singh, G. (2023). *Disruptive Technologies in International Business: Challenges and Opportunities for Emerging Markets*. Walter de Gruyter GmbH & Co KG. doi:10.1515/9783110734133

Naved, M., Devi, V. A., Gaur, L., & Elngar, A. A. (2023). *IoT-Enabled Convolutional Neural Networks: Techniques and Applications*. CRC Press. doi:10.1201/9781003393030

Protic, D., Gaur, L., Stankovic, M., & Rahman, M. A. (2022). Cybersecurity in smart cities: Detection of opposing decisions on anomalies in the computer network behavior. *Electronics MDPI*, *11*(22), 3718. doi:10.3390/electronics11223718

Rana, J., Gaur, L., & Santosh, K. (2022). Classifying Customers' Journey from Online Reviews of Amazon Fresh via Sentiment Analysis and Topic Modelling. *2022 3rd International Conference on Computation, Automation and Knowledge Management (ICCAKM)*, (pp. 1–6). IEEE. 10.1109/ICCAKM54721.2022.9990124

Sahu, G., Gaur, L., & Singh, G. (2023). Investigating the impact of Personality Tendencies and Gratification Aspects on OTT Short Video Consumption: A case of YouTube Shorts. *2023 3rd International Conference on Innovative Practices in Technology and Management (ICIPTM)*, (pp. 1–6). IEEE. 10.1109/ICIPTM57143.2023.10118122

Santosh, K. C., & Gaur, L. (2021). AI in Sustainable Public Healthcare. In K. C. Santosh & L. Gaur (Eds.), *Artificial Intelligence and Machine Learning in Public Healthcare: Opportunities and Societal Impact* (pp. 33–40). doi:10.1007/978-981-16-6768-8_4

Santosh, K. C., Gaur, L., Santosh, K. C., & Gaur, L. (2021). Societal Impact:- AI in Public Health Issues. In *Artificial Intelligence and Machine Learning in Public Healthcare: Opportunities and Societal Impact* (pp. 49–54). Springer. doi:10.1007/978-981-16-6768-8_6

Sharma, S., Singh, G., Gaur, L., & Afaq, A. (2022). Exploring customer adoption of autonomous shopping systems. *Telematics and Informatics*, *73*, 101861. doi:10.1016/j.tele.2022.101861

Solanki, A., Jain, V., & Gaur, L. (2022). *Applications of Blockchain and Big IoT Systems: Digital Solutions for Diverse Industries*. CRC Press. doi:10.1201/9781003231332

Chapter 2
Metaverse:
Virtual Gyms and Sports

Siva Raja Sindiramutty
Taylor's University, Malaysia

Navid Ali Khan
Taylor's University, Malaysia

Noor Zaman Jhanjhi
 https://orcid.org/0000-0001-8116-4733
Taylor's University, Malaysia

Loveleen Gaur
 https://orcid.org/0000-0002-0885-1550
University of the South Pacific, Fiji

Sayan Kumar Ray
Taylor's University, Malaysia

Abdalla Gharib
Zanzibar University, Tanzania

Husin Jazri
 https://orcid.org/0009-0005-3940-2351
Taylor's University, Malaysia

Amaranadha Reddy Manchuri
 https://orcid.org/0000-0002-3873-0469
Kyungpook National University, South Korea

ABSTRACT

In recent years, the concept of the metaverse has garnered substantial attention as an emerging digital realm that combines virtual reality, augmented reality, and various interactive technologies to create immersive and interconnected digital spaces. As traditional fitness routines and sports activities transform due to technological advancements, virtual gyms and sports have emerged as innovative solutions to engage individuals in physical activities within the metaverse. Dive into the dynamic realm of the metaverse with this chapter on virtual gyms and sports. The metaverse's business models, user experience design, and scaling strategies are explored, as are its applications in healthcare, therapy, and sports training. As the curtain falls, the authors delve into virtual fan engagement, community building, and future trends. The dynamic landscape of the metaverse awaits your exploration within these pages. Join the researchers in navigating the boundless possibilities of virtual gyms and sports, unraveling their impact on society, industry, and beyond.

DOI: 10.4018/978-1-6684-9823-1.ch002

1. INTRODUCTION TO THE METAVERSE

1.1 Definition and Evolution of the Metaverse

The metaverse concept has garnered substantial attention in recent times, owing to technological advancements and the increasing fusion of virtual and VR within our daily routines. The metaverse, characterized as a unified virtual communal realm arising from the intersection of physical and VR, encompasses a range of interconnected digital domains, including AR and VR platforms (Barbera, 2023; Humayun et al., 2020). Neal Stephenson originally coined the term "metaverse" in his 1992 science fiction novel "Snow Crash," wherein it denoted a VR-oriented successor to the internet. However, this notion has undergone notable evolution since its inception. As technological progress unfolded, the metaverse began crystallizing in the shape of online multiplayer games and virtual realms (Yilmaz et al., 2023; Almusaylim et al., 2018). The 2000s witnessed the emergence of platforms like Second Life, affording users the ability to craft avatars, engage with fellow users, and participate in diverse undertakings. These nascent endeavors to construct a metaverse laid the foundational framework for subsequent advancements.

In recent times, the metaverse's advancement has been fueled by remarkable technological strides. The fusion of VR and VR technologies has emerged as a pivotal force, engendering more captivating and participatory virtual realms. Industry giants such as Facebook (now Meta), Microsoft, and Apple have made substantial investments in the development of AR and VR hardware and software, thereby further obfuscating the demarcation between the tangible and digital domains (Parcu et al., 2023). The widespread proliferation of smartphones and cost-effective VR headsets has democratized access to these encounters (Pizzo, 2023). The maturation of the metaverse carries profound implications across multifarious sectors. In the realm of entertainment, the metaverse has orchestrated a paradigm shift in our interaction with media and content. Virtual concerts, art galleries, and interactive narrative experiences are gaining prevalence (Rejeb et al., 2023; Chatrati et al., 2022). Furthermore, the metaverse possesses the potential to overhaul the landscape of education. Virtual classrooms and immersive pedagogical encounters have the capacity to render education more engrossing and attainable for students across the globe (Soni & Kaur, 2023).

The metaverse's impact extends beyond cultural and social dimensions, encompassing economic prospects as well. A thriving digital economy has taken root within the metaverse, characterized by the trade of virtual commodities and services facilitated by digital currencies such as cryptocurrencies (Şanlisoy & Çiloğlu, 2023). This phenomenon has catalyzed the emergence of the "creator economy," enabling individuals to monetize their digital innovations and proficiencies. Concurrently, businesses are delving into metaverse-centric marketing approaches, introducing novel methods to connect with consumers (Arya et al., 2023). Figure 1 shows the timeline evolution of metaverse.

Figure 1. Evolution of Metaverse
Source: Glen (2023)

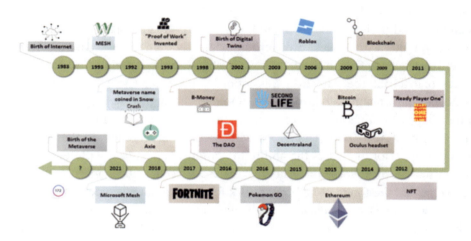

1.2 Role of Virtual Gyms and Sports in the Metaverse

Virtual fitness centers have garnered attention as an innovative approach to partake in physical fitness endeavors within the metaverse. These virtual domains harness the capabilities of VR and AR technologies to replicate workout settings and apparatuses, enabling individuals to engage in exercise regimens and physical activities from the confines of their own abodes (Suh et al., 2023). Within these virtual realms, virtual personal trainers assume the role of guides, leading participants through workout routines, providing immediate insights, and curating bespoke fitness plans. Empirical investigations have indicated that the virtual gym experience can be comparably efficacious to conventional gymnasium sessions in terms of enhancing cardiovascular endurance and muscular potency (Thamrongrat et al., 2023). Moreover, the geographical barriers are dismantled by virtual fitness centers, thus extending fitness opportunities to a global demographic.

Prominently embedded within the metaverse's fabric is its potential to cultivate interpersonal connections and cultivate a sense of community, a facet that extends even to the domain of physical fitness. Within this context, virtual fitness establishments serve as conduits for collective exercise encounters, enabling individuals to engage in workouts alongside acquaintances, kin, or even individuals hailing from diverse corners of the globe. This communal ambiance imbues a profound sense of social presence, fostering an elevated drive and commitment to adhering to prescribed exercise routines (Ose et al., 2023). Furthermore, the metaverse's expansive framework facilitates the establishment of virtual fitness cohorts, wherein individuals can partake in amicable rivalries, exchange advancements, and extend mutual support – an emulation of the camaraderie typically witnessed in conventional fitness centers (Mozumder et al., 2023).

Extending far beyond individualized fitness pursuits, the metaverse stands poised on the precipice of a revolutionary transformation of the sports and recreational landscape. At the vanguard of this transformation lie virtual sports, a paradigm facilitated by the synergy of motion-tracking apparatuses and immersive technologies. This novel dimension empowers individuals to immerse themselves in activities such as basketball, soccer, and tennis without departing the confines of their domestic spaces. This amalgamation of corporeal exertion and digital interaction yields an unparalleled encounter, resonating compellingly with both athletes and non-athletes alike (Höner et al., 2023). Notably, a burgeoning realm of virtual sports leagues and tournaments has emerged, presenting a global arena for competitive engagement that artfully blurs the demarcation between corporeal and virtual sportsmanship, thus auguring an evolutionary leap in the world of sports (Benti, 2023).

In conclusion, the integration of virtual gyms and sports in the metaverse has the potential to reshape how individuals engage in physical fitness, socialize, and experience sports. As the metaverse continues to expand, the opportunities for immersive and interconnected fitness experiences will grow. The current landscape is characterized by innovative virtual fitness solutions, shared workout experiences, and the emergence of virtual sports leagues. However, challenges related to technology, privacy, and safety must be addressed to ensure the successful integration of these experiences into daily lives. With careful consideration and ongoing development, virtual gyms and sports are set to play a pivotal role in shaping the metaverse of the future

Figure 2. VR in the martial arts
Source: Crew (2023)

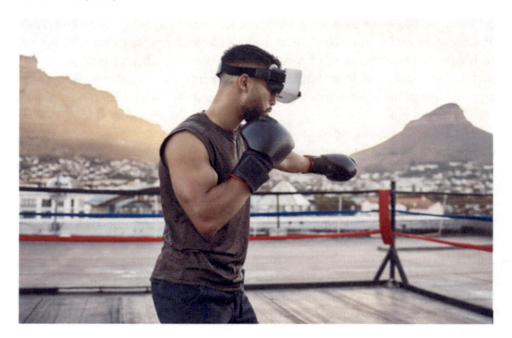

1.3 Scope and Objectives Research

The scope of this research chapter encompasses an in-depth exploration of the intersection between the metaverse, virtual gyms, and sports. The research will delve into the various dimensions of virtual fitness experiences and sports activities within the digital realm, considering their impact on health, entertainment, technology, and society at large. The scope also encompasses the integration of immersive technologies such as VR and AR to create engaging and personalized fitness and sports environments. Additionally, the chapter will examine the potential implications of these developments for the sports industry, healthcare, and society, while addressing the associated benefits, challenges, and ethical considerations.

    This research chapter is designed with several core objectives in mind. Firstly, it seeks to provide a thorough comprehension of the metaverse concept, its historical development, and its intricate interplay with virtual gyms and sports. The exploration extends to virtual gyms, encompassing an analysis of their merits, limitations, and the transformative role played by VR and AR technologies in elevating fitness encounters. Similarly, the study scrutinizes diverse manifestations of virtual sports, spanning esports to VR-based sports simulations, shedding light on their significance within the metaverse.

Secondly, the research scrutinizes the health, fitness, and social benefits arising from participation in virtual gym workouts and sports activities, while simultaneously addressing the challenges posed by digital environments. The investigation encompasses the technological innovations propelling virtual fitness and sports experiences, encompassing immersive technologies, AI-guided coaching, haptic feedback, and motion tracking. Additionally, it delves into the pragmatic dimensions of the virtual fitness and sports landscape, contemplating business models, scalability strategies, and the broader transformation of the conventional sports industry. Furthermore, the research explores the transformative potential of integrating virtual fitness and sports into healthcare and therapy contexts, fostering rehabilitation, mental health support, and skill cultivation. The study also assesses the sociocultural dynamics at play in metaverse sports, encompassing fan involvement, diversity promotion, virtual gatherings, and collaborative teamwork. Ultimately, the research culminates in identifying emerging trends, ethical considerations, and furnishing recommendations for stakeholders and researchers in the pursuit of effectively integrating virtual fitness and sports into the expanding metaverse landscape

1.4 Key Concepts and Terminology

Metaverse: A collective virtual shared space, merging physical and VR, where users can interact with each other and digital environments in real time.

Virtual Gym: A digital space within the metaverse that offers fitness and exercise activities using VR technology.

Virtual Sports: Sports and athletic activities that take place in virtual environments, often using augmented or VR technology.

Immersive Fitness: A workout experience that fully engages participants through sensory stimulation and interactive elements.

Augmented Reality Sports: Sports experiences that blend virtual elements with the real world using VR technology.

Virtual Coaching: Personalized guidance and instruction provided by virtual trainers or coaches in the metaverse.

E-sports: Competitive video gaming where players or teams compete against each other in various video games.

Gamification of Exercise: Applying game design elements, such as rewards and challenges, to fitness routines to enhance motivation.

Avatar: A virtual representation of a user within the metaverse, often customizable and used for social interactions.

Physical Activity in Virtual Worlds: Engaging in exercise and movement-based activities within digitally created environments.

Athlete Training in the Metaverse: Sports training and skill development carried out through VR simulations.

VR Fitness Platforms: Online platforms that offer VR-based fitness programs and workouts.

Social Interactions in Virtual Sports: Communication and interaction between users while participating in virtual sports or fitness activities.

VR Technology in Sports Training: Incorporating VR technology to enhance training techniques and strategies in sports.

Virtual Trainers: AI-powered or human-controlled virtual characters that guide users through workouts and exercises.

VR Wellness: Using VR experiences to promote mental and emotional well-being.

Sports Simulation in VR: Simulating real sports scenarios and matches within VR environments.

Virtual Sports Events: Competitive sports events conducted in virtual environments, often with real-world counterparts.

1.5 Research Contribution

This book chapter makes a significant research contribution by thoroughly exploring and analyzing the interplay between the metaverse and the domains of fitness and sports. It seeks to offer a comprehensive comprehension of the evolving landscape of virtual gyms and sports within the metaverse, investigating their potential impact on diverse aspects like society, technology, health, and business. Through an extensive examination of existing literature, case studies, and emerging trends, the chapter provides an in-depth exploration of virtual gyms and sports, incorporating insights from varied fields to present a holistic understanding. It also evaluates the latest technological advancements influencing virtual fitness and sports, while addressing ethical concerns and considering their broader effects. By examining the transformation of conventional fitness and sports industries, the chapter underscores the potential for virtual platforms to reshape established norms and introduce new business models. Additionally, it highlights the role of metaverse sports in fostering social engagement, collaboration, and inclusiveness, and points out promising research directions for future innovation at the convergence of the metaverse, fitness, and sports.

Metaverse

1.6 Chapter Organization

The chapter follows a coherent and systematic structure, progressing logically from foundational principles to more advanced themes, culminating in implications and recommendations. It begins by introducing the metaverse, tracing its evolution, and spotlighting virtual gyms and sports in this immersive digital domain. Subsequently, it examines virtual fitness experiences, incorporating VR and AR technologies, personalized approaches, and gamification for heightened engagement. The discussion extends to virtual sports, encompassing esports, VR sports encounters, and the fusion of real-world and virtual athletics. Benefits like improved health and community involvement, alongside challenges related to ethics and accessibility, are explored in depth. Technological strides, such as immersive technologies, AI coaching, haptic feedback, and motion tracking, shaping the landscape of virtual fitness and sports, are investigated. Business strategies, user experience design, community expansion, and strategic partnerships in metaverse fitness platforms are addressed, followed by a look at applications in healthcare and therapy. The transformative impact on traditional fitness and sports industries is analyzed, alongside metaverse sports' social dimensions and collaboration potential. Future possibilities are speculated, including integration with physical fitness, ethical considerations, and emerging research avenues. The chapter concludes by summarizing crucial insights and implications, offering guidance to industry stakeholders and prospective researchers, resulting in a comprehensive comprehension of virtual gyms and sports in the metaverse.

Figure 3. Virtual gym

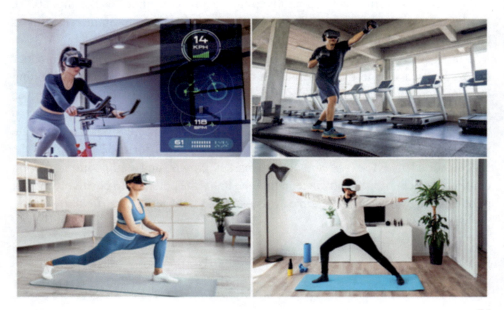

2. VIRTUAL GYMS IN THE METAVERSE

2.1 Overview of Virtual Gyms and Fitness Experiences

In recent years, the fitness industry has undergone a significant transformation with the advent of virtual gyms and fitness experiences. These innovative platforms leverage technology to provide individuals with flexible and convenient ways to engage in physical activity, offering a range of benefits that cater to modern lifestyles. Virtual gyms and fitness experiences refer to online platforms and applications that offer a diverse range of fitness-related activities, classes, and workouts to users. These platforms harness various technologies, such as livestreaming, on-demand videos, interactive interfaces, and wearable devices, to create an immersive and engaging fitness environment. Virtual fitness experiences encompass a wide array of activities, including yoga, cardio workouts, strength training, dance classes, and meditation sessions, among others (Villa-García et al., 2023). The appeal of virtual fitness lies in its accessibility, enabling users to engage in exercise routines from the comfort of their homes or other convenient locations.

The success of virtual gyms and fitness experiences is predominantly attributed to the underlying technological advancements that drive these platforms. By utilizing livestreaming and on-demand videos, these platforms offer real-time remote fitness classes and flexible workout access (Zhu et al., 2023). The integration of wearable devices, encompassing fitness trackers and smartwatches, becomes instrumental in monitoring users' performance metrics like heart rate and calorie expenditure (Jerath et al., 2023). Incorporating gamification elements, such as rewards, challenges, and leaderboards, enhances user motivation and engagement levels (Zhang, 2023). Furthermore, the utilization of VR and AR technologies generates immersive fitness encounters, simulating diverse environments and scenarios for users.

The rise of virtual gyms and fitness experiences has deeply influenced the broader fitness landscape. These platforms have democratized fitness access, transcending location and socioeconomic status barriers, while the surge of virtual fitness has given rise to hybrid models that merge in-person and virtual options, catering to diverse user preferences. This shift has prompted fitness professionals to innovate workout designs for engagement and efficacy in virtual formats. Moreover, the success of virtual fitness has spurred market growth and competition, driving continuous technological advancements, and holds the potential to positively impact public health by offering accessible avenues for physical activity, particularly during periods of limited mobility.

2.2 Advantages and Limitations of Virtual Gym Workouts

The emergence of virtual fitness centers and fitness encounters has ushered in a multitude of advantages tailored to address the shifting inclinations of individuals in search of streamlined and effective means to sustain their physical well-being. By affording adaptability and convenience, these immersive experiences facilitate personalized exercise regimens, accommodating individuals grappling with demanding or erratic schedules (Jo et al., 2023). These platforms proffer an extensive spectrum of workout routines, spanning the gamut from high-intensity interval training (HIIT) to specialized yoga sessions. This diversity empowers users to delve into a myriad of exercise modalities, thus staving off tedium and ensuring sustained engagement (Batrakoulis et al., 2023). Through synergistic collaborations with proficient fitness instructors on a global scale, virtual fitness hubs furnish access to expertise that may otherwise be scarce within local environs. Notably, they often present economically viable subscription models, undercutting conventional gym memberships while simultaneously negating the need for travel and ancillary expenditures. Moreover, the realm of virtual fitness safeguards personal privacy and comfort, permitting workout sessions within familiar settings and thereby mitigating self-consciousness. An additional attribute lies in its capacity to foster a worldwide community by means of interactive features that nurture social interplay, thereby engendering a shared sense of accountability and camaraderie among users.

In spite of the myriad advantages inherent in virtual gyms and fitness encounters, it is imperative to acknowledge the salient challenges and contemplations they bring forth. The absence of a tangible gymnasium milieu and the lack of direct interaction with fitness instructors can engender impediments for individuals, notably in terms of sustaining motivation and upholding a consistent regimen. The presence of technical hindrances, such as constrained access to dependable internet connectivity and compatible devices, can potentially curtail engagement within specific geographical regions (Stocker et al., 2023). Even with the guidance of seasoned trainers, these digital platforms might not seamlessly replicate the tailored direction synonymous with in-person sessions. The emulation of specialized equipment or the supervision requisite for certain workout modalities in a virtual space can be a multifaceted endeavor, characterized by intricacies (Purdy et al., 2023). Furthermore, notwithstanding concerted endeavors aimed at fostering a sense of communal belonging, it is noteworthy that virtual fitness experiences may occasionally exhibit limitations with regard to engendering the sociable interplay and companionship inherent in face-to-face group fitness sessions.

2.3 VR and AR Applications in Virtual Gyms

Virtual fitness centers can be characterized as online platforms that leverage VR and AR technologies to replicate exercise settings, granting participants a participatory and captivating physical training encounter. These platforms are designed to tackle several constraints associated with conventional workout regimens, such as monotony and motivational deficits. Through the amalgamation of VR and AR capabilities, virtual fitness centers present users with the chance to immerse themselves in diverse scenarios, surroundings, and hurdles, thereby transmuting their fitness endeavors into dynamic and stimulating pursuits. The immersive attributes inherent to these technologies empower individuals to liberate themselves from the confines of their immediate physical milieu, allowing them to interact within virtual landscapes that span from picturesque panoramas to competitive trials.

2.3.1 Improve Engagement and Motivation

The integration of VR and AR technologies into virtual gyms furnishes a prominent advantage in terms of heightened engagement and motivation encountered by users. Conventional exercise regimens frequently succumb to the pitfall of monotony and repetition, resulting in waning interest and compliance. Nevertheless, the interactive attributes inherent to VR and AR applications within virtual gyms introduce an innovative paradigm to physical fitness, sustaining user engagement through immersive visual experiences and interactive components (Li et al., 2023). These technological advancements facilitate user participation in activities that seamlessly blend amusement with physical exertion, thereby amplifying their inclination to partake in exercise (Doskarayev et al., 2023).

2.3.2 Diverse Exercise Options

Leveraging the capabilities of VR and AR, virtual gyms furnish an extensive array of exercise modalities tailored to diverse preferences and proclivities. Within the virtual realm, users can immerse themselves in activities encompassing virtual cycling, interactive dance routines, and lifelike sports simulations, thereby transcending the boundaries of physical constraints (Khan et al., 2023). This multifaceted repertoire of exercise options serves to surmount the constraints encountered in conventional fitness centers, characterized by limited choices available to users. The provision of such diverse activities within virtual gyms serves as an impetus for users to delve into novel exercise modalities, contributing synergistically to a comprehensive and all-encompassing fitness regimen (Da Silva Schlickmann et al., 2023).

Metaverse

2.3.3 Social Interaction and Communication

The infusion of VR and AR functionalities into virtual gyms introduces an intriguing facet: the prospect of social interaction and competitive engagement. Through these technological conduits, users are afforded the opportunity to forge connections with friends or fellow participants within immersive virtual domains, nurturing a shared sense of community and mutual encouragement (Mejtoft et al., 2023). The gamut of possibilities encompasses participatory involvements in virtual races, interactive challenges, and collaborative workout endeavors, thereby amplifying user motivation by harnessing the impetus of friendly rivalry. This social dimension inherent to virtual gyms engenders an environment that is both captivating and gratifying, mirroring the conviviality emblematic of conventional group exercise sessions.

Figure 4. Other benefits of virtual gym

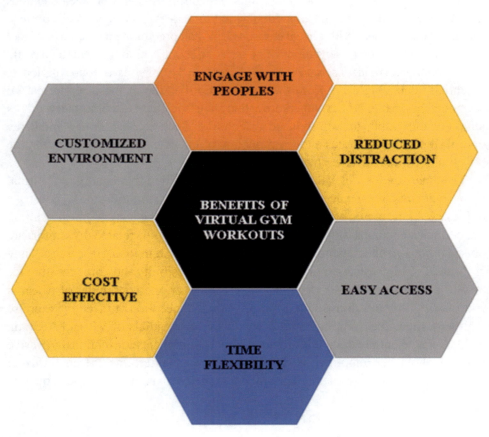

2.4 Personalization and Gamification for Enhanced Virtual Fitness

The incorporation of VR and AR technologies within the realm of virtual gyms presents an avenue for furnishing users with bespoke workout encounters. Achieved through the amalgamation of sensors and tracking devices, these systems have the capability to meticulously observe users' movements, subsequently making real-time adjustments to exercises contingent upon their performance metrics and existing fitness thresholds (Menhas et al., 2023). This adaptive paradigm ensures the provision of exercise regimens attuned to the idiosyncratic requisites of each user, thereby enhancing the efficacy of their pursuit of fitness objectives. Moreover, these technological frameworks are poised to provide instantaneous feedback and precise guidance, thereby fostering the cultivation of accurate form and concurrently diminishing the susceptibility to exercise-related injuries.

An aspect warranting consideration within the realm of VR and AR implementations in virtual gyms is the potential for inducing motion sickness and physical discomfort. Extended engagement with virtual environments can precipitate motion-associated ailments, manifesting as sensations of nausea or dizziness among users (Yun et al., 2023). Such occurrences can serve as impediments to the holistic workout experience, potentially deterring users from the continued utilization of these platforms. To surmount this challenge, developers are called upon to institute strategic interventions aimed at mitigating motion-induced discomfort. Such strategies may entail the optimization of frame rates and the reduction of latency, thereby ameliorating the potential for these adverse physical sensations.

The amalgamation of VR and AR technologies within the paradigm of virtual gyms augments the auspices for transformative prospects in the fitness industry's trajectory. As the march of these technologies persists in its evolution, the prevailing impediments encompassing hardware requisites and motion-related discomfort are poised to wane, a phenomenon anticipated in light of contemporary research (Chang et al., 2023). This trajectory portends heightened accessibility and a broader embrace of virtual gyms across user demographics. Moreover, the continuum of research endeavors within this domain holds promise for the inception of inventive exercise regimens, ingeniously capitalizing on the intrinsic potentials of VR and AR (An, 2023). VR's potential extends to the emulation of environments conventionally evasive to physical reach, exemplified by subaquatic or celestial terrains, thereby infusing the spectrum of exercise encounters with unparalleled diversity and dimensionality.

3. SPORTS IN THE METAVERSE

3.1 Virtual Sports: Overview and Types

The landscape of virtual sports has unfolded as a captivating and swiftly burgeoning domain nestled within the expansive arena of online entertainment and gaming. Manifesting as digital emulations of authentic sports events, these simulations proffer participants and spectators an engrossing and immersive journey that artfully blurs the demarcation between time-honored athletic pursuits and contemporary technological innovations. The realm of virtual sports encompasses an eclectic assortment of sporting disciplines, each harboring distinctive attributes and allure, thereby orchestrating an inclusive reach across a wide spectrum of enthusiasts. This segment undertakes a comprehensive scrutiny of virtual sports, elucidates their sundry typologies, and delves into their transformative ramifications on the landscape of the entertainment industry.

Virtual sports are characterized as intricate computer-generated recreations of genuine sports occurrences. These simulations meticulously emulate the multifaceted intricacies underpinning conventional sports, encapsulating facets such as regulations, teams, athletes, and even the venues, thereby fabricating an environment replete with authenticity and realism for users. The conceptual underpinning of virtual sports resides in the adept utilization of sophisticated algorithms and data inputs to mimic the trajectories of matches or races, engendering outcomes that are imbued with both randomness and impartiality. These virtual enactments are masterminded to mirror with remarkable fidelity the capriciousness and exhilaration intrinsic to live sports scenarios, thereby presenting users with a conduit to interact with their favored sporting pursuits, irrespective of the temporal absence of live events (Afsar et al., 2023).

A manifold of virtual sports genres exists, thoughtfully curated to cater to an expansive spectrum of interests. Prominently featured among these categories is virtual soccer—an arena wherein participants engage in wagers and observe the unfolding of meticulously simulated soccer matches. These virtual renditions deliver an immersive engagement akin to the dynamics of real-world soccer, a sentiment corroborated by Yaqoob et al. (2023). Notably, users are afforded the capacity to scrutinize team metrics, prevailing form, and strategic inclinations, facilitating informed betting decisions. Another notable genre is virtual horse racing, accentuated by Cameron and Ride (2023), where players are afforded the chance to stake their bets on virtual horse races embellished with lifelike animations and accompanying commentary, thereby ameliorating the intensity of thrill. Furthermore, the realm of virtual motorsports has garnered significant traction, with simulations such as Formula 1 and NASCAR captivating the interest of racing aficionados who aspire for an authentic driving experience, harnessed from the haven of their own abodes (Pontin, 2023).

The ascent of virtual sports is propelled by a convergence of influential factors. Foremost among these is the stride of technological progress, culminating in the inception of intricately detailed and visually captivating simulations. As emphasized by Miljković et al. (2023), the integration of cutting-edge graphics, authentic physics engines, and sophisticated artificial intelligence precipitates an environment steeped in immersion within virtual sports. Moreover, the pivotal element of convenience bears potent significance. Virtual sports embrace the attribute of round-the-clock accessibility, affording users the latitude to partake in their favored sporting engagements independent of temporal constraints dictated by real-world schedules (Torrance et al., 2022).

The repercussions of virtual sports on the entertainment landscape are resounding. These virtual realms furnish an alternative entertainment avenue, seamlessly harmonizing with established conventional sports, thereby ensnaring the interest of a burgeoning youthful demographic attuned to the contours of digital experiences (Wang & Wen-Guang, 2023). In consonance with Waitt et al. (2023), the fusion of virtual sports within online betting platforms has engendered transformative ripples across the gambling realm, bequeathing users with an interactive and absorbing medium to indulge in sports wagering. This symbiotic fusion has engendered augmented revenue streams that redound favorably upon both the gaming and gambling sectors alike.

Nevertheless, the emergence of virtual sports also propels forward a tapestry of ethical and regulatory apprehensions. The effortless accessibility and potentially enthralling propensity of virtual sports betting kindle apprehensions regarding its influence on susceptible demographics, including individuals grappling with gambling addiction and minors, who may be more susceptible to its allure (Synnott, 2023). The amalgamation of sports and gambling elements within the virtual sports domain begets inquiries pertaining to the implementation of responsible gambling paradigms and safeguards to ensure consumer protection.

To conclude, virtual sports have arisen as a salient and captivating facet of the entertainment panorama, providing users with a realm of immersive encounters that deftly replicate the vivacity synonymous with traditional sports. Via a diverse spectrum of virtual sports genres, enthusiasts can indulge in a spectrum encompassing simulated soccer duels, equestrian contests, motorsport escapades, and beyond. The genesis of these simulations has been underpinned by technological strides, conferring an expedient and engrossing avenue of amusement. However, the nexus between virtual sports and the domain of gambling engenders ethical qualms, mandating scrupulous contemplation of measures that embrace responsible gaming protocols. As the landscape of virtual sports continues its dynamic evolution, stakeholders are summoned to strike an equipoise between innovation and ethical contemplations, thus guaranteeing a sustainable and gratifying experience for all stakeholders involved. Figure 4 shows type of sports in Metaverse.

Figure 5. Type of virtual sports in metaverse

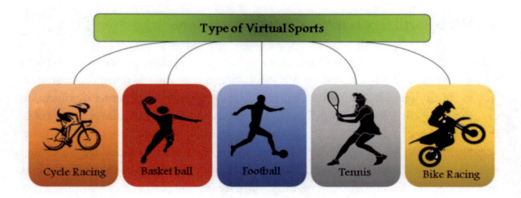

3.2 Esports and Competitive Gaming in the Metaverse

The virtual realm has transcended its role merely as a domain of social interactions and entertainment; it has burgeoned into a flourishing arena for esports and competitive gaming. Termed as "esports," which abbreviates electronic sports, this domain encompasses meticulously orchestrated competitive video gaming events where professional players or teams vie for supremacy. The convergence of esports within the metaverse, an all-encompassing digital universe, begets novel prospects and complexities that reverberate across both domains.

In the recent continuum, esports has undergone a remarkable metamorphosis, transcending the confines of niche fascination to burgeon into a mainstream facet of amusement. The advent of the metaverse unfurls an exhilarating juncture wherein esports can embark upon an augmented trajectory of expansion, wielding the potential to redefine the panorama of competitive gaming. The metaverse unfurls platforms characterized by distinct virtual arenas meticulously tailored to an array of games, immersing spectators within heightened and enriched environs (Salem et al., 2023). Moreover, the metaverse shatters geographical confines, unshackling players and enthusiasts across the globe to partake in and witness esports spectacles, thus culminating in an expansion of the esports aficionado base (Sun, 2023). This fertile ground has served as a crucible for the gestation of innovative tournament paradigms, sculpted within the metaverse's contours. Through harnessing the capabilities of VR technologies, novel gameplay mechanics and challenges hitherto implausible in the physical realm can be woven into these innovative tournament structures (Zoe, 2023). In conclusion, the metaverse's emergence as a platform for esports and competitive gaming presents a transformative opportunity. This digital realm provides a canvas for new forms of engagement and interaction, bringing players, fans, and brands together in unprecedented ways.

3.3 VR Sports Experiences and Simulations

An eminent facet of VR's application in the realm of sports resides in its prowess within training and skill cultivation. VR simulations usher athletes into an environment that faithfully emulates authentic game scenarios, thereby furnishing a controlled crucible for skill honing and refinement. This dynamic is particularly apparent in instances where basketball players can engage in simulated high-pressure free-throw scenarios, while their soccer counterparts can fine-tune penalty kicks against virtual goalkeepers. This granulated and focused training regime augments facets such as muscle memory, astute decision-making, and overarching performance amplification (Parry & Giesbrecht, 2023).

Beyond the realm of player development, VR has wrought a paradigm shift in how spectators and enthusiasts interact with sporting endeavors. By means of VR transmissions, fans traverse the threshold of mere observation and immerse themselves within games, akin to the ambiance within a stadium. This immersive and interactive viewing vista is tailored through a myriad of camera perspectives, real-time statistics, and the unique capacity to toggle between players' viewpoints (T. Wang, 2023). This heightened level of engagement fosters an unassailable sense of presence and exhilaration, metamorphosing the act of remotely viewing sports events into a more captivating and encompassing venture.

In conjunction with athlete training and fostering fan involvement, VR assumes a pivotal role in the comprehensive assessment of athletes' performance. This transformative technology empowers coaches and sports analysts to leverage VR simulations for the meticulous scrutiny of athletes' kinematics, decision-making processes, and overarching game-time performance dynamics. Such meticulous dissection not only affords the identification of intrinsic strengths but also discerns areas warranting refinement, thereby contributing substantively to the formulation of judicious coaching paradigms (Van Biemen et al., 2023).

The assimilation of VR within the realm of sporting experiences and simulated scenarios confers a multitude of advantages upon athletes and aficionados alike. Principal among these is the capacity of VR to facilitate efficient and secure training regimens, thereby mitigating the inherent injury risks associated with high-intensity training protocols. Furthermore, the immersive fabric of VR simulations augments intrinsic motivation and engenders heightened engagement, thereby imbuing practice sessions with heightened efficacy and enjoyment (Alsem et al., 2023). Beyond this, enthusiasts are afforded novel vistas through which to partake in sporting events, transcending geographical confines and ushering in unprecedented access to global athletic spectacles.

3.4 Integration of Real-World Sports With Virtual Platforms

The convergence of tangible sports events with digital realms has been significantly propelled by the progressions in technology. The widespread availability of smartphones, high-speed internet connectivity, and VR innovations has effectively empowered enthusiasts to seamlessly access sports-related content irrespective of their geographic location. Furthermore, the integration of AR has tactically heightened the proximity of sporting exhilaration for fans by superimposing computer-generated elements onto the actual sports milieu (Shen et al., 2023). An illustrative instance can be found in applications such as Snapchat, wherein users can employ AR filters to encapsulate moments during live sports spectacles, thereby augmenting their interactive involvement with the ongoing match. This fusion of genuine sports encounters with virtual platforms has, undeniably, brought about a paradigm shift in the landscape of fan engagement.

Social media platforms have evolved into indispensable facets of the sports encounter, serving as conduits that establish a direct nexus between aficionados and athletes (Adrian et al., 2023). Platforms like Instagram and Twitter, for instance, offer aficionados the opportunity to trail their beloved athletes, gain access to exclusive backstage glimpses, and even engage in real-time dialogues. This form of interaction significantly contributes to the amplification of the communal sentiment and emotional affinities that patrons harbor for their respective teams and sports personalities.

Figure 6. Training in VR
Source: Pastel et al. (2022)

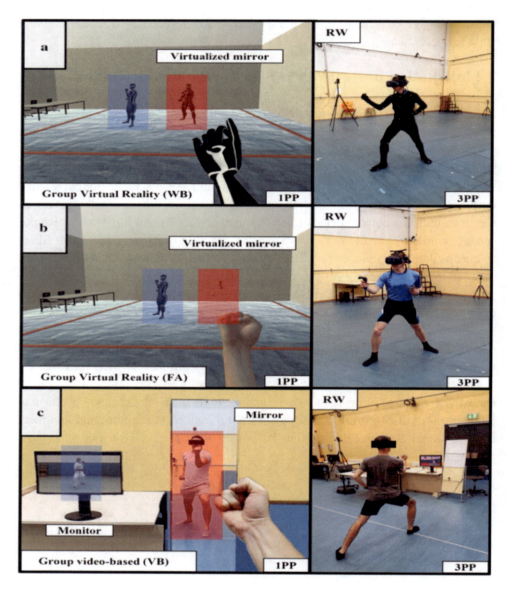

The integration of tangible sports experiences with virtual platforms has exerted a profound influence not only on the realm of fan engagement but also on the transformative reconfiguration of how athletes and teams assess and scrutinize their performance dynamics. The advent of advanced data analytics tools has furnished the means for a comprehensive dissection of player kinetics, strategic gameplay intricacies, and multifaceted performance metrics (Van Rijmenam, 2022). Virtual platforms adeptly aggregate and process data in real-time, thereby furnishing coaches and athletes with invaluable insights that are pivotal in the refinement of tactical approaches and the elevation of overall performance benchmarks. Notably, the penetration of VR technologies into the domain of athlete training regimens stands as a testament to its pioneering impact. Through VR simulations, athletes are endowed with the capacity to engage in iterative practice sessions and envision diverse scenarios, a practice that substantially augments their aptitude for astute decision-making across variable contexts (Murakawa, 2023). The strategic integration of VR within the sphere of physical training holds the potential to expedite the maturation of skillsets and the augmentation of overall athletic prowess.

The emergence of live streaming has, in a similar vein, emerged as a pivotal facet in the amplification of fan engagement. Prominent platforms such as Twitch and YouTube have metamorphosed into veritable epicenters for the real-time dissemination of sports events, thereby affording enthusiasts the dual privilege of witnessing gameplay while concurrently partaking in dynamic exchanges with co-viewers (B. Li et al., 2021). This synchronous mode of interaction engenders a profound sense of collective participation and nurtures a digital fraternity that is intrinsically linked by their shared encounter with the sporting spectacle.

4. BENEFITS AND CHALLENGES OF VIRTUAL GYMS AND SPORTS IN THE METAVERSE

4.1 Health and Fitness Benefits of Virtual Gym Workouts

Physical fitness and well-being are essential components of a healthy lifestyle. Traditional gym workouts have long been a popular choice for individuals seeking to improve their fitness levels. However, with the emergence of virtual gym workouts, individuals now have the option to engage in exercise routines without the constraints of location and time. Virtual gym workouts refer to guided fitness sessions that are conducted remotely through online platforms, providing participants with access to a wide range of workouts led by professional trainers. This report will delve into the numerous health and fitness benefits associated with virtual gym workouts.

Virtual gym workout programs offer an extensive spectrum of exercise modalities, encompassing disciplines such as yoga, high-intensity interval training (HIIT), strength training, and dance, thereby adeptly catering to a diverse range of fitness inclinations (Wedig et al., 2023). This diverse repertoire serves to thwart the encroachment of workout monotony and to perpetuate the motivation levels of participants. The salient attributes characterizing virtual gym platforms, namely personalized features encompassing live coaching, instructive video resources, and real-time performance feedback, collectively function to engender optimal exercise technique, mitigate the prospect of injuries, and amplify the overall effectiveness of workouts (Zikas et al., 2023). The act of engaging in these virtual exercise regimens has been empirically linked to the enhancement of psychological well-being, occasioned by a reduction in levels of stress, anxiety, and depression as a corollary of consistent participation (Turoń-Skrzypińska, 2023).

Furthermore, the virtual workout milieu fosters a heightened sense of accountability and motivation through mechanisms like social interactivity, digital communities, and goal-oriented challenges (Jamshidi, 2023). The inherent convenience and adaptability of these digital fitness routines contribute decisively to the sustenance of long-term adherence by seamlessly integrating physical activity within the contours of daily routines (Hasson et al., 2023). In summation, virtual gym workouts furnish an expansive spectrum of health and fitness benefits that seamlessly harmonize with the contemporary exigencies of the individual's lifestyle. The juxtaposition of convenience, adaptability, diversity, and unfettered accessibility collectively engender improvements in physiological well-being, psychological equilibrium, and the holistic status of one's fitness quotient. The weight of evidence elucidated within the confines of this discourse substantially underscores the inherent potential of virtual gym workouts as a efficacious and enduring modality for the pursuit and perpetuation of a healthy lifestyle. Figure 6 and Figure 7 show the disadvantages and advantages of VR games.

4.3 Accessibility and Inclusivity in the Metaverse

Incorporating principles of accessibility and inclusivity is of paramount significance during the developmental phases of any technological platform, and this tenet holds true for the burgeoning concept of the metaverse as well. The metaverse, with its expansive potential encompassing work, social engagement, leisure, and education, must be architected in a manner that embraces individuals of diverse abilities and backgrounds. As elucidated by Meena et al. in their recent study (2023), the assurance of accessibility within the metaverse transcends beyond a mere legal and ethical obligation; it stands as a strategic advantage within the business realm. Analogous to the legal requisites dictating physical spaces' accessibility, virtual domains must similarly adhere to analogous principles. By ascribing precedence to accessibility, developers can unlock a more expansive user demographic and effectively cater to the heterogeneous array of potential users.

The realization of an accessible and inclusive metaverse hinges upon collaborative efforts among a constellation of stakeholders, encompassing technology enterprises,

Metaverse

policymakers, advocacy cohorts, and the populace at large. Essential to this endeavor is the integration of accessibility features as an intrinsic facet of the developmental trajectory, rather than relegating them to an auxiliary consideration, as stipulated by Radanliev (2023). The active engagement of governmental entities and policymakers is pivotal in fostering a climate of inclusivity within the metaverse. These stakeholders possess the capacity to institute and enforce regulations that stipulate specific accessibility benchmarks for virtual landscapes, mirroring the precedent set by the Americans with Disabilities Act in the physical realm (Dwivedi et al., 2023).

In addition, educational endeavors assume a crucial role in the propagation of awareness concerning matters of accessibility and inclusivity within the metaverse. Academic institutions, in particular, hold the potential to offer curricula tailored to instruct developers in the techniques for crafting accessible virtual domains. Furthermore, initiatives such as consciousness-raising campaigns and immersive workshops serve to sensitize the general populace to the intricacies of challenges encountered by individuals with disabilities within virtual spheres (AbuKhousa et al., 2023).

Figure 7. VR disadvantages

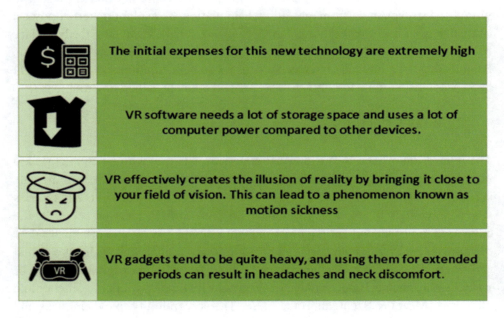

4.4 Ethical Considerations and Safety Concerns in Virtual Environments

4.4.1 Ethical Consideration

In virtual realms, a paramount ethical concern revolves around the gathering and exploitation of personal data (Dhiman, 2023). As users engage within these digital landscapes, their actions, inclinations, and even physiological reactions can be meticulously traced and evaluated. While this data holds value for corporations seeking precise marketing strategies, it concurrently triggers inquiries about consent, possession, and the potential for its misuse. The extent of data amassed and its utilization often remains concealed from users, leading to potential privacy breaches. Furthermore, virtual environments introduce a unique facet of digital identity and representation, as users craft avatars or digital personas to inhabit the virtual realm (Yoo et al., 2023). This practice sparks inquiries about authenticity, as individuals might embrace attributes distinct from their real-world selves. This division between genuine and virtual identities can offer both constructive and adverse outcomes, ranging from amplified self-expression to the possibility of deceit and impersonation. Alongside these concerns, the diversity of content present in virtual spaces, spanning from educational simulations to explicit material, poses a challenge in terms of regulation (Carr & England, 2023). Balancing the boundary between freedom of expression and safeguarding vulnerable users becomes intricate. Establishing apt guidelines and mechanisms for content curation and user oversight becomes indispensable to cultivate a secure and ethically sound environment.

4.4.2 Safety Concerns

The immersion offered by VR and AR experiences comes with a potential risk to physical safety, as users may become disoriented and unaware of their immediate surroundings (Cho et al., 2023). This detachment can lead to accidents and injuries when individuals inadvertently collide with real-world objects or people while engrossed in virtual content. To avert such incidents, it's crucial to establish safety measures like physical boundaries and pass-through cameras that bridge the virtual and real environments, enhancing user awareness. However, the digital landscape of virtual environments is not immune to cybersecurity threats, similar to other online platforms (Mezei & Szentgáli-Tóth, 2023). The susceptibility to cyberattacks and unauthorized access poses risks of data breaches, disruptions to experiences, and the introduction of malicious elements. Maintaining robust cybersecurity protocols, encompassing encryption and authentication mechanisms, becomes imperative in safeguarding users' data and ensuring a secure virtual realm. Alongside these technical challenges, virtual environments can also perpetuate social issues, including harassment and toxic behavior (Javed et al., 2023). The anonymity inherent in such spaces can embolden individuals to engage in harmful conduct. To address this, implementing comprehensive reporting avenues, effective user moderation tools, and clear community guidelines is vital to cultivate a virtual social sphere that prioritizes safety and inclusivity.

5. TECHNOLOGICAL INNOVATIONS IN VIRTUAL GYMS AND SPORTS

5.1 Immersive Technologies and Their Role in Virtual Fitness

The integration of immersive technologies into the realm of fitness regimens not only amplifies engagement and commitment but also constitutes a contributive factor to overarching enhancements in health. A comprehensive examination conducted by X. Li et al. (2023) underscores that VR-based exercise routines manifest demonstrable enhancements in cardiovascular endurance, muscular robustness, and suppleness. Furthermore, applications grounded in VR furnish real-time evaluative insights into posture and kinetics, thereby mitigating the risk of exercise-related injuries (Solas-Martínez et al., 2023). This technological domain facilitates bespoke workout regimens that align precisely with individualized levels of fitness, thereby engendering outcomes of paramount efficacy.

Integral to the quest for enduring health dividends is the concept of exercise adherence, denoting the capacity to sustain a regular workout regimen. Immersive technologies assume a seminal role in elevating adherence rates. As substantiated by the inquiry conducted by Smith et al. (2023), participants who immersed themselves in virtual fitness programs demonstrated higher proclivities to adhere to their prescribed exercise routines, eclipsing their counterparts following conventional protocols. The immersive character of these technologies functions as a salient diversion from the physical exertion, thereby imbuing workout sessions with a diminished perception of strenuousness and an augmented sense of gratification.

Immersive technologies have introduced a paradigm shift in the fitness industry by merging physical activity with virtual environments. The role of these technologies in virtual fitness goes beyond novelty; they significantly enhance engagement, motivation, and exercise adherence. Moreover, they contribute to a wide range of health benefits by providing personalized and interactive workout experiences. As the field of virtual fitness continues to evolve, addressing challenges and refining applications will be pivotal in ensuring that immersive technologies remain an effective tool for promoting active and healthy lifestyles.

5.2 Haptic Feedback and Sensory Integration in Virtual Sports

Within the realm of virtual sports, the intricate interplay of sensory integration assumes a pivotal role in shaping an experience that is both captivating and credible for its users. As individuals partake in physical engagements, their cerebral faculties engage in an incessant process of amalgamating inputs from a myriad of senses—ranging from vision and audition to touch—thus fashioning a cohesive apprehension of their surroundings. The augmentation of haptic feedback in conjunction with visual and auditory cues serves to elevate this cognitive undertaking, bestowing upon the virtual sports milieu an aura of authenticity and immersive allure (T. Sun et al., 2023).

In the context of virtual sports, haptic feedback mechanisms transpire through the utilization of devices engineered to emulate tactile perceptions encompassing vibrations, resistive forces, and textural sensations. These mechanisms effectively mimic the tactile sensations that might arise from interactions with virtual entities—be they objects, adversaries, or equipment. For instance, envision a virtual tennis encounter where a player experiences the vibrational resonance of a racket making contact with a ball. This tactile input substantially fortifies the user's affiliation with their actions within the virtual expanse, nurturing a heightened symbiosis between individual behavior and the simulated surroundings (Van Wegen et al., 2023).

The landscape of virtual sports harbors a spectrum of devices devised to deliver haptic feedback, encompassing wearable haptic vests, gloves, and controllers. Endowed with actuators primed to engender tactile sensations in concordance with in-game occurrences, these devices operate as conduits to convey tactile experiences mirroring real-world phenomena. Consider, for instance, the emulation of a gust of wind or the sensation of resistance during a virtual skiing escapade, which serves not solely to amplify verisimilitude, but concurrently augments the user's capacity to execute precision-laden movements and decisions (L. Zhang et al., 2022).

Metaverse

Figure 8. VR advantages

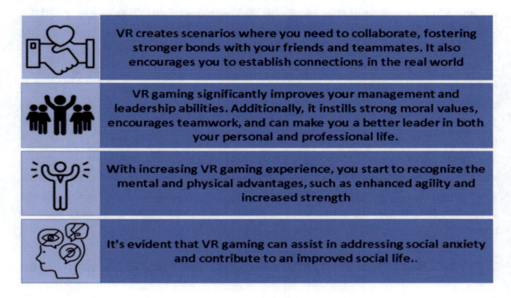

5.3 Artificial Intelligence (AI) in Personalized Fitness Coaching

The infusion of Artificial Intelligence (AI) across diverse spheres of human existence has engendered profound paradigm shifts, extending its transformative influence to the realm of fitness coaching. The domain of fitness instruction is undergoing a radical metamorphosis as AI technology becomes instrumental in furnishing bespoke guidance, thereby revolutionizing the modus operandi individuals adopt to pursue their health and well-being aspirations. The ensuing discourse delves into the substantive import of AI within the context of personalized fitness coaching, elucidating its attendant merits, confronting impediments, and auguring its latent prospects for the unfolding future.

Traditional paradigms of fitness coaching have typically adhered to a standardized approach, proffering universally applicable directives that may inadvertently overlook the idiosyncrasies intrinsic to each individual. In stark contradistinction, AI emboldens the domain of fitness coaching to transcend the conventional boundaries of homogeneity. Operationalized through intricate computational systems, AI algorithms meticulously scrutinize an extensive array of salient data points, encompassing an individual's medical chronicle, prevailing physical acumen, dietary proclivities, and even contemporaneous health metrics gleaned from wearable technologies. This multifaceted assimilation of information equips AI-driven platforms with the acumen to meticulously customize workout regimes, dietary schemas, and holistic well-being stratagems calibrated in meticulous tandem with the distinct contours of an individual's exigencies (Bays et al., 2023; Singhal et al., 2020; Dogra et al., 2022).

The assimilation of AI into the fabric of personalized fitness coaching bequeaths a panoply of discernible advantages. Foremost, it engenders an elevated adherence quotient to fitness regimens. By recalibrating exercise routines in consonance with individual inclinations and physiological capacities, AI engenders the creation of engaging and sustainable fitness protocols, thereby amplifying the propensity for sustained commitment and tangible results (Lee & Lin, 2023). Secondly, the integration of AI technology furnishes real-time surveillance and appraisal. Wearable apparatuses that incorporate AI-driven algorithms adeptly track pivotal metrics encompassing heart rate dynamics, caloric expenditures, and even nuances of movement biomechanics. The upshot is an immediate and granulated feedback loop, thereby endowing users with expeditious insights into their performance trajectories (Kim & Baek, 2023; Shafiq et al., 2021).

5.4 Advancements in Motion Tracking and Gesture Recognition

The evolution of motion tracking and gesture recognition technologies has exhibited rapid progression, propelled by the refinement of sensory apparatus, machine learning algorithms, and computational potency. These advancements have engendered the emergence of avant-garde applications that hitherto resided within the realm of futuristic speculation. As posited by N. Li (2023), motion tracking entails the meticulous capture and subsequent analysis of object or human movements, facilitated by an amalgam of sensors and cameras. Conversely, gesture recognition is concerned with the discernment and interpretation of specific gestures or actions executed by human agents. These technological strides have invariably laid the foundation for pioneering user interfaces and an elevated echelon of user engagement.

The domains of motion tracking and gesture recognition have ushered in a paradigm shift within the expanse of the gaming industry, furnishing players with a heightened sphere of immersive and physically dynamic gameplay. The advent of instrumental contrivances such as the Microsoft Kinect and Sony PlayStation Move has afforded gamers the capacity to dictate the actions of in-game avatars through corporeal maneuvers (Mabary, 2023). Beyond this, the precincts of gesture recognition technology have unfurled a vista of opportunities in the form of interactive VR escapades. Within this context, users are empowered to manipulate virtual objects and surroundings via instinctual gestures, amplifying the sense of tangibility and agency within virtual environments (Lopes, 2023).

Within the domain of healthcare, the assimilation of motion tracking and gesture recognition technologies has engendered noteworthy applications, particularly within the purview of physical therapy and rehabilitation. Diligent scholarship has yielded the development of intricate frameworks that meticulously scrutinize the locomotive maneuvers of patients during therapeutic exercises. Consequent to this, instantaneous feedback is proffered to both patients and healthcare practitioners, thus engendering a symbiotic loop of responsiveness (Monge et al., 2023). These technological modalities stand as catalysts for the augmentation of the efficacy and engrossment quotient intrinsic to rehabilitation regimens, thereby culminating in the amelioration of patient prognoses.

The trajectory of advancements witnessed within motion tracking and gesture recognition technologies has profoundly impacted the landscape of human-robot interactivity. Robots, endowed with the compendium of these technological features, have acquired the adeptness to comprehend and reciprocate to human gestures, thus conferring an augmented layer of intuition upon their operability (Qi et al., 2023). This paradigm shift holds palpable significance within sectors such as manufacturing, where robots can seamlessly harmonize their functions with those of human laborers, thereby heralding a nexus of efficiency and safety.

6. BUILDING AND SCALING VIRTUAL GYM AND SPORTS PLATFORMS

6.1 Business Models and Monetization Strategies for Metaverse Fitness

The incorporation of fitness activities into the metaverse unveils fresh possibilities for businesses to craft inventive business models and approaches to generating revenue. This segment delves into the diverse business models and revenue-generation methods applicable in the realm of metaverse fitness.

One notable business model within the metaverse fitness sector revolves around subscription-based virtual fitness platforms. Users commit to a monthly fee in exchange for access to an array of virtual fitness classes, personalized training sessions, and interactive fitness encounters within the metaverse. This approach extends users a steady and varied fitness regimen while ensuring a reliable income stream for the platform providers (Shuai et al., 2023). Such platforms commonly feature elements like customizable avatars, social engagements, and tracking of progress to enhance user involvement and motivation.

An additional approach for revenue generation involves the pay-per-class or experience model. Within this structure, users make payments for individual fitness classes or experiences within the metaverse. This setup affords users flexibility in selecting specific activities that align with their preferences and schedules (Morrison & Buhalis, 2023). Fitness instructors or virtual fitness centers can present an assortment of classes, spanning from yoga to high-intensity interval training, granting users the freedom to only pay for their chosen engagements.

Virtual personal trainers and coaches provide another avenue for revenue. Fitness experts can offer tailored guidance, workout plans, and feedback to users through virtual interactions within the metaverse. This strategy caters to individuals in pursuit of individualized fitness solutions and empowers fitness professionals to transcend physical constraints. Generating revenue can be accomplished via subscription models or fees for one-on-one sessions.

A distinctive monetization strategy comes in the form of in-app purchases for virtual fitness attire and equipment. Users can enhance their virtual fitness experiences by acquiring virtual workout apparel, gear, and accessories for their avatars (Cennamo et al., 2023). This approach blends the emotional gratification of personalization with a revenue avenue for platform providers. Beyond being a means of revenue, virtual fitness gear adds to the sense of immersion for users within the metaverse environment.

Figure 9. Business model for metaverse gym and spots

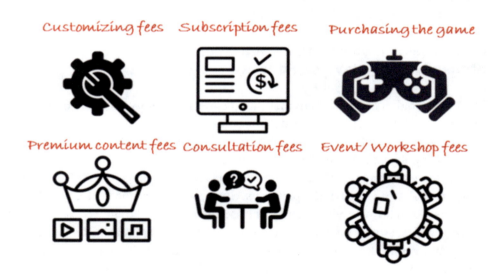

6.2 User Experience Design and User Interface in Virtual Gyms and Sports

Virtual fitness facilities and sports platforms have garnered significant attention, offering users an alternative avenue for partaking in physical endeavors and maintaining their fitness regimens. The pivotal underpinning of these platforms' success resides in the meticulous deliberation of User Experience (UX) design and User Interface (UI) components. This exposition delves into the profound importance of UX design and UI within the realm of virtual fitness facilities and sports platforms, elucidating their far-reaching implications on user engagement, motivational dynamics, and overarching contentment.

The pertinence of User Experience Design materializes as an instrumental determinant in the efficacy of virtual fitness facilities and sports platforms. A judiciously conceived UX framework revolves around ensuring that users encounter an interface that is inherently user-friendly, pleasurable to interact with, and facile to traverse. As posited by Ferreira et al. (2023), a cardinal tenet of UX design lies in the doctrine of "user-centered design," wherein the crux involves custom-tailoring the user experience to seamlessly align with their requisites, predilections, and behavioral patterns. Within the contours of virtual fitness facilities and sports platforms, this doctrine translates to the creation of interfaces that transcend visual allure, encompassing functional efficiency as well.

The quintessence of efficacious UX design instigates heightened user engagement through the facilitation of an unimpeded progression of activities and interactions. As underscored by Deng et al. (2023), the fostering of a heightened sense of immersion and presence within a virtual milieu augments user engagement dynamics. Constituents such as interactive workout regimens, real-time feedback mechanisms, and judicious integration of gamification stratagems collectively contribute to an augmented sense of user connection and motivation for active participation. This tenet finds reinforcement in the investigations conducted by Johnson et al. (2020), wherein discernment of the virtual fitness facility experience as an enjoyable and interactive encounter correlates positively with elevated levels of user engagement. Figure 9 shows types and categories of haptic feedback in metaverse gym and sports.

6.3 Scaling and Managing Virtual Communities and Events

To efficiently expand virtual communities and events, organizations must embrace several pivotal strategies. Firstly, the critical role lies in selecting a suitable platform. This platform should be aligned with the community's objectives and should cater to desired functionalities, including real-time communication, content sharing, and participant engagement (Hughes et al., 2023). Secondly, nurturing user-generated content and interactions heightens the sense of belonging and ownership within the community (Lister, 2023). Achieving this entails motivating members to contribute ideas, discussions, and pertinent content. Thirdly, implementing moderation mechanisms ensures that interactions maintain a respectful and relevant nature

(Brown, n.d.). Collaborative efforts between automated content filters and human moderators uphold a positive and secure environment.

Technological advancements have furnished tools and solutions for the efficient management and expansion of virtual communities and events. The integration of artificial intelligence (AI) and machine learning (ML) algorithms can automate specific tasks such as content curation, moderation, and tailored recommendations (Gupta & Kumar, 2023). Furthermore, harnessing the capabilities of cloud computing resources can offer the requisite scalability to accommodate growing participant numbers. Cloud-based solutions facilitate the seamless expansion of server capacities, capable of managing heightened traffic during peak periods.

6.4 Partnerships and Collaborations in the Metaverse Fitness Industry

Partnerships between fitness experts and VR developers have facilitated the creation of a diverse and captivating array of fitness content. These collaborations yield a multitude of workout routines and wellness experiences designed to suit various fitness levels and preferences. Fitness trainers and studios have teamed up with VR companies to offer interactive classes that harness the immersive potential of the Metaverse (Høeg et al., 2023). Collaborations between manufacturers of wearable technology and Metaverse fitness platforms have made real-time tracking and monitoring of users' physical activity possible. Wearable devices seamlessly integrate into virtual fitness experiences, providing users with precise data about their heart rate, calories expended, and exercise intensity (Letafati & Otoum, 2023). The alignment of Metaverse fitness platforms with social media networks through collaborations has nurtured a sense of community among users. Integration with social platforms empowers users to connect, share their accomplishments, and partake in friendly competitions, thereby elevating motivation and responsibility (Brayshaw et al., 2023). Educational institutions partnering with Metaverse fitness platforms have contributed to the research and advancement of inventive fitness technologies. These collaborations result in practices grounded in evidence, ensuring that virtual workouts are both effective and safe for users (Arpaci & Bahari, 2023).

7. VIRTUAL GYM AND SPORTS APPLICATIONS IN HEALTHCARE AND THERAPY

7.1 Virtual Rehabilitation and Physical Therapy

Virtual rehabilitation, an inventive approach that merges technology with therapy, has garnered substantial interest within the realm of physical therapy. This method harnesses the capabilities of VR and AR technologies to craft immersive and interactive settings, enabling individuals to partake in therapeutic activities. Virtual rehabilitation presents several advantages compared to conventional methods. It furnishes a motivating and captivating environment for patients, elevating their commitment to treatment plans. Findings from Nath et al.'s research (2023) highlight that VR interventions led to enhanced functional outcomes among stroke patients. Furthermore, virtual rehabilitation empowers therapists to tailor exercises to each patient's specific requirements and to more effectively monitor progress (Maskeliūnas et al., 2023; Placidi et al., 2023). This personalized approach augments treatment results and contributes to patient contentment.

The applications of virtual rehabilitation span a wide range of medical conditions. Patients grappling with neurological disorders like Parkinson's disease can reap benefits from VR-based exercises targeting balance and coordination (Kwon et al., 2023). In orthopedic rehabilitation, virtual environments can simulate real-life scenarios to facilitate functional recovery (Kato, 2023). Cardiac rehabilitation programs can leverage VR to bolster cardiovascular health through engaging activities (Brewer et al., 2022). Additionally, individuals recuperating post-surgery can engage in virtual exercises aimed at enhancing range of motion and muscle strength (Vaccaro et al., 2016).

Figure 10. Types and categories of haptic feedback in Metaverse

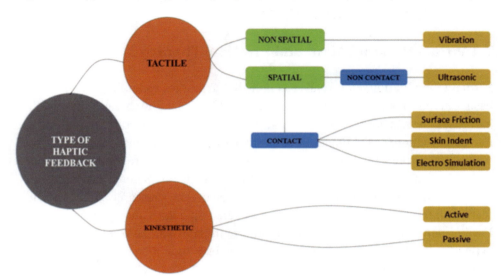

7.2 Mental Health and Wellness Applications in the Metaverse

The emergence of the metaverse has introduced fresh avenues for approaching mental health and wellness challenges in innovative manners. The metaverse, a shared virtual space that arises from the convergence of physical and VR, provides a distinct platform for conceiving and deploying mental health and wellness applications.

Within the metaverse, a diverse and inventive terrain has evolved to champion mental well-being and offer crucial support. Central to this landscape are virtual support groups, which facilitate connections among individuals wrestling with similar mental health struggles. These groups foster an environment of empathy and confidentiality, creating a secure space for exchanging experiences without fear (Ezawa et al., 2023). Moreover, the metaverse serves as a sanctuary for mindfulness and meditation, presenting serene settings that guide users through relaxation practices, contributing to a balanced mental state (Ahuja et al., 2023). The digital realm also hosts online counseling services, enabling users to access licensed therapists within virtual therapy offices, transcending geographical barriers and furnishing convenient avenues for obtaining professional mental health assistance (Ahuja et al., 2023).

Within these immersive digital domains, artistic expression and therapeutic interventions flourish. Virtual art studios and interactive music spaces act as outlets for self-expression, allowing individuals to channel creativity for emotional release and self-discovery (Kępińska & Wiśniewski, 2023). Furthermore, VR exposure therapy (VRET) emerges as a groundbreaking method for addressing phobias and anxiety disorders. This approach utilizes controlled environments to guide individuals in confronting their fears within a secure and controlled framework (Jonathan et al., 2023; Hawajri et al., 2023). The metaverse also champions social connectedness through customizable environments, enabling users to craft their social spaces, thereby diminishing feelings of isolation and fostering meaningful interactions (Xie et al., 2023).

Functioning as a hub of comprehensive growth, the metaverse offers an array of psychoeducational resources and skill-building sessions. Interactive workshops and seminars augment mental health understanding and impart coping mechanisms, bolstering users' mental well-being (Kamaruddin et al., 2023). The metaverse's potential for stress alleviation is harnessed through engaging games that incorporate biofeedback and relaxation techniques, aiding users in managing stress and anxiety levels (Dias et al., 2023; Champion, 2022). Within this evolving digital expanse, the fusion of technology and mental health initiatives presents a transformative paradigm that transcends physical confines and nurtures emotional well-being on a profound scale.

As the metaverse's promise in mental health and wellness garners recognition, ethical concerns like data privacy, accessibility, and the qualifications of virtual therapists necessitate attention. Concurrently, ongoing research is scrutinizing the lasting efficacy of metaverse-based interventions and their integration with traditional therapeutic approaches. In conclusion, the metaverse offers a promising domain for reshaping mental health and wellness interventions. Through virtual support groups, mindfulness spaces, therapeutic simulations, and an array of other applications, individuals gain access to innovative tools for addressing mental health challenges. Nevertheless, prudent deliberation must be accorded to ethical and practical ramifications, ensuring the responsible and effective execution of these interventions.

7.3 Virtual Sports for Training and Skill Development

Virtual sports have emerged as an innovative and effective method for enhancing training and skill development across various domains. These virtual environments offer engaging and interactive platforms that replicate real-world scenarios, enabling individuals to acquire and refine essential competencies. Incorporating elements of gamification, simulations, and immersive technologies, virtual sports provide a dynamic learning experience with numerous benefits.

Virtual sports are increasingly utilized in fields such as healthcare, aviation, and military training. Through simulated medical scenarios, medical professionals can practice critical decision-making and procedural skills in a risk-free environment (Smith et al., 2020). Similarly, aviation personnel can undergo virtual flight training, enabling them to acquire complex flying skills and emergency responses (Jones & Williams, 2018). In sports education, virtual platforms contribute to skill development. Soccer players, for instance, use VR to analyze and improve their performance through immersive match simulations (Renshaw & Chow, 2019). Basketball players train using VR systems that track movements and provide real-time feedback for refining shooting techniques (Johnson et al., 2021).

The education sector also benefits from virtual sports. Chemistry students employ gamified simulations to grasp complex molecular interactions (Brown et al., 2017), while history learners engage in virtual reconstructions of historical events, deepening their understanding (Davis, 2016). Virtual sports offer inclusivity and accessibility. Individuals with physical disabilities can engage in sports simulations tailored to their abilities, enhancing their self-esteem and physical well-being (Shapiro et al., 2019). Furthermore, remote training and collaboration are facilitated, breaking geographical barriers (Miller & Smith, 2022). However, challenges exist, including the cost of VR equipment and the need for sophisticated software. Moreover, individual experiences may vary due to differing levels of technological familiarity (Wilson & Lee, 2020). Ensuring the balance between engagement and accurate skill representation also remains a concern (Garcia et al., 2018).

In conclusion, virtual sports have revolutionized training and skill development across diverse fields. With their potential for experiential learning and broad applicability, these platforms offer a promising future for education and professional growth.

7.4 Telehealth and Telemedicine Integration With Virtual Fitness

The convergence of telehealth and telemedicine with virtual fitness has emerged as a transformative strategy within the healthcare sector. This innovative synergy offers convenient and easily accessible solutions for both patients and healthcare providers, leveraging technology to elevate healthcare provision, enhance patient outcomes, and encourage overall well-being. Telehealth pertains to the remote delivery of healthcare services, whereas telemedicine concentrates specifically on clinical diagnosis and treatment. On the other hand, virtual fitness encompasses digital platforms designed for exercise and wellness endeavors. The fusion of telehealth and telemedicine with virtual fitness exhibits great potential in tackling various healthcare challenges. Through remote consultations, patients can promptly receive medical advice and monitoring, consequently reducing the necessity for in-person appointments (Ullah et al., 2023). Virtual fitness platforms offer guided workouts and personalized exercise routines, fostering physical activity and preemptively addressing chronic conditions (Hang, 2023).

This integration fosters patient engagement and bolsters adherence to treatment regimens. The ability to track vital signs and exercise data in real time empowers healthcare providers to tailor interventions more effectively (Dogheim, 2023). Interactive virtual fitness sessions motivate patients to maintain an active lifestyle, which synergizes with their medical care (Ștefan et al., 2023). Furthermore, the integration of telehealth and telemedicine with virtual fitness greatly amplifies access to healthcare services, particularly for marginalized populations (Norman et al., 2023). Individuals residing in rural areas or facing limited mobility can reap benefits from virtual consultations and guided fitness sessions, transcending geographical barriers (Jones et al., 2023). Nevertheless, certain challenges such as technological literacy and privacy concerns necessitate attention (D. B. Dhiman, 2023). Healthcare providers require training to proficiently navigate virtual platforms and ensure effective communication (Chengoden et al., 2023). Additionally, safeguarding patient data and upholding regulatory compliance emerge as pivotal considerations (Saha, n.d.).

In conclusion, the amalgamation of telehealth and telemedicine with virtual fitness showcases substantial potential in reshaping healthcare provision. By amalgamating remote consultations with virtual fitness platforms, this approach heightens patient engagement, adherence, and accessibility while also confronting specific challenges. As technology forges ahead, further exploration and collaboration stand as imperative components for optimizing this integration and magnifying its impact on global healthcare. Figure 10 shows metaverse application in other industries.

Figure 11. Metaverse application in other industry

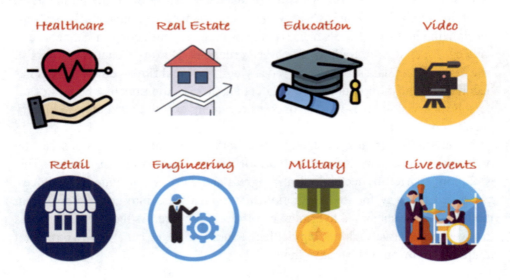

8. IMPACT OF VIRTUAL GYMS AND SPORTS ON SPORTS INDUSTRY

8.1 Transformation of the Fitness and Sports Industry

The fitness and sports sector has undergone a substantial makeover with the emergence of virtual gyms. Virtual gyms encompass online platforms that grant access to fitness classes, training sessions, and workout routines through digital devices, thereby enabling remote engagement. This shift in approach has been propelled by advancements in technology and shifts in consumer inclinations.

Virtual gyms present the advantages of convenience and accessibility, empowering individuals to partake in workouts from the comfort of their own homes. As outlined by Miyoung et al. (2023), the ascent of virtual fitness solutions gained momentum during the COVID-19 pandemic, as individuals sought alternatives to traditional gym settings. This trend is corroborated by research conducted by Soilemezi et al. (2022), which underscores the growing demand for flexible fitness alternatives. The influence of virtual gyms goes beyond mere convenience. The study by Bannell et al. (2023) suggests that virtual fitness platforms often incorporate interactive elements like real-time feedback and social interaction, elevating user motivation and adherence. Furthermore, the convergence of VR technology with fitness has started to create immersive experiences simulating outdoor activities (Settimo et al., 2023). The business landscape has also adjusted to this transformation. Established players in the fitness industry have seamlessly integrated virtual offerings into their array of services (Kaihua, 2023). This strategic maneuver has allowed traditional gyms to retain members seeking hybrid workout experiences. Simultaneously, startups specializing in virtual fitness have risen in prominence, attracting investments and causing disruptions in traditional market structures. However, challenges persist. The assurance of data security and privacy within virtual fitness environments has become of utmost importance (H. Ullah et al., 2023). Additionally, the lack of in-person supervision gives rise to concerns regarding exercise technique and injury prevention.

In summary, virtual gyms have revolutionized the fitness and sports sector by presenting convenient, interactive, and all-encompassing workout options. This evolution, spurred by technological progress and shifting consumer preferences, has paved the way for the integration of virtual fitness into conventional gym models, thereby shaping a hybrid trajectory for the future. As the sector continues to advance, effectively addressing challenges and optimizing benefits will be pivotal in upholding this transformative trend.

8.2 New Business Opportunities and Revenue Streams

The dynamic landscape of virtual gyms and sports has ushered in a realm of exciting business prospects and potential avenues for generating revenue. This transformative shift in the fitness and sports sector revolves around the accessibility, convenience, and novel experiences virtual platforms bring to users. One avenue for capitalizing on this shift is through subscription models, which provide users with access to an array of on-demand workouts, personalized training regimens, and virtual classes (Schneider et al., 2023). By adopting this approach, businesses can establish a reliable income stream while granting users the flexibility to engage on their terms.

Live virtual classes present another alluring opportunity. Hosting real-time fitness sessions led by seasoned trainers can attract a dedicated user base that values interactive, engaging workouts (Belt & Lowenthal, 2022). These classes not only foster a sense of community but also promote accountability among participants. Additionally, tapping into the virtual personal training sphere can prove lucrative. By offering tailor-made guidance remotely, fitness professionals can cater to individuals in search of personalized attention (Siricharoen, 2023). This premium service not only caters to specific needs but also contributes to augmented revenue streams. Beyond individual endeavors, orchestrating virtual events and competitions—such as fitness challenges, tournaments, and races—can draw a global participant base, with entry fees bolstering overall revenue (Lee et al., 2018). Lastly, capitalizing on the rising demand for workplace health initiatives, businesses can collaborate with corporations to provide virtual wellness programs to employees, offering a strategic pathway into corporate wellness programs (Huang & Kim, 2020). Figure 11 shows the transformation in learning using metaverse technology.

8.3 Disruptive Potential and Challenges for Traditional Sports

Virtual sports have emerged as a formidable and transformative presence, challenging the established prominence of traditional sports within the realm of entertainment. These virtual alternatives offer distinct advantages that disrupt the conventional sports landscape. They present accessibility and convenience, enabling individuals to partake in sports experiences unrestricted by physical limitations (Xu, 2023). This accessibility holds particular appeal for the younger, digitally native generation (Singh & Kumar, 2023). Additionally, virtual sports introduce immersive encounters through technologies such as VR and AR, elevating fan engagement (Jiang et al., 2023). These immersive encounters blur the boundaries between the real and the virtual, captivating audiences in unprecedented ways.

The ascendancy of virtual sports poses significant challenges for traditional sports. The ease of accessibility and engagement in virtual sports diverts attention from conventional sports events (Chen et al., 2023). By offering innovative modes of competition, virtual sports capture a portion of the sports enthusiast demographic, potentially impacting viewership of traditional sports (Desbordes, 2023). Moreover, the captivating virtual experiences may lead to reduced attendance at physical sports venues, thereby affecting revenue streams (Greenhalgh & Goebert, 2023). The monetization strategies employed by virtual sports present additional hurdles for traditional sports. Virtual sports open avenues for inventive revenue generation through in-game purchases, virtual merchandise, and microtransactions (Kesavan & N, 2023). These revenue channels have the potential to rival the traditional sports' reliance on ticket sales and broadcasting rights. The disruptive potential of virtual sports is undeniable, driven by factors like accessibility, immersive interactions, and innovative monetization models. In response, traditional sports must adapt to these challenges by embracing technological innovations, amplifying fan engagement, and exploring novel revenue sources. The coexistence of conventional and virtual sports is likely to mold the future sports landscape, necessitating all stakeholders to adeptly navigate this evolving and dynamic scenario.

Figure 12. Transforming learning skill using metaverse

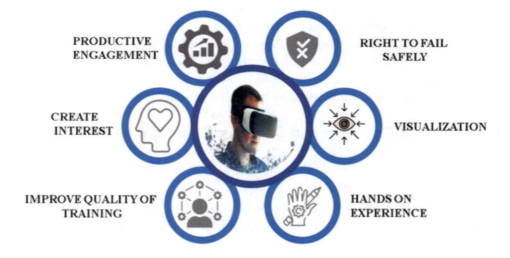

9. SOCIAL AND COMMUNITY ASPECTS OF METAVERSE SPORTS

9.1 Virtual Fan Engagement and Spectatorship

Enhancing fan engagement within metaverse sports has become a central focus for elevating the viewer experience. Through the utilization of VR and AR technologies, enthusiasts can now immerse themselves in highly realistic stadiums, creating an unparalleled sense of being present (Koohang et al., 2023). This interactive digital realm facilitates fan interaction, enabling them to connect with fellow supporters, digitally cheer for their teams, and even participate in sport-related mini-games. This type of engagement has the potential to redefine the conventional boundaries of fanhood, establishing stronger emotional ties between fans and their favorite teams and athletes (Buhalis et al., 2023).

The advent of metaverse sports has also prompted a reimagination of how spectators engage with events. The traditional passive observation is evolving into active involvement through virtual platforms. Fans have the capability to craft personalized avatars to attend matches, virtually interacting with others and engaging in real-time discussions. These avatars are able to convey emotions, intensifying the feeling of unity and passion commonly experienced during in-person events. Furthermore, the metaverse allows for a broader global reach, eliminating geographical limitations and making sports events accessible to a wider audience (Ning et al., 2023).

Additionally, metaverse sports offer monetization possibilities for both sports organizations and technology developers (Zalan & Barbesino, 2023). By means of virtual merchandise and experiences, revenue streams can expand beyond traditional methods. Virtual fan engagement also unlocks potential for targeted advertising and partnerships, as insights derived from user interactions can shape personalized marketing approaches.

However, this revolutionary transition comes with certain challenges. Privacy concerns emerge as personal data is collected to create tailored experiences, necessitating robust security measures (Q. Zhang, 2023). Technical glitches and differences in access could impede inclusivity (D. P. Radanliev, 2023). Striking a balance between seamlessly integrating metaverse engagement while upholding the authenticity of the sport is also of utmost importance.

In conclusion, metaverse sports have ushered in a new era of fan engagement and spectatorship. Through the implementation of VR and AR technologies, fans are now active participants, forging deeper connections with their cherished sports. The metaverse introduces unprecedented avenues for revenue generation, while also demanding careful attention to privacy and accessibility concerns. Finding a harmonious equilibrium between innovation and tradition will be pivotal as the realm of sports continues to evolve within the metaverse.

9.2 Creating Inclusive and Diverse Virtual Sports Communities

The rapidly evolving digital landscape has given rise to a notable phenomenon: the emergence of virtual sports communities. In these dynamic spaces, ensuring inclusivity and diversity stands as a crucial pillar for nurturing a positive and rewarding experience for all participants (Ferraro et al., 2022). Diversity in this context encompasses a wide array of dimensions, including but not limited to race, ethnicity, gender, and abilities, each contributing uniquely to the vibrant tapestry of these communities. At the heart of these virtual sports communities lies the importance of fostering inclusiveness, where individuals from all walks of life are not only represented but actively encouraged to engage, fostering a deep sense of belonging and acceptance (X. Chen et al., 2023).

A cornerstone of this endeavor is the creation of an accessible metaverse, particularly catering to individuals with disabilities. The incorporation of features like text-to-speech capabilities and customizable avatars serves to extend meaningful engagement to people with diverse abilities, thereby solidifying the commitment to an all-encompassing environment (Mogavi et al., 2023). By thoughtfully addressing accessibility concerns, virtual sports communities demonstrate their dedication to ensuring that no participant is left behind. Authentic representation plays an integral role in shaping the character of these digital realms. The provision of a diverse range of avatars and virtual sports content empowers users to express their identities authentically, offering a profound sense of validation and resonance (Baker et al., 2023). This aspect not only enriches the virtual experience but also resonates deeply with individuals, cultivating a sense of belonging that bridges the gap between the digital and physical realms.

In these virtual sports communities, cultural sensitivity is of utmost importance. Acknowledging and respecting cultural differences becomes a foundational principle, guarding against inadvertent offense and fostering an atmosphere of inclusivity (Villalonga-Gómez et al., 2023). By embracing the intricacies of diverse cultures, developers contribute to an environment where participants feel respected and understood, culminating in a harmonious space where collaboration thrives. In summation, the ongoing journey towards establishing inclusive and diverse virtual sports communities within the metaverse is a collaborative endeavor that involves developers, users, and experts. Prioritizing diversity and inclusion is not just a theoretical concept; it shapes the very fabric of these digital interactions, mirroring the richness and complexity of real-world experiences, and creating a more enriching and fulfilling engagement for all (Abdusatarov, 2023).

9.3 Virtual Sports Events and Tournaments

One of the standout elements within metaverse sports events involves the fusion of VR and AR technologies. These technologies enable participants to engage with sports in a manner that replicates a physical presence. By utilizing VR headsets and AR devices, both athletes and spectators can immerse themselves in realistic settings, facilitating interactions with one another and their surroundings, regardless of geographical distances. This blending of real and virtual realms has resulted in the creation of extraordinary and captivating spectator experiences (Hadi et al., 2023).

Metaverse sports events extend beyond the boundaries of traditional sports, encompassing unconventional and imaginative sports encounters. Participants can partake in activities like anti-gravity racing and hyperrealistic simulations that challenge the limits of human capabilities (Czegledy, 2023). Furthermore, metaverse sports provide avenues for cross-disciplinary competitions, where participants combine athletic prowess with innovative problem-solving, underscoring the metaverse's capacity for multidimensional engagement (Inwood, 2022). The interactive nature of the metaverse fosters a deeper level of engagement by granting spectators the ability to impact the outcomes of events. The concept of the "spectator-as-participant" is reshaping the perception and enjoyment of sports events. Audiences can interact with athletes, objects, and even influence the course of a game through real-time inputs (Beng et al., 2023). This participatory aspect adds an additional layer of excitement and unpredictability to the sports experience. Nevertheless, metaverse sports also introduce ethical concerns, particularly in regard to data privacy, digital security, and fair competition. The virtual realm of these events introduces the potential for cheating through digital enhancements or manipulation (Fiske, 2023). Striking a harmonious balance between innovations and upholding the integrity of sports stands as a significant challenge.

In conclusion, metaverse sports events and competitions are reshaping the landscape of competitive sports, offering opportunities for unmatched spectator engagement and pushing the boundaries of the integration between physical and digital realms. While delivering futuristic and imaginative sports encounters, addressing ethical considerations is of utmost importance to ensure a just and secure environment for all participants and spectators.

9.4 Leveraging Social VR for Team Building and Collaboration

Social VR is emerging as a promising method for enhancing team cohesion and collaboration across a range of fields. This technology enables individuals to interact and communicate within shared virtual environments, breaking down geographical barriers and distances. With the capability to replicate in-person interactions, Social VR presents a distinctive platform for nurturing teamwork and cooperative efforts.

The immersive quality of Social VR cultivates a sense of presence and involvement among team participants (Tan et al., 2023b). As users feel as though they are physically situated in a virtual realm, their interactions carry greater authenticity and significance. This heightened sense of presence serves to facilitate candid communication and establish confidence among team members. Numerous studies have showcased the positive outcomes of Social VR on collaborative undertakings. Through real-time engagement, team members can partake in impromptu discussions and collaborative brainstorming sessions (Grech et al., 2023). Additionally, the visual and auditory cues conveyed by avatars within Social VR settings mirror nonverbal communication, enriching the quality of interactions (Wieland et al., 2023).

Furthermore, Social VR revolutionizes team-building exercises. Virtual team-building activities, such as interactive problem-solving games and shared escapades, encourage cooperation and a sense of camaraderie (Knoll et al., 2023). These activities cultivate a feeling of unity and shared involvement, even when team members are situated in different geographic locations.

In summary, the potential of Social VR for fostering team unity and collaborative efforts is vast. Its immersive characteristics and capacity to surmount physical barriers facilitate authentic interactions and nurture trust among team members. The impact of this technology on collaborative tasks and team-building exercises finds support in various research studies. Nonetheless, it will be crucial to address technical and privacy obstacles to ensure its widespread adoption.

Figure 13. The development of metaverse

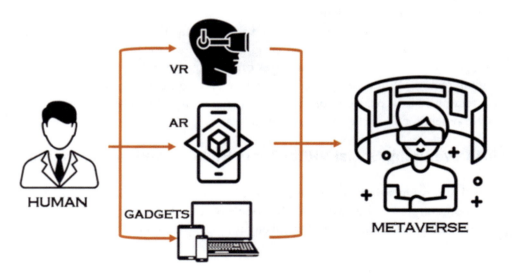

10. FUTURE TRENDS AND RESEARCH DIRECTIONS IN VIRTUAL GYMS AND SPORTS

10.1 Evolving Technologies and Innovations in the Metaverse

The metaverse, an interconnected collection of virtual digital spaces, is rapidly progressing due to the advancement of evolving technologies and groundbreaking developments. This dynamic environment is being molded by the convergence of AR, VR, artificial intelligence (AI), blockchain, and other innovations.

The evolution of the metaverse is significantly influenced by AR and VR technologies. VR enriches real-world experiences by superimposing digital content onto physical surroundings, enhancing user interactions across diverse sectors (P. T. Kumar et al., 2023; Zaman et al., 2022). Conversely, VR provides immersive digital environments that users can engage with (Ozacar et al., 2023). Artificial intelligence contributes intelligence and autonomy to the metaverse, enabling virtual entities to replicate human-like behaviors and interactions (Huynh-The et al., 2023). AI algorithms analyze user behaviors, adapting experiences in real-time. Blockchain technology ensures security and trust within the metaverse. Utilizing decentralized ledgers, users can securely own and trade digital assets (S. Ali et al., 2023). Smart contracts automate transactions, reducing the need for intermediaries Figure 12 shows the evolution of metaverse..

The metaverse is also influenced by the Internet of Things (IoT), as interconnected devices gather and exchange data (D. Wang et al., 2023). This amplifies the metaverse's potential for interactions that are real-time and contextually aware. Social interaction stands as a pivotal aspect of the metaverse. Social VR platforms permit users to socialize, collaborate, and create together (Goel et al., 2023). These platforms are evolving to mirror real-world interactions and enable communication across different platforms (Almeida, 2023). Education and training are undergoing a transformation through the metaverse. Immersive learning environments facilitate experiential education, intensifying engagement and retention (Rachmadtullah et al., 2022; Alenizi et al., 2021). Virtual laboratories and simulations provide practical hands-on experiences. Commerce is also transitioning to the metaverse. Virtual marketplaces allow users to purchase virtual goods and services using cryptocurrencies (Purcarea, 2023). Brands are exploring metaverse advertising to captivate users in innovative ways (Nagarajan, 2023; Gill et al., 2022).

In conclusion, the metaverse is experiencing a remarkable evolution propelled by advancing technologies and revolutionary innovations. AR, VR, AI, blockchain, IoT, and social platforms are propelling its expansion across various domains. As the metaverse continues to develop, its potential impact on communication, education, commerce, and society as a whole is increasingly evident.

10.2 Ethical and Privacy Considerations in Metaverse Sports

The emergence of sports within the metaverse has brought forth a range of ethical and privacy considerations that require thorough examination. As virtual and real-world athletic realms converge, matters concerning data security, virtual identity, and fair competition take center stage. Privacy, often an overlooked aspect in virtual spaces, gains prominence, necessitating vigilant efforts to protect users' personal data. The risk of data breaches and unauthorized access underscores the need for robust security measures (Blowers et al., 2023; Hamid et al., 2019). Additionally, the introduction of virtual athletes raises ethical queries regarding ownership and exploitation (Hutson, n.d.). Companies can profit from the likeness and achievements of virtual athletes, yet concerns arise regarding the authenticity of representation and the fair compensation of the real individuals inspiring these avatars. Such scenarios challenge conventional concepts of intellectual property and the rights of virtual entities (Berggren, 2023; Tayyab et al., 2023)

A further ethical issue pertains to addiction and potential mental health repercussions (Muslihati, 2023). The immersive experiences offered by metaverse sports might encourage compulsive behavior and divert attention from real-world responsibilities, potentially aggravating preexisting mental health challenges. Striking a balance between engagement and responsible usage becomes a crucial consideration. Lastly, the aspect of surveillance within metaverse sports raises concerns about personal liberties (Dwivedi et al., 2023; Humayan et al., 2020b). In the pursuit of maintaining fair gameplay and preventing cheating, the extent of monitoring users' activities could encroach upon their privacy. Developers must establish transparent policies regarding data collection and surveillance to alleviate potential ethical infringements.

In summary, the emergence of metaverse sports introduces an array of ethical and privacy concerns that demand careful deliberation. As this virtual realm intertwines with real-world experiences, safeguarding personal data, addressing ownership matters, ensuring inclusivity, promoting mental well-being, and maintaining a balance with surveillance become critical imperatives. The resolution of these concerns will shape the ethical landscape of metaverse sports and determine their potential as a positive and equitable platform for athletes and enthusiasts alike.

10.3 Emerging Research Areas in the Field

The concept of the metaverse, which blends physical and digital realities in a shared virtual space, is rapidly evolving and has captured significant attention across various fields. Scholars are exploring various facets of this phenomenon, uncovering new dimensions that carry important implications for technology, society, and the economy.

Within the realm of Education and Training, there is a focus on leveraging the capabilities of the metaverse to enrich learning and training experiences. Researchers are investigating how immersive virtual environments can transform education. An example is the work by S. Lee (2023), who delves into the idea of virtual classrooms that replicate traditional educational settings within the metaverse. These virtual classrooms offer a distinctive environment for both students and educators to interact, collaborate, and engage with content in dynamic and innovative ways. This approach has the potential to create more interactive, captivating, and easily accessible learning experiences, overcoming geographical barriers and providing diverse educational opportunities. As experts in education and research delve further into this field, they are actively exploring ways to optimize virtual classrooms for various subjects, student demographics, and learning objectives. This exploration paves the way for a significant transformation in the paradigms of education and training.

In the realm of Virtual Economy and Commerce, the focus shifts towards the economic dimensions of the metaverse. Researchers are examining how economies can thrive within virtual spaces, encompassing the creation and exchange of virtual commodities, services, and currencies. Torky et al. (2023) delve into the importance of blockchain technology in ensuring secure transactions within the metaverse. The decentralized and transparent nature of blockchain holds the potential to establish trust and mitigate fraud in virtual economies.

In the realm of Social Dynamics and Identity, scholars are actively investigating how individuals interact and form relationships within the metaverse. Avatars, which are virtual representations of users, hold a pivotal role in shaping how people present themselves and engage with others. Dwivedi et al. (2023) underscore the psychological implications of adopting diverse identities in virtual environments. This inquiry illuminates the potential influence of these digital interactions on individuals' behaviors and self-perception in the real world. Within the domain of Healthcare and Well-being, researchers are examining how the metaverse could contribute to healthcare and overall well-being. E. J. Kim and Kim (2023) are among those exploring the effectiveness of metaverse applications for therapeutic purposes. These applications have the potential to provide support for mental health and physical rehabilitation. By utilizing immersive experiences, these interventions aim to create captivating and impactful approaches that might elevate individuals' well-being. In the effort to conserve cultural heritage within the metaverse, endeavors are focused on digitizing artifacts, artworks, and other cultural components. Museums and institutions are actively seeking methods to craft virtual renditions of physical spaces and items. This allows users to engage with cultural heritage in novel and immersive manners. Mousazadeh et al. (2023) emphasize the importance of this initiative in ensuring the perpetuity and accessibility of cultural heritage for forthcoming generations. These emerging research areas collectively contribute to understanding the metaverse's multidimensional nature, offering insights that guide its responsible development and integration into society

11. CONCLUSION

11.1 Recapitulation of Key Findings

In this comprehensive exploration of the interplay between the metaverse and physical activity, we delved into the transformative landscape of virtual gyms and sports. Throughout this chapter, we have uncovered a multitude of insights that shed light on the present and future of this dynamic synergy. We started by defining the metaverse and its evolution, setting the stage for the emergence of virtual gyms and sports as pivotal components of this digital realm. Examining virtual gyms, we identified their advantages such as convenience and customization, while acknowledging limitations such as potential disconnection from physicality. The integration of immersive technologies like VR and AR offered new dimensions to fitness experiences, enhanced by personalization and gamification for motivational gains.

Turning to virtual sports, we recognized their diverse forms, from esport competitions to realistic simulations. These virtual endeavors showcased their potential to transcend traditional sporting boundaries, even as they integrated with real-world counterparts. Exploring the benefits and challenges, we found that virtual fitness and sports offered health and social advantages, yet ethical and safety concerns in virtual spaces necessitate careful consideration. Technological innovation, including AI-guided coaching and haptic feedback, has poised the metaverse as a hub of novel fitness experiences. With a focus on scaling and user experience, we examined potential monetization strategies and the significance of partnerships in fostering community growth.

This journey extended to applications in healthcare, revealing the potential of virtual environments in rehabilitation, mental wellness, and training. We also envisioned the transformative impact of metaverse sports on the industry, creating new avenues for business and reshaping traditional paradigms. The social dimensions of metaverse sports highlighted fan engagement, inclusivity, and collaborative potential through VR. As we looked ahead, the integration of evolving technologies, ethical considerations, and emerging research areas stood as significant waypoints in this evolving landscape. In summation, this chapter has presented a panoramic view of the metaverse's convergence with physical activity, underlining its capacity to revolutionize fitness, sports, and social interaction in ways that invite excitement, introspection, and further exploration.

11.2 Summary of Virtual Gyms and Sports in the Metaverse

The emergence of the metaverse has ushered in a paradigm shift in our approach to fitness and sports, leading to the emergence of virtual gyms and sports experiences that are reshaping the conventional landscape. Within the metaverse, virtual gyms offer users the chance to partake in workouts and wellness routines within immersive digital settings. These environments present a spectrum of customizable options, ranging from tranquil natural backdrops to futuristic urban vistas, thereby enhancing the overall exercise experience.

Furthermore, virtual sports experiences within the metaverse have redefined the realm of competitive gaming and athletic involvement. Established sports like basketball, soccer, and racing have been reenvisioned within virtual arenas, where users take control of avatars and compete either individually or in teams. This fusion of physical and digital realms extends accessibility to a worldwide audience, enabling participation regardless of geographical constraints.

These advancements have also paved the way for enhanced social interaction. Users have the ability to connect with both acquaintances and strangers, fostering a sense of community through shared fitness objectives or collaborative gameplay. The virtual gyms and sports experiences within the metaverse hold the potential to elevate physical activity and engagement, while simultaneously pushing the boundaries of technological advancement. As the metaverse continues to evolve, its influence on the fitness and sports industry is poised to revolutionize how we engage in exercise, compete, and establish connections in entirely unprecedented ways.

11.3 Implications and Recommendations for Industry and Research

The advent of the metaverse is ushering in transformative changes across industries, offering unique opportunities and presenting challenges that necessitate comprehensive research efforts. One significant implication is the heightened level of customer engagement it offers businesses. By creating immersive brand experiences, companies can forge deeper connections with their target audience, fostering increased loyalty and brand advocacy (Wongkitrungrueng & Suprawan, 2023). Additionally, the metaverse provides fertile ground for new business models to flourish. This includes monetization avenues such as virtual goods sales, digital real estate transactions, and in-world services, enabling enterprises to diversify revenue streams beyond conventional approaches (Marabelli & Newell, 2023).

Another critical impact of the metaverse is its ability to facilitate global collaboration by transcending geographical barriers. The seamless cross-border collaboration it enables holds the potential to enhance international business operations, thus unlocking novel markets and opportunities (Y. Li et al., 2023). However, as the metaverse accumulates substantial user data, concerns regarding data privacy and security are amplified. Ensuring robust data protection measures becomes paramount to safeguard personal information against potential breaches (Zhao et al., 2023). This shift toward the metaverse also necessitates a recalibration of skill requirements, creating demand for professionals skilled in virtual world development, management, and maintenance (Anshari et al., 2023).

From a research perspective, several critical avenues emerge for investigation. The impact of extensive metaverse use on individuals' mental health, social interactions, and overall well-being requires rigorous examination to foster the development of responsible virtual environments (Chakraborty et al., 2023). Moreover, the economic viability and growth potential of metaverse-operating businesses warrant careful analysis, shedding light on their sustainability and profitability (Papamichael et al., 2023). Ethical considerations arising from the metaverse, encompassing digital identity, intellectual property rights, and virtual ethics, demand nuanced exploration to establish guidelines and best practices (Kaddoura & Husseiny, 2023).

The metaverse's capacity to spur innovation and creativity across diverse sectors beckons researchers to delve into its transformative potential (Wider et al., 2023). Additionally, the metaverse's role in revolutionizing education delivery is a crucial area deserving comprehensive study, uncovering how immersive learning experiences can elevate educational outcomes (Muthmainnah et al., 2023). In essence, the metaverse is reshaping industries and research in tandem. By understanding and addressing its multifaceted implications, both enterprises and individuals can harness its potential responsibly and innovatively.

REFERENCES

Abdusatarov, J. (2023, April 26). *Issues That Need To Be Resolved When Developing The Legal Framework Of International Private Law Relations In Metaverse*. Scholar Express. https://www.scholarexpress.net/index.php/wbml/article/view/2626

AbuKhousa, E., El-Tahawy, M. S., & Atif, Y. (2023). Envisioning architecture of Metaverse Intensive Learning Experience (MILEX): Career readiness in the 21st century and collective intelligence development scenario. *Future Internet*, *15*(2), 53. doi:10.3390/fi15020053

Adrian, D., Frances, D., & Burns, A. (2023). *An Examination of the Virtual Event Experience of Cyclists Competing on Zwift*. Ingenta Connect., doi:10.3727/152599523X16907613842110

Afsar, M. M., Saqib, S., Alarfaj, M., Alatiyyah, M. H., Alnowaiser, K., Aljuaid, H., Jalal, A., & Park, J. (2023). Body-Worn sensors for recognizing physical sports activities in exergaming via deep learning model. *IEEE Access: Practical Innovations, Open Solutions*, *11*, 12460–12473. doi:10.1109/ACCESS.2023.3239692

Ahuja, A. S., Polascik, B. W., Doddapaneni, D., Byrnes, E. S., & Sridhar, J. (2023). The digital metaverse: Applications in artificial intelligence, medical education, and integrative health. *Integrative Medicine Research*, *12*(1), 100917. doi:10.1016/j.imr.2022.100917 PMID:36691642

Alenizi, B. A., Humayun, M., & Jhanjhi, N. Z. (2021). Security and privacy issues in cloud computing. *Journal of Physics: Conference Series*, *1979*(1), 012038. doi:10.1088/1742-6596/1979/1/012038

Ali, S., Abdullah, N., Armand, T. P. T., Athar, A., Hussain, A., Ali, M., Muhammad, Y., Joo, M., & Kim, H. C. (2023). Metaverse in Healthcare Integrated with Explainable AI and Blockchain: Enabling Immersiveness, Ensuring Trust, and Providing Patient Data Security. *Sensors (Basel)*, *23*(2), 565. doi:10.339023020565 PMID:36679361

Almeida, L. G. G. (2023). *Innovating Industrial Training with Immersive Metaverses: A Method for Developing Cross-Platform Virtual Reality Environments*. MDPI., doi:10.3390/app13158915

Almusaylim, Z. A., Jhanjhi, N. Z., & Jung, L. T. (2018). Proposing A Data Privacy Aware Protocol for Roadside Accident Video Reporting Service Using 5G In *Vehicular Cloud Networks Environment. 2018 4th International Conference on Computer and Information Sciences (ICCOINS)*. IEEE. 10.1109/ICCOINS.2018.8510588

Alsem, S. C., Van Dijk, A., Verhulp, E., Dekkers, T. J., & De Castro, B. O. (2023). Treating children's aggressive behavior problems using cognitive behavior therapy with virtual reality: A multicenter randomized controlled trial. *Child Development*, cdev.13966. Advance online publication. doi:10.1111/cdev.13966 PMID:37459452

An, N. (2023, May 2). *Toward learning societies for digital aging*. arXiv.org. https://arxiv.org/abs/2305.01137

Anshari, M., Syafrudin, M., & Alfian, G. (2023). *Metaverse applications for new business models and disruptive innovation*. IGI Global. doi:10.4018/978-1-6684-6097-9

Arpaci, I., & Bahari, M. (2023). Investigating the role of psychological needs in predicting the educational sustainability of Metaverse using a deep learning-based hybrid SEM-ANN technique. *Interactive Learning Environments*, 1–13. doi:10.1080/10494820.2022.2164313

Arya, V., Sambyal, R., Sharma, A., & Dwivedi, Y. K. (2023). Brands are calling your AVATAR in Metaverse–A study to explore XR-based gamification marketing activities & consumer-based brand equity in virtual world. *Journal of Consumer Behaviour*, cb.2214. doi:10.1002/cb.2214

Baker, J., Nam, K., & Dutt, C. (2023). *A user experience perspective on heritage tourism in the metaverse: Empirical evidence and design dilemmas for VR*. Spinger. https://link.springer.com/article/10.1007/s40558-023-00256-x

Bannell, D. J., France-Ratcliffe, M., Buckley, B. J. R., Crozier, A., Davies, A., Hesketh, K., Jones, H., Cocks, M., & Sprung, V. S. (2023). Adherence to unsupervised exercise in sedentary individuals: A randomised feasibility trial of two mobile health interventions. *Digital Health*, 9, 20552076231183552. doi:10.1177/20552076231183552 PMID:37426588

BarberaS. (2023). Navigating the Virtual Frontier: The Convergence of Decentralized Finance and the Metaverse. *Preprint.org*. doi:10.20944/preprints202307.1734.v1

Batrakoulis, A., Veiga, O. L., Franco, S., Thomas, E., Alexopoulos, A., Torrente, M. V., Santos-Rocha, R., Ramalho, F., Di Credico, A., Vitucci, D., Ramos, L., Simões, V., Romero-Caballero, A., Vieira, I., Mancini, A., & Bianco, A. (2023). Health and fitness trends in Southern Europe for 2023: A cross-sectional survey. *AIMS Public Health*, *10*(2), 378–408. doi:10.3934/publichealth.2023028 PMID:37304589

Bays, H., Fitch, A., Cuda, S., Rickey, E., Hablutzel, J., Coy, R., & Censani, M. (2023). Artificial intelligence and obesity management: An Obesity Medicine Association (OMA) Clinical Practice Statement (CPS) 2023. *Obesity Pillars*, *6*, 100065. doi:10.1016/j.obpill.2023.100065

Belt, E. S., & Lowenthal, P. R. (2022). Synchronous video-based communication and online learning: An exploration of instructors' perceptions and experiences. *Education and Information Technologies*, *28*(5), 4941–4964. doi:10.100710639-022-11360-6 PMID:36320822

Beng, C. O., Gang, C., Shou, Z. M., Tan, K.-L., Tung, A., Xiao, X., James, W. L. Y., Bingxue, Z., & Meihui, Z. (2023). The Metaverse Data Deluge: What Can We Do About It? In *2023 IEEE 39th International Conference on Data Engineering (ICDE)*. IEEE. 10.1109/ICDE55515.2023.00296

BentiB. S. (2023). Sports and eSports: A structural comparison based on the B|Orders in Motion Framework. opus4.kobv.de. doi:10.11584/opus4-1293

Berggren, N. (2023). *Unlocking the Fashion Metaverse: Exploring the impact of external factors on innovation diffusion in the metaverse fashion industry*. DIVA. https://www.diva-portal.org/smash/record.jsf?pid=diva2%3A1761437&dswid=-6051

Blowers, M., Jaimes, N., & Williams, J. (2023). *Benefits and challenges of a military metaverse*. SPIE. doi:10.1117/12.2663772

Brayshaw, M., Gordon, N., Kambili-Mzembe, F., & Jaber, T. A. (2023). Why the Educational Metaverse Is Not All About Virtual Reality Apps. In Lecture Notes in Computer Science (pp. 22–32). doi:10.1007/978-3-031-34550-0_2

Brewer, L. C., Abraham, H., Kaihoi, B., Leth, S., Egginton, J. S., Slusser, J. P., Scott, R. J., Penheiter, S. G., Albertie, M., Squires, R. W., Thomas, R. J., Scales, R., Trejo-Gutiérrez, J. F., & Kopecky, S. L. (2022). A Community-Informed Virtual World-Based cardiac rehabilitation program as an extension of Center-Based cardiac rehabilitation. *Journal of Cardiopulmonary Rehabilitation and Prevention*, 43(1), 22–30. doi:10.1097/HCR.0000000000000705 PMID:35881503

Brown, L. (n.d.). *From Coffee Houses to Internet Speech: Civility and Moderation within The Contemporary Public Sphere*. Works. https://works.swarthmore.edu/theses/323/

Buhalis, D., Leung, D., & Lin, M. (2023). Metaverse as a disruptive technology revolutionising tourism management and marketing. *Tourism Management*, 97, 104724. doi:10.1016/j.tourman.2023.104724

Cameron, L., & Ride, J. (2023). The role of mental health in online gambling decisions: A discrete choice experiment. *Social Science & Medicine*, 326, 115885. doi:10.1016/j.socscimed.2023.115885 PMID:37087972

Carr, K., & England, R. (2023). *Simulated And Virtual Realities: Elements Of Perception*. CRC Press.

Cennamo, C., Dagnino, G. B., & Zhu, F. (2023). *Research Handbook on Digital Strategy*. Edward Elgar Publishing. doi:10.4337/9781800378902

Chakraborty, D., Patre, S., & Tiwari, D. (2023). Metaverse mingle: Discovering dating intentions in metaverse. *Journal of Retailing and Consumer Services*, 75, 103509. Advance online publication. doi:10.1016/j.jretconser.2023.103509

Champion, E. (2022). Mixed histories, augmented pasts. In Human-computer interaction series (pp. 163–184). doi:10.1007/978-3-031-10932-4_7

Chatrati, S. P., Hossain, G., Goyal, A., Bhan, A., Bhattacharya, S., Gaurav, D., & Tiwari, S. (2022). Smart home health monitoring system for predicting type 2 diabetes and hypertension. *Journal of King Saud University - Computer and Information Sciences, 34*(3), 862–870. doi:10.1016/j.jksuci.2020.01.010

Chen, G., Peachey, J. W., & Stodolska, M. (2023). Sense of community among virtual race participants: The case of the Illinois Marathon. *Managing Sport and Leisure*, 1–23. doi:10.1080/23750472.2023.2239246

Chen, X., Zou, D., Xie, H., & Wang, F. L. (2023). Metaverse in Education: Contributors, cooperations, and research themes. *IEEE Transactions on Learning Technologies*, 1–18. doi:10.1109/TLT.2023.3277952

Chengoden, R., Victor, N., Huynh-The, T., Yenduri, G., Jhaveri, R. H., Alazab, M., Bhattacharya, S., Hegde, P., Maddikunta, P. K. R., & Gadekallu, T. R. (2023). Metaverse for Healthcare: A survey on potential applications, challenges and future directions. *IEEE Access : Practical Innovations, Open Solutions, 11*, 12765–12795. doi:10.1109/ACCESS.2023.3241628

Cho, Y., Park, M., & Kim, J. (2023). XAVE: Cross-platform based Asymmetric Virtual Environment for Immersive Content. *IEEE Access : Practical Innovations, Open Solutions, 1*, 71890–71904. doi:10.1109/ACCESS.2023.3294390

Crew, E. (2023, April 20). How can virtual reality sports training help athletes? *4Experience.* https://4experience.co/how-virtual-reality-sports-training-helps-athletes/

Czegledy, P. K. (2023). Crystal Ball Gazing: The future of sports betting. *Gaming Law Review, 27*(2), 65–70. doi:10.1089/glr2.2022.0046

Da Silva Schlickmann, D., Molz, P., Uebel, G. C., Santos, C. D., Brand, C., Colombelli, R. W., Da Silva, T. G., Steffens, J. P., Da Silva Limberger Castilhos, E., Benito, P. J., Rieger, A., & Franke, S. I. R. (2023). The moderating role of macronutrient intake in relation to body composition and genotoxicity: A study with gym users. *Mutation Research, 503660*, 503660. doi:10.1016/j.mrgentox.2023.503660 PMID:37567647

Deng, J., Tajuddin, R. B. M., Chen, Z., Ren, B., & Shariff, S. M. (2023). *The impact of virtual presence on the behavior of live E-Commerce consumers.* Atlantis Press. doi:10.2991/978-94-6463-210-1_47

Desbordes, M. (2023). Analysis of the sport ecosystem and its value chain, What lessons in an uncertain world? In Sports economics, management and policy (pp. 109–142). doi:10.1007/978-981-19-7010-8_6

DhimanB. (2023). Ethical Issues and Challenges in social Media: A current scenario. *Social Science Research Network*. doi:10.2139/ssrn.4406610

Dhiman, D. B. (2023, March 10). *Key issues and New Challenges in New Media Technology in 2023: A Critical review*. https://papers.ssrn.com/sol3/papers.cfm?abstract_id=4387353

DiasS. B.JelinekH. F.HadjileontiadisL. (2023). Wearable Neurofeedback Acceptance Model: An Investigation within Academic Settings to Explore a Multimodal Framework for Student Stress and Anxiety Management. SSRN. doi:10.2139/ssrn.4485826

Dogheim, G. M. (2023, June 5). *Patient Care through AI-driven Remote Monitoring: Analyzing the Role of Predictive Models and Intelligent Alerts in Preventive Medicine*. DL Press. https://publications.dlpress.org/index.php/jcha/article/view/20

Dogra, V., Verma, S., Kavita, K., Jhanjhi, N. Z., Ghosh, U., & Le, D. (2022). A comparative analysis of machine learning models for banking news extraction by multiclass classification with imbalanced datasets of financial news: Challenges and solutions. *International Journal of Interactive Multimedia and Artificial Intelligence*, *7*(3), 35. doi:10.9781/ijimai.2022.02.002

Doskarayev, B., Omarov, N., Omarov, B., Ismagulova, Z., Kozhamkulova, Z., Nurlybaeva, E., & Kasimova, G. (2023). Development of computer vision-enabled augmented reality games to increase motivation for sports. *International Journal of Advanced Computer Science and Applications*, *14*(4). doi:10.14569/IJACSA.2023.0140428

Dwivedi, Y. K., Kshetri, N., Hughes, L., Rana, N. P., Baabdullah, A. M., Kar, A. K., Koohang, A., Ribeiro-Navarrete, S., Belei, N., Balakrishnan, J., Basu, S., Behl, A., Davies, G. H., Dutot, V., Dwivedi, R., Evans, L., Felix, R., Foster-Fletcher, R., Giannakis, M., & Yan, M. (2023). Exploring the Darkverse: A Multi-Perspective Analysis of the negative societal impacts of the Metaverse. *Information Systems Frontiers*, *25*(5), 2071–2114. doi:10.100710796-023-10400-x PMID:37361890

Ezawa, I. D., Hollon, S. D., & Robinson, N. J. (2023). Examining Predictors of Depression and Anxiety Symptom change in Cognitive Behavioral Immersion: Observational study. *JMIR Mental Health*, *10*, e42377. doi:10.2196/42377 PMID:37450322

Ferraro, C., Hemsley, A., & Sands, S. (2022). Embracing diversity, equity, and inclusion (DEI): Considerations and opportunities for brand managers. *Business Horizons*. doi:10.1016/j.bushor.2022.09.005

Ferreira, M. S. L., Antão, J., Pereira, R., Bianchi, I. S., Tovma, N., & Shurenov, N. (2023). Improving real estate CRM user experience and satisfaction: A user-centered design approach. *Journal of Open Innovation*, *9*(2), 100076. doi:10.1016/j.joitmc.2023.100076

Fiske, J. (2023, June 1). *Identity Assurance in an era of Digital Disruption: Planning a Controlled transition*. Harvard Press. https://dash.harvard.edu/handle/1/37376453

Gill, S. H., Razzaq, M. A., Ahmad, M., Almansour, F. M., Haq, I. U., Jhanjhi, N. Z., Alam, M. Z., & Masud, M. (2022). Security and privacy aspects of cloud Computing: A Smart Campus case study. *Intelligent Automation and Soft Computing*, *31*(1), 117–128. doi:10.32604/iasc.2022.016597

Glen, S. (2023). History of the metaverse in one picture. *Data Science Central*. https://www.datasciencecentral.com/history-of-the-metaverse-in-one-picture/

Goel, R., Baral, S. K., Mishra, T., & Jain, V. (2023). *Augmented and Virtual Reality in Industry 5.0*. Walter de Gruyter GmbH & Co KG. doi:10.1515/9783110790146

Grech, A., Mehnen, J., & Wodehouse, A. (2023). An extended AI-Experience: Industry 5.0 in Creative Product innovation. *Sensors (Basel)*, *23*(6), 3009. doi:10.339023063009 PMID:36991718

Greenhalgh, G. P., & Goebert, C. (2023). From Gearshifts to Gigabytes: An analysis of how NASCAR used iRacing to engage fans during the COVID-19 shutdown. *International Journal of Sport Communication*, 1–15. doi:10.1123/ijsc.2023-0145

Gupta, N. S., & Kumar, P. (2023). Perspective of artificial intelligence in healthcare data management: A journey towards precision medicine. *Computers in Biology and Medicine*, *162*, 107051. doi:10.1016/j.compbiomed.2023.107051 PMID:37271113

Hadi, R., Melumad, S., & Park, E. S. (2023). The Metaverse: A new digital frontier for consumer behavior. *Journal of Consumer Psychology*, jcpy.1356. doi:10.1002/jcpy.1356

Hamid, B., Jhanjhi, N. Z., Humayun, M., Khan, A. F., & Alsayat, A. (2019). Cyber Security Issues and Challenges for Smart Cities: A survey. In *2019 13th International Conference on Mathematics, Actuarial Science, Computer Science and Statistics (MACS)*. ACM. 10.1109/MACS48846.2019.9024768

Hang, Y. (2023). Research on the problems and countermeasures in the In-Person Fitness industry in the post-pandemic era. *Highlights in Business, Economics and Management*, *13*, 29–38. doi:10.54097/hbem.v13i.8618

Hasson, H., Rundgren, E. H., & Schwarz, U. V. T. (2023). *The adaptation and fidelity tool to support social service practitioners in balancing fidelity and adaptations: Longitudinal, mixed-method evaluation study.* SIRC. doi:10.1177/26334895231189198

Hawajri, O., Lindberg, J., & Suominen, S. (2023). Virtual Reality Exposure Therapy as a Treatment Method Against Anxiety Disorders and Depression-A Structured Literature Review. *Issues in Mental Health Nursing*, 1–25. 10.1080/01612840.2023.2190051

Høeg, E. R., Andersen, N. B., Malmkjær, N., Vaaben, A. H., & Uth, J. (2023). Hospitalized older adults' experiences of virtual reality-based group exercise therapy with cycle ergometers: An early feasibility study. *Computers in Human Behavior Reports*, *11*, 100301. doi:10.1016/j.chbr.2023.100301

Höner, O., Dugandzic, D., Hauser, T., Stügelmaier, M., Willig, N., & Schultz, F. (2023). Do you have a good all-around view? Evaluation of a decision-making skills diagnostic tool using 360° videos and head-mounted displays in elite youth soccer. *Frontiers in Sports and Active Living*, *5*, 1171262. doi:10.3389/fspor.2023.1171262 PMID:37342613

Hughes, J., Martin, T., Gladwell, T. D., Akiyode, O., Purnell, M. C., Shahid, M., Moultry, A. M., Rapp, K. I., & Unonu, J. (2023). Lessons from a cross-institutional online professional development pilot. *Currents in Pharmacy Teaching & Learning*, *15*(5), 534–540. doi:10.1016/j.cptl.2023.05.004 PMID:37202331

Humayun, M., Jhanjhi, N. Z., Alruwaili, M., Amalathas, S. S., Balasubramanian, V., & Selvaraj, B. (2020). Privacy protection and energy optimization for 5G-Aided industrial internet of things. *IEEE Access : Practical Innovations, Open Solutions*, *8*, 183665–183677. doi:10.1109/ACCESS.2020.3028764

Humayun, M., Niazi, M., Jhanjhi, N. Z., Alshayeb, M., & Mahmood, S. (2020b). Cyber Security Threats and Vulnerabilities: A Systematic Mapping study. *Arabian Journal for Science and Engineering*, *45*(4), 3171–3189. doi:10.100713369-019-04319-2

Hutson, J. (n.d.). *Life, death, and AI: Exploring digital necromancy in popular culture—Ethical considerations, technological limitations, and the pet cemetery conundrum.* Digital Commons@Lindenwood University. https://digitalcommons.lindenwood.edu/faculty-research-papers/478/

Huynh-The, T., Pham, Q., Pham, X., Nguyen, T., Han, Z., & Kim, D. (2023). Artificial intelligence for the metaverse: A survey. *Engineering Applications of Artificial Intelligence*, *117*, 105581. doi:10.1016/j.engappai.2022.105581

Inwood, H. (2022). Towards Sinophone Game Studies. *Apollo (London. 1925), 12*(2), 1–10. doi:10.51661/bjocs.v12i2.219

Jamshidi, M. (2023). *The Meta-Metaverse: Ideation and future Directions.* MDPI., doi:10.3390/fi15080252

Javed, N., Ahmed, T., Faisal, M., Sadia, H., & Sidaine-Daumiller, E. Z. J. (2023). Workplace cyberbullying in the Remote-Work era. In Advances in human and social aspects of technology book series (pp. 166–177). doi:10.4018/978-1-6684-8133-2.ch009

JerathR.SyamM.AhmedS. Z. (2023). *The Future of Stress Management: Integration Smartwatches and HRV Technology.* doi:10.20944/preprints202307.1283.v2

Jiang, X., Deng, N., & Zheng, S. (2023). Understanding the core technological features of virtual and augmented reality in tourism: A qualitative and quantitative review. *Current Issues in Tourism*, 1–21. doi:10.1080/13683500.2023.2198118

Jo, H., Seidel, L., Pahud, M., Sinclair, M., & Bianchi, A. (2023). *FlowAR: How Different Augmented Reality Visualizations of Online Fitness Videos Support Flow for At-Home Yoga Exercises.* ACM. doi:10.1145/3544548.3580897

Jonathan, N. T., Bachri, M. R., Wijaya, E., Ramdhan, D., & Chowanda, A. (2023). The efficacy of virtual reality exposure therapy (VRET) with extra intervention for treating PTSD symptoms. *Procedia Computer Science, 216*, 252–259. doi:10.1016/j.procs.2022.12.134

Jones, L., Lee, M., & Gomes, R. S. M. (2023). Remote rehabilitation (telerehabilitation) in the sight loss sector: Reflections on challenges and opportunities from service providers in the United Kingdom. *British Journal of Visual Impairment*, 02646196231188634. doi:10.1177/02646196231188634

Kaddoura, S., & Husseiny, F. A. (2023). The rising trend of Metaverse in education: Challenges, opportunities, and ethical considerations. *PeerJ, 9*, e1252. doi:10.7717/peerj-cs.1252 PMID:37346578

Kaihua, N. (2023, June 1). *Disruptive Innovation in Finnish hospitality: An analysis and mapping of incumbent perceptions.* Osuva. https://osuva.uwasa.fi/handle/10024/15987

Kamaruddin, I. K., Ma'rof, A. M., Nazan, A. I. N. M., & Jalil, H. A. (2023). A systematic review and meta-analysis of interventions to decrease cyberbullying perpetration and victimization: An in-depth analysis within the Asia Pacific region. *Frontiers in Psychiatry, 14*, 1014258. doi:10.3389/fpsyt.2023.1014258 PMID:36778634

Kato, N. (2023). *Comparison of Smoothness, Movement Speed and Trajectory during Reaching Movements in Real and Virtual Spaces Using a Head-Mounted Display.* MDPI. doi:10.3390/life13081618

Kępińska, A., & Wiśniewski, R. (2023). Metaverse and its creative potential for visual arts. *Acta Universitatis Lodziensis*, *85*(85), 57–75. doi:10.18778/0208-600X.85.04

Kesavan, D., & N, M. A. (2023). *Emerging insights on the relationship between cryptocurrencies and decentralized economic models.* IGI Global.

Khan, S., Kannapiran, T., Muthiah, A., & Shetty, S. (2023). *Exergaming intervention for children, adolescents, and elderly people.* IGI Global. doi:10.4018/978-1-6684-6320-8

Kim, E. J., & Kim, J. (2023). The Metaverse for Healthcare: Trends, applications, and future directions of digital therapeutics for Urology. *International Neurourology Journal*, *27*(Suppl 1), S3–S12. doi:10.5213/inj.2346108.054 PMID:37280754

Kim, K. B., & Baek, H. J. (2023). Photoplethysmography in Wearable Devices: A comprehensive review of technological advances, current challenges, and future directions. *Electronics (Basel)*, *12*(13), 2923. doi:10.3390/electronics12132923

Knoll, T., Liaqat, A., & Monroy-Hernández, A. (2023). *ARctic Escape: Promoting Social Connection, Teamwork, and Collaboration Using a Co-Located Augmented Reality Escape Room.* ACM Digital Library. doi:10.1145/3544549.3585841

Koohang, A., Nord, J. H., Ooi, K., Tan, G. W., Al-Emran, M., Aw, E. C., Baabdullah, A. M., Buhalis, D., Cham, T., Dennis, C., Dutot, V., Dwivedi, Y. K., Hughes, L., Mogaji, E., Pandey, N., Phau, I., Raman, R., Sharma, A., Sigala, M., & Wong, L. (2023). Shaping the Metaverse into Reality: A Holistic Multidisciplinary Understanding of Opportunities, Challenges, and Avenues for Future Investigation. *Journal of Computer Information Systems*, *63*(3), 735–765. doi:10.1080/08874417.2023.2165197

KumarP. T.MohamedJ. S.PadmajaR. (2023). *Contrasting virtual reality and augmented reality in the health care system - Briefing.* Zenodo. doi:10.5281/zenodo.8068117

Kwon, S., Park, J. K., & Koh, Y. H. (2023). A systematic review and meta-analysis on the effect of virtual reality-based rehabilitation for people with Parkinson's disease. *Journal of Neuroengineering and Rehabilitation*, *20*(1), 94. doi:10.118612984-023-01219-3 PMID:37475014

Labbaf, S., Abbasian, M., Azimi, I., Dutt, N., & Rahmani, A. M. (2023). *ZotCare: a flexible, personalizable, and affordable MHealth service provider.* https://doi.org//arxiv.2307.01905 doi:10.48550

Lee, J. C., & Lin, R. (2023). The continuous usage of artificial intelligence (AI)-powered mobile fitness applications: The goal-setting theory perspective. *Industrial Management & Data Systems*, *123*(6), 1840–1860. doi:10.1108/IMDS-10-2022-0602

Lee, S. (2023). *Sustainable Vocational Preparation for Adults with Disabilities: A Metaverse-Based Approach.* MDPI. doi:10.3390u151512000

Letafati, M., & Otoum, S. (2023). *On the privacy and security for e-health services in the metaverse: An overview.* ScienceDirect. doi:10.1016/j.adhoc.2023.103262

Li, B., Naraine, M. L., Liang, Z., & Li, C. (2021). A magic "Bullet": Exploring sport fan usage of On-Screen, ephemeral posts during live stream sessions. *Communication & Sport*, *11*(2), 334–355. doi:10.1177/21674795211038949

Li, H.-H., Lian, J.-J., & Liao, Y.-H. (2023). *Design an Adaptive Virtual Reality Game to Promote Elderly Health.* IEEE Explore. doi:10.1109/CITS58301.2023.10188784

Li, N. (2023). Application of motion tracking technology in movies, television production and photography using big data. *Soft Computing*, *27*(17), 12787–12806. doi:10.100700500-023-08963-7

Li, X., Huang, J., Kong, Z., Sun, F., Sit, C. H. P., & Li, C. (2023). Effects of Virtual Reality-Based Exercise on Physical Fitness in People with Intellectual Disability: A Systematic Review of Randomized Controlled Trials. *Games for Health Journal*, *12*(2), 89–99. doi:10.1089/g4h.2022.0168 PMID:36716183

Li, Y., Ma, Z., & Zhang, L. L. (2023). Research on interaction design based on artificial intelligence technology in a metaverse environment. In Lecture Notes in Computer Science (pp. 193–209). doi:10.1007/978-3-031-35699-5_15

Lister, P. (2023). Opening up smart learning cities - building knowledge, interactions and communities for lifelong learning and urban belonging. In Lecture Notes in Computer Science (pp. 67–85). doi:10.1007/978-3-031-34609-5_5

Lopes, F. (2023). *Exploring the features and benefits of Mixed Reality Toolkit 2 for developing immersive games : a reflective study.* Theseus. https://www.theseus.fi/handle/10024/803207

Mabary, J. (2023). *Analyzing compositional strategies in video game music.* MoSpace. https://mospace.umsystem.edu/xmlui/handle/10355/96145

Marabelli, M., & Newell, S. (2023). Responsibly strategizing with the metaverse: Business implications and DEI opportunities and challenges. *The Journal of Strategic Information Systems*, *32*(2), 101774. doi:10.1016/j.jsis.2023.101774

Maskeliūnas, R., Damaševičius, R., Blažauskas, T., Canbulut, C., Adomavičienė, A., & Griškevičius, J. (2023). BioMacVR: A virtual Reality-Based system for precise human posture and motion analysis in rehabilitation exercises using depth sensors. *Electronics (Basel)*, *12*(2), 339. doi:10.3390/electronics12020339

Meena, S. D., Mithesh, G. S. S., Panyam, R., Chowdary, M. S., Sadhu, V. S., & Sheela, J. (2023). *Advancing Education through Metaverse: Components, Applications, Challenges, Case Studies and Open Issues*. IEEE Explore. doi:10.1109/ICSCSS57650.2023.10169535

Mejtoft, T., Lindahl, H., Norberg, O., Andersson, M., & Söderström, U. (2023). *Enhancing Digital Social Interaction Using Augmented Reality in Mobile Fitness Applications*. ACM. doi:10.1145/3591156.3591170

Menhas, R., Luo, Q., Saqib, Z. A., & Younas, M. (2023). The association between COVID-19 preventive strategies, virtual reality exercise, use of fitness apps, physical, and psychological health: Testing a structural equation moderation model. *Frontiers in Public Health*, *11*, 1170645. doi:10.3389/fpubh.2023.1170645 PMID:37483921

Mezei, K., & Szentgáli-Tóth, B. (2023). Some comments on the legal regulation on misinformation and cyber attacks conducted through online platforms. *Lexonomica*, *15*(1), 33–52. doi:10.18690/lexonomica.15.1.33-52.2023

Miljković, I., Shlyakhetko, O., & Fedushko, S. (2023). Real estate app development based on AI/VR technologies. *Electronics (Basel)*, *12*(3), 707. doi:10.3390/electronics12030707

Miyoung, R., Choi, Y., & Park, H. (2023). Analysis of Issues in Fitness Centers through News Articles before and after the COVID-19 Pandemic in South Korea: Applying Big Data Analysis. *Sustainability (Basel)*, *15*(3), 2660. doi:10.3390u15032660

Mogavi, R. H., Hoffman, J., Deng, C., Yihang, D., Haq, E., & Hui, P. (2023). *Envisioning an Inclusive Metaverse: Student Perspectives on Accessible and Empowering Metaverse-Enabled Learning*. doi:10.1145/3573051.3596185

Monge, J., Ribeiro, G., Raimundo, A., Postolache, O., & Santos, J. F. D. (2023). AI-Based Smart Sensing and AR for GAIT Rehabilitation Assessment. *Information (Basel)*, *14*(7), 355. doi:10.3390/info14070355

Morrison, A. M., & Buhalis, D. (2023). *Routledge Handbook of Trends and Issues in Global Tourism Supply and Demand*. Routledge. doi:10.4324/9781003260790

Mousazadeh, H., Ghorbani, A., Azadi, H., Almani, F. A., Ali, Z., Zhu, K., & Dávid, L. D. (2023). Developing sustainable behaviors for underground heritage tourism management: The case of Persian Qanats, a UNESCO World Heritage property. *Land (Basel)*, *12*(4), 808. doi:10.3390/land12040808

Mozumder, M. I., Armand, T. P. T., Uddin, S. M. I., Athar, A., Sumon, R. I., Hussain, A., & Kim, H. C. (2023). Metaverse for Digital Anti-Aging Healthcare: An overview of potential use cases based on artificial intelligence, blockchain, IoT technologies, its challenges, and future directions. *Applied Sciences (Basel, Switzerland)*, *13*(8), 5127. doi:10.3390/app13085127

Murakawa D. (2023). Decision making under virtual environment triggers more aggressive tactical solutions. *2023 株式会社産経デジタル*. doi:10.51015/jdl.2023.3.9

Muslihati, M. (2023). *How to prevent student mental health problems in metaverse era?* Muslihati | Jurnal Kajian Bimbingan Dan Konseling. http://journal2.um.ac.id/index.php/jkbk/article/view/37598

Muthmainnah, Y., Al Yakin, A., & Ibna Seraj, P. M. (2023). Impact of metaverse technology on student engagement and academic performance: The Mediating role of learning motivation. *International Journal of Computations. Information and Manufacturing*, *3*(1), 10–18. doi:10.54489/ijcim.v3i1.234

Nagarajan, G. (2023, July 15). *The Role Of The Metaverse In Digital Marketing*. Universidad De Granada. https://digibug.ugr.es/handle/10481/84077

Nath, D., Singh, N., Saini, M., Banduni, O., Kumar, N., Srivastava, M. V. P., & Mehndiratta, A. (2023). Clinical potential and neuroplastic effect of targeted virtual reality based intervention for distal upper limb in post-stroke rehabilitation: A pilot observational study. *Disability and Rehabilitation*, 1–10. doi:10.1080/09638288.2023.2228690 PMID:37383015

Ning, H., Wang, H., Lin, Y., Wang, W., Dhelim, S., Farha, F., Ding, J., & Daneshmand, M. (2023). A survey on the metaverse: The State-of-the-Art, technologies, applications, and challenges. *IEEE Internet of Things Journal*, *1*(16), 14671–14688. doi:10.1109/JIOT.2023.3278329

Norman, K., French, A., Lake, A., Tchuisseu, Y. P., Repka, S., Vasudeva, K., Dong, C., Whitaker, R., & Bettger, J. P. (2023). Describing Perspectives of Telehealth and the Impact on Equity in Access to Health Care from Community and Provider Perspectives: A Multimethod Analysis. *Telemedicine Journal and e-Health*, tmj.2023.0036. doi:10.1089/tmj.2023.0036 PMID:37410525

Ose, S. O., Thaulow, K., Færevik, H., Hoffmann, P. L., Lestander, H., Stiles, T. C., & Lindgren, M. (2023). Development of a social skills training programme to target social isolation using virtual reality technology in primary mental health care. *Journal of Rehabilitation and Assistive Technologies Engineering*, 10. doi:10.1177/20556683231187545 PMID:37456950

Ozacar, K., Ortakci, Y., & Küçükkara, M. Y. (2023). VRArchEducation: Redesigning building survey process in architectural education using collaborative virtual reality. *Computers & Graphics*, 113, 1–9. doi:10.1016/j.cag.2023.04.008

Papamichael, I., Pappas, G., Siegel, J. E., Inglezakis, V. J., Demetriou, G., Zorpas, A. A., & Hadjisavvas, C. (2023). Metaverse and circular economy. *Waste Management & Research*, 41(9), 1393–1398. doi:10.1177/0734242X231180406 PMID:37313976

Parcu, P. L., Rossi, M. A., Innocenti, N., & Carrozza, C. (2023). How real will the metaverse be? Exploring the spatial impact of virtual worlds. *European Planning Studies*, 31(7), 1466–1488. doi:10.1080/09654313.2023.2221323

Parry, J., & Giesbrecht, J. (2023). Esports, real sports and the Olympic Virtual Series. *Journal of the Philosophy of Sport*, 50(2), 1–21. doi:10.1080/00948705.2023.2216883

Pastel, S., Petri, K., Chen, C. H., Cáceres, A. M. W., Stirnatis, M., Nübel, C., Schlotter, L., & Witte, K. (2022). Training in virtual reality enables learning of a complex sports movement. *Virtual Reality (Waltham Cross)*, 27(2), 523–540. doi:10.100710055-022-00679-7

Pizzo, A. D. (2023). Hypercasual and Hybrid-Casual Video Gaming: A Digital Leisure perspective. *Leisure Sciences*, 1–20. doi:10.1080/01490400.2023.2211056

Placidi, G., Di Matteo, A., Lozzi, D., Polsinelli, M., & Theodoridou, E. (2023). Patient–Therapist Cooperative Hand Telerehabilitation through a Novel Framework Involving the Virtual Glove System. *Sensors (Basel)*, 23(7), 3463. doi:10.339023073463 PMID:37050523

Pontin, S. (2023). *AI-Based Race StrategyAssistant and Car data Monitor*. DIVA. https://www.diva-portal.org/smash/record.jsf?pid=diva2%3A1756880&dswid=-6708

Purcarea, I. M. (2023). *E-Commerce Business Under Pressure To Grow*. https://ideas.repec.org/a/hmm/journl/v13y2023i2p24-30.html

Purdy, G. M., Sobierajski, F., Onazi, M. M. A., Effa, C., Venner, C. P., Tandon, P., & McNeely, M. L. (2023). Exploring participant perceptions of a virtually supported home exercise program for people with multiple myeloma using a novel eHealth application: A qualitative study. *Supportive Care in Cancer*, *31*(5), 298. doi:10.100700520-023-07762-y PMID:37097319

Qi, J., Ma, L., Cui, Z., & Yu, Y. (2023). Computer vision-based hand gesture recognition for human-robot interaction: A review. *Complex & Intelligent Systems*. doi:10.100740747-023-01173-6

Rachmadtullah, R., Setiawan, B., Setiawan, B., & Wicaksono, J. W. (2022). Elementary school teachers' perceptions of the potential of metaverse technology as a transformation of interactive learning media in Indonesia. *International Journal of Innovative Research and Scientific Studies*, *6*(1), 128–136. doi:10.53894/ijirss.v6i1.1119

RadanlievD. P. (2023, August 1). *Accessibility and inclusiveness of new information and communication technologies for disabled users and content creators in the metaverse*. https://arxiv.org/abs/2308.01925

RadanlievP. (2023). *Accessibility and inclusiveness of new information and communication technologies for disabled users and content creators in the metaverse*. doi:10.2139/ssrn.4528363

Rejeb, A., Rejeb, K., & Treiblmaier, H. (2023). Mapping Metaverse research: Identifying future research areas based on bibliometric and topic modeling techniques. *Information (Basel)*, *14*(7), 356. doi:10.3390/info14070356

Saha, B. (n.d.). *Analysis of the adherence of MHealth applications to HIPAA Technical Safeguards*. DigitalCommons@Kennesaw State University. https://digitalcommons.kennesaw.edu/msit_etd/14/

Salem, S. F., Lawry, C. A., Alanadoly, A., & Li, J. (2023). Branded experiences in the immersive spectrum: How will fashion consumers react to the Metaverse? *ResearchGate*. https://www.researchgate.net/publication/372782798_Branded_experiences_in_the_immersive_spectrum_How_will_fashion_consumers_react_to_the_Metaverse

Şanlisoy, S., & Çiloğlu, T. (2023). A View of the Future of the Metaverse Economy on the Basis of The Global Financial System: New Opportunities and Risks. *Journal of Corporate Governance, Insurance and Risk Management*, *10*(1), 28–41. doi:10.56578/jcgirm100104

Schneider, M., Woodworth, A., Arumalla, S., Gowder, C., Hernandez, J., Kim, A., & Moorthy, B. (2023). Development of a tool for quantifying need-supportive coaching in technology-mediated exercise classes. *Psychology of Sport and Exercise*, *64*, 102321. doi:10.1016/j.psychsport.2022.102321 PMID:37665807

Settimo, C., De Cola, M. C., Pironti, E., Muratore, R., Giambò, F. M., Alito, A., Tresoldi, M., La Fauci, M., De Domenico, C., Tripodi, E., Impallomeni, C., Quartarone, A., & Cucinotta, F. (2023). Virtual Reality Technology to Enhance Conventional Rehabilitation Program: Results of a Single-Blind, Randomized, Controlled Pilot Study in Patients with Global Developmental Delay. *Journal of Clinical Medicine*, *12*(15), 4962. doi:10.3390/jcm12154962 PMID:37568364

Shafiq, D. A., Jhanjhi, N. Z., & Abdullah, A. (2021). Machine Learning Approaches for Load Balancing in Cloud Computing Services. *2021 National Computing Colleges Conference (NCCC)*. 10.1109/NCCC49330.2021.9428825

Shen, J., Wang, J., & Zhang, J. (2023). *The Development of Digital Technology Efficiency in the Communication of Large-Scale Events*. European Union Digital Library. doi:10.4108/eai.6-1-2023.2330328

Shuai, Q., Li, Z., & Zhang, Y. (2023). E-Commerce Channels and Platforms. In Spinger Link (pp. 283–318). Springer. doi:10.1007/978-981-99-0043-5_8

Singh, M., & Kumar, A. (2023). A Critical Political Economy Perspective on Indian Television: STAR, Hotstar, and Live Sports Streaming. *TripleC*, *21*(1), 18–32. doi:10.31269/triplec.v21i1.1395

Singhal, V., Jain, S. P., Anand, D., Singh, A., Verma, S., Kavita, Rodrigues, J. J. P. C., Jhanjhi, N. Z., Ghosh, U., Jo, O., & Iwendi, C. (2020). Artificial Intelligence Enabled Road Vehicle-Train Collision Risk Assessment Framework for Unmanned railway level crossings. *IEEE Access : Practical Innovations, Open Solutions*, *8*, 113790–113806. doi:10.1109/ACCESS.2020.3002416

Siricharoen, N. (2023). Creative Brain Training Apps and Games Can Help Improve Memory, Cognitive Abilities, and Promote Good Mental Health for The Elderly. *EAI Endorsed Transactions on Context-aware Systems and Applications*, *9*(1). doi:10.4108/eetcasa.v9i1.3524

Smith, M. J., Mark, R., Nette, H., & Rhodes, R. E. (2023). Correlates and participation in community-based exercise programming for cancer patients before and during COVID-19. *Supportive Care in Cancer*, *31*(6), 319. doi:10.100700520-023-07725-3 PMID:37148447

Soilemezi, D., Roberts, H., Navarta-Sánchez, M. V., Kunkel, D., Ewings, S., Reidy, C., & Portillo, M. C. (2022). Managing Parkinson's during the COVID-19 pandemic: Perspectives from people living with Parkinson's and health professionals. *Journal of Clinical Nursing*, *32*(7–8), 1421–1432. doi:10.1111/jocn.16367 PMID:35581711

Solas-Martínez, J. L., Suárez-Manzano, S., De La Torre-Cruz, M. J., & Ruiz-Ariza, A. (2023). Artificial Intelligence and Augmented Reality in Physical Activity: A Review of Systems and Devices. In Spinger Link (pp. 245–270). doi:10.1007/978-3-031-27166-3_14

Soni, L., & Kaur, A. (2023). *Strategies for Implementing Metaverse in Education*. IEEE Explore. doi:10.1109/ICDT57929.2023.10150886

Ştefan, S. C., Popa, I., & Mircioiu, C. (2023). Lessons Learned from Online Teaching and Their Implications for Students' Future Careers: Combined PLS-SEM and IPA Approach. *Electronics (Basel)*, *12*(9), 2005. doi:10.3390/electronics12092005

Stocker, V., Whalley, J., & Lehr, W. (2023). Beyond the pandemic: towards a digitally enabled society and economy. In Emerald Publishing Limited eBooks (pp. 245–265). doi:10.1108/978-1-80262-049-820231012

Suh, I. H., McKinney, T., & Siu, K. (2023). Current Perspective of Metaverse Application in Medical Education, Research and Patient Care. *MDPI*, *2*(2), 115–128. doi:10.3390/virtualworlds2020007

Sun, P. (2023). *A Guidebook for 5GTOB and 6G Vision for Deep Convergence*. Springer Nature. doi:10.1007/978-981-99-4024-0

Sun, T., Jin, T., Huang, Y., Meng, L., Yun, W., Jiang, Z., & Fu, X. (2023). Restoring Dunhuang Murals: Crafting Cultural Heritage Preservation Knowledge into Immersive Virtual Reality Experience Design. *International Journal of Human-Computer Interaction*, 1–22. doi:10.1080/10447318.2023.2232976

SynnottC. K. (2023). Gambling companies' contracts in higher education raise concerns. *Social Science Research Network*. doi:10.2139/ssrn.4394642

Tan, M. C. C., Chye, S., & Min, T. J. (2023). Teaching Social-Emotional Learning with Immersive Virtual Technology: Exploratory Considerations. In Spinger Link (pp. 169–195). doi:10.1007/978-981-99-2107-2_10

Tayyab, M., Marjani, M., Jhanjhi, N. Z., Hashem, I. T., Usmani, R. S. A., & Qamar, F. (2023). A comprehensive review on deep learning algorithms: Security and privacy issues. *Computers & Security*, *131*, 103297. doi:10.1016/j.cose.2023.103297

Thamrongrat, P., Khundam, C., Pakdeebun, P., & Nizam, D. M. (2023). Desktop vs. Headset: A Comparative Study of User Experience and Engagement for Flexibility Exercise in. *ResearchGate*. doi:10.28991/ESJ-2023-07-04-03

Torky, M., Darwish, A., & Hassanien, A. E. (2023). Blockchain technology in metaverse: opportunities, applications, and open problems. In Springer eBooks (pp. 225–246). doi:10.1007/978-3-031-29132-6_13

Torrance, J., O'Hanrahan, M., Carroll, J., & Newall, P. (2022). *The structural characteristics of online sports betting: a scoping review of current product features and utility patents as indicators of potential future developments.* Taylor Francis Online. doi:10.1080/16066359.2023.2241350

Turoń-Skrzypińska, A., Tomska, N., Mosiejczuk, H., Rył, A., Szylińska, A., Marchelek-Myśliwiec, M., Ciechanowski, K., Nagay, R., & Rotter, I. (2023). Impact of virtual reality exercises on anxiety and depression in hemodialysis. *Nature*, *13*(1), 12435. doi:10.103841598-023-39709-y PMID:37528161

Ullah, H., Manickam, S., Obaidat, M., Laghari, S. A., & Uddin, M. (2023). Exploring the potential of metaverse technology in healthcare: Applications, challenges, and future directions. *IEEE Access : Practical Innovations, Open Solutions*, *11*, 69686–69707. doi:10.1109/ACCESS.2023.3286696

Ullah, M., Hamayun, S., Wahab, A., Khan, S. U., Qayum, M., Ullah, A., Rehman, M. U., Mehreen, A., Awan, U. A., & Naeem, M. (2023). Smart Technologies used as Smart Tools in the Management of Cardiovascular Disease and their Future Perspective. *Current Problems in Cardiology*, *101922*(11), 101922. doi:10.1016/j.cpcardiol.2023.101922 PMID:37437703

Vaccaro, A., Koerner, J. D., & Kim, D. H. (2016). *Recent advances in spinal surgery*. JP Medical Ltd.

Van Biemen, T., Müller, D., & Mann, D. L. (2023). Virtual reality as a representative training environment for football referees. *Human Movement Science*, *89*, 103091. doi:10.1016/j.humov.2023.103091 PMID:37084551

Van Rijmenam, M. (2022). *Step into the Metaverse: How the Immersive Internet Will Unlock a Trillion-Dollar Social Economy*. John Wiley & Sons.

Van Wegen, M., Herder, J. L., Adelsberger, R., Pastore-Wapp, M., Van Wegen, E. E. H., Bohlhalter, S., Nef, T., Krack, P., & Vanbellingen, T. (2023). An overview of wearable haptic technologies and their performance in virtual object exploration. *Sensors (Basel)*, *23*(3), 1563. doi:10.339023031563 PMID:36772603

Villa-García, L., Davey, V., Pérez, L. M., Soto-Bagaria, L., Risco, E., Díaz, P., Kuluski, K., Giné-Garriga, M., Castellano-Tejedor, C., & Inzitari, M. (2023). Co-designing implementation strategies to promote remote physical activity programs in frail older community-dwellers. *Frontiers in Public Health*, *11*, 1062843. doi:10.3389/fpubh.2023.1062843 PMID:36960372

Villalonga-Gómez, C., Ortega-Fernández, E., & Borau-Boira, E. (2023). Fifteen years of metaverse in Higher Education: A systematic literature review. *IEEE Transactions on Learning Technologies*, 1–14. doi:10.1109/TLT.2023.3302382

Waitt, G. R., Gordon, R., Harada, T., Gurrieri, L., Reith, G., & Ciorciari, J. (2023). Towards relational geographies of gambling harm: Orientation, affective atmosphere, and intimacy. *Progress in Human Geography*, (5), 627–644. doi:10.1177/03091325231177278

Wang, D., Yang, Z., Zhang, P., Wang, R., Yang, B., & Ma, X. (2023). Virtual-Reality Inter-Promotion Technology for Metaverse: A survey. *IEEE Internet of Things Journal*, *1*(18), 15788–15809. doi:10.1109/JIOT.2023.3265848

Wang, N., & Wen-Guang, C. (2023). The effect of playing e-sports games on young people's desire to engage in physical activity: Mediating effects of social presence perception and virtual sports experience. *PLoS One*, *18*(7), e0288608. doi:10.1371/journal.pone.0288608 PMID:37498937

Wang, T. (2023, January 3). *Augmented Reality in Sports Event Videos: A Qualitative Study on Viewer experience*. Scholar Space. https://scholarspace.manoa.hawaii.edu/items/00382afd-df6e-4ece-8b84-21e7922dad76

Wedig, I. J., Phillips, J. J., Kamm, K., & Elmer, S. J. (2023). Promoting Physical Activity in Rural Communities During COVID-19 with Exercise is Medicine® on Campus. *ACSM's Health & Fitness Journal*, *27*(2), 33–40. doi:10.1249/FIT.0000000000000849

Wieland, M., Sedlmair, M., & Machulla, T. (2023). *VR, Gaze, and Visual Impairment: An Exploratory Study of the Perception of Eye Contact across different Sensory Modalities for People with Visual Impairments in Virtual Reality*. ACM. doi:10.1145/3544549.3585726

Wongkitrungrueng, A., & Suprawan, L. (2023). Metaverse Meets Branding: Examining consumer responses to immersive brand experiences. *International Journal of Human-Computer Interaction*, 1–20. doi:10.1080/10447318.2023.2175162

Xu, Y. (2023). The evolving eSports landscape: Technology empowerment, intelligent embodiment, and digital ethics. *Sport, Ethics and Philosophy*, *17*(3), 356–368. doi:10.1080/17511321.2023.2168039

Yaqoob, I., Salah, K., Jayaraman, R., & Omar, M. (2023). Metaverse applications in smart cities: Enabling technologies, opportunities, challenges, and future directions. *Internet of Things*, *100884*, 100884. doi:10.1016/j.iot.2023.100884

Yilmaz, M., O'Farrell, E., & Clarke, P. M. (2023). Examining the training and education potential of the metaverse: Results from an empirical study of next generation SAFe training. *Journal of Software (Malden, MA)*, *35*(9), e2531. doi:10.1002mr.2531

Yoo, K., Welden, R., Hewett, K., & Haenlein, M. (2023). The merchants of meta: A research agenda to understand the future of retailing in the metaverse. *Journal of Retailing*, *99*(2), 173–192. doi:10.1016/j.jretai.2023.02.002

Yun, S. J., Hyun, S. E., Oh, B. M., & Seo, H. G. (2023). Fully immersive virtual reality exergames with dual-task components for patients with Parkinson's disease: A feasibility study. *Journal of Neuroengineering and Rehabilitation*, *20*(1), 92. doi:10.118612984-023-01215-7 PMID:37464349

Zalan, T., & Barbesino, P. (2023). Making the metaverse real. *Digital Business*, *3*(2), 100059. doi:10.1016/j.digbus.2023.100059

Zaman, N., Gaur, L., & Humayun, M. (2022). *Approaches and applications of deep learning in virtual medical care*. IGI Global. doi:10.4018/978-1-7998-8929-8

Zhang, J. (2023, June 1). *Gamification in marketing to increase customer retention*. MIT. https://dspace.mit.edu/handle/1721.1/151418

Zhang, L., He, W., Cao, Z., Wang, S., Bai, H., & Billinghurst, M. (2022). HapticProxy: Providing positional vibrotactile feedback on a physical proxy for Virtual-Real interaction in augmented reality. *International Journal of Human-Computer Interaction*, 1–15. doi:10.1080/10447318.2022.2041895

Zhang, Q. (2023). Secure preschool education using machine learning and metaverse technologies. *Applied Artificial Intelligence*, *37*(1), 2222496. doi:10.1080/08839514.2023.2222496

Zhao, R., Zhang, Y., Zhu, Y., Lan, R., & Hua, Z. (2023). Metaverse: Security and Privacy Concerns. *Dergi Park*, *3*(2), 93–99. doi:10.57019/jmv.1286526

Zhu, Q., Zhang, X., Dai, S., Satake, N., & Wang, H. (2023). ZoomBaTogether: a video conference add-on for generating interactive visual feedback for online group exercise through On-The-Fly pose tracking. *Designing Interactive Systems Conference*. 10.1145/3563703.3596653

Zikas, P., Protopsaltis, A., Lydatakis, N., Kentros, M., Geronikolakis, S., Kateros, S., Kamarianakis, M., Evangelou, G., Filippidis, A., Grigoriou, E., Angelis, D., Tamiolakis, M., Dodis, M., Kokiadis, G., Petropoulos, J., Pateraki, M., & Papagiannakis, G. (2023). MAGES 4.0: Accelerating the world's transition to VR training and democratizing the authoring of the medical metaverse. *IEEE Computer Graphics and Applications*, *43*(2), 43–56. doi:10.1109/MCG.2023.3242686

Zikas, P., Protopsaltis, A., Lydatakis, N., Kentros, M., Geronikolakis, S., Kateros, S., Kamarianakis, M., Evangelou, G., Filippidis, A., Grigoriou, E., Angelis, D., Tamiolakis, M., Dodis, M., Kokiadis, G., Petropoulos, J., Pateraki, M., & Papagiannakis, G. (2023). MAGES 4.0: Accelerating the world's transition to VR training and democratizing the authoring of the medical metaverse. *IEEE Computer Graphics and Applications*, *43*(2), 43–56. doi:10.1109/MCG.2023.3242686

Zoe, V. R. (2023, July 17). *Development of a therapy game proof of concept using the Virtual Reality technology*. Repostori. https://repositori.uji.es/xmlui/handle/10234/203631

Chapter 3
Metaverse:
Virtual Meditation

Siva Raja Sindiramutty
Taylor's University, Malaysia

Noor Zaman Jhanjhi
https://orcid.org/0000-0001-8116-4733
Taylor's University, Malaysia

Sayan Kumar Ray
Taylor's University, Malaysia

Husin Jazri
https://orcid.org/0009-0005-3940-2351
Taylor's University, Malaysia

Navid Ali Khan
Taylor's University, Malaysia

Loveleen Gaur
https://orcid.org/0000-0002-0885-1550
University of the South Pacific, Fiji

ABSTRACT

The rise of the metaverse as a digital domain for diverse activities has birthed an innovative application known as 'metaverse virtual meditation.' This concept seamlessly merges technology and mindfulness, employing virtual reality (VR) and augmented reality (AR) to craft serene digital landscapes. These immersive settings, ranging from natural vistas to abstract spaces, enable users to overcome physical constraints and distractions, facilitating mindfulness, stress reduction, and emotional resilience. The chapter navigates the fusion of technology and contemplative practices, from traditional meditation to modern VR and AR experiences. Stress reduction, heightened focus, and inclusivity are among the advantages highlighted. The convergence of visuals, biofeedback, brain-computer interfaces (BCIs), and AI-driven personalization is explored for tailored meditation. Design principles, interactive elements, and natural components play a crucial role in shaping tranquil virtual environments.

DOI: 10.4018/978-1-6684-9823-1.ch003

1. INTRODUCTION TO METAVERSE VIRTUAL MEDITATION

1.1 Definition and Concept of the Metaverse

The metaverse stands as a virtual realm encompassing interconnected digital spaces, enabling users to engage, communicate, and partake in activities through avatars and digital representations of themselves. It's a fusion of AR, VR, and the internet, resulting in a shared virtual space. This concept encapsulates an expansive virtual universe where people can interact socially, conduct economic transactions, pursue education, find entertainment, and more. As discussed by Uddin et al. (2023), the metaverse aims to seamlessly bridge the gap between the physical and digital realms, allowing users to navigate various virtual domains effortlessly.

An essential aspect of the metaverse is immersion, where users are deeply engrossed within the digital environment. This immersive encounter is accomplished through advanced technologies like VR headsets, haptic feedback systems, and spatial computing (Richter & Richter, 2023). By integrating these technologies, the metaverse provides an elevated sense of presence and interactivity. A crucial characteristic of the metaverse is its enduring nature. In contrast to conventional online platforms, the metaverse maintains its continuity, with virtual spaces persisting and evolving even when users log out (Jo, 2023). Interconnectedness is a foundational feature of the metaverse. Users can smoothly navigate between diverse virtual realms and spaces, encouraging cross-platform social interactions (Aljanabi, 2023). This interconnected nature facilitates a smooth exchange of information, assets, and experiences.

Moreover, the metaverse encourages user-generated content and personalization. Users possess the capability to generate, modify, and trade virtual assets, resulting in a thriving digital economy (Zhi et al., 2023). The metaverse's influence isn't limited to entertainment; it encompasses various sectors. In the realm of education, it provides immersive learning encounters through simulations and collaborative settings (Soni & Kaur, 2023; Shafiq et al., 2021)). Concerning healthcare, it facilitates applications for telemedicine and medical training simulations (Suh et al., 2023; Zaman et al., 2022; Chatrati et al., 2022). Businesses are also delving into the metaverse for virtual conferences, product launches, and collaborative workspaces (Nagarajan, 2023).

In summation, the metaverse symbolizes a transformative digital domain that merges VR, AR, and the internet. It encourages immersion, interconnectedness, durability, and user-driven content generation. As technology progresses, the metaverse's potential applications across various domains are becoming increasingly apparent Figure 1 and Figure 2 show the example of VR and AR devices.

Metaverse

Figure 1. VR device
DeGuzman (2021b)

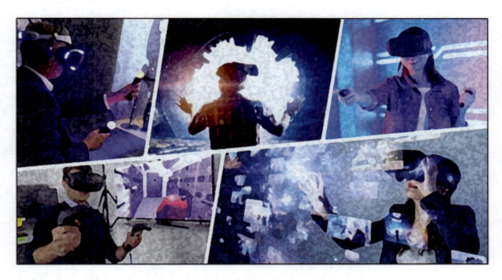

Figure 2. AR devices

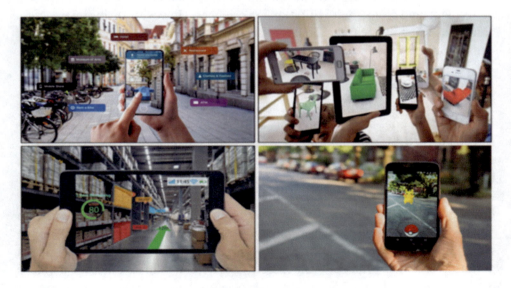

95

1.2 Virtual Meditation and its Role in the Metaverse

The fusion of technology and mindfulness, known as virtual meditation, has garnered significant attention in the burgeoning world of the metaverse. The metaverse, an interconnected digital realm comprised of virtual environments, provides a distinctive platform for incorporating meditation techniques. This section delves into the role of virtual meditation in the metaverse, emphasizing its potential advantages and implications.

Virtual meditation blends age-old mindfulness practices with immersive digital encounters, providing a fresh approach to meditation. It harnesses technologies like VR and AR to fashion serene and customizable meditation settings. Research suggests that these technologies can heighten relaxation and alleviate stress (Bhumika et al., 2023). Additionally, studies propose that virtual meditation can bolster concentration and cognitive performance (Chuanhua, 2023). The metaverse's interconnected nature enables shared meditation experiences, regardless of physical distance. Individuals can meditate together in virtual spaces, fostering a sense of community and connection. This communal aspect aligns with the social essence of the metaverse, potentially magnifying the emotional advantages of meditation (Ahuja et al., 2023).

In conclusion, the integration of virtual meditation into the metaverse introduces inventive prospects for enhancing mindfulness practices. The convergence of meditation and technology opens doors to relaxation, cognitive betterment, and collective meditation experiences. However, as this intersection continues to evolve, careful contemplation of potential drawbacks and ethical considerations remains pivotal.

1.3 Importance and Benefits of Virtual Meditation

Virtual meditation, an amalgamation of time-honoured mindfulness techniques and contemporary technology, has garnered substantial attention due to its myriad advantages for one's mental, emotional, and physical welfare. This segment delves into the significance and merits of virtual meditation, drawing from a variety of investigations and scholarly work. Virtual meditation presents a convenient avenue for individuals to partake in mindfulness rituals, which have been correlated with diminished stress and heightened mental lucidity (Adam et al., 2023). Through virtual platforms, individuals can engage in guided meditation sessions aimed at nurturing relaxation and self-awareness (Stockly & Wildman, 2022). This holds particular relevance in today's fast-paced society, where adept stress management is of paramount importance.

Moreover, virtual meditation brings about flexibility and accessibility, permitting users to join in from the comforts of their homes or any location of their choice

(Hopkins & Bardoel, 2023). This facet is especially advantageous for those with restricted mobility or demanding schedules. Notably, virtual meditation has shown the potential in boosting concentration and attentiveness, thereby potentially enhancing overall productivity (Claisse & Durrant, 2023). Numerous studies underscore the affirmative influence of virtual meditation on mental well-being. Research suggests that regular engagement can alleviate symptoms of anxiety and depression (Jin et al., 2023). Additionally, virtual meditation has been associated with heightened emotional regulation and an increased sense of self-compassion (Banerji, 2023). These findings accentuate the potential of virtual meditation as a tool to foster psychological equilibrium. From a physical health perspective, virtual meditation has exhibited advantages such as reduced blood pressure and enhanced sleep quality (Bai, 2023). Participation in virtual meditation sessions can also contribute to pain management and a bolstered immune system (Demeco et al., 2023).

In sum, virtual meditation presents an expedient and efficacious avenue to cultivate mindfulness, alleviate stress, amplify mental well-being, and nurture physical health. Through guided sessions made accessible via virtual platforms, individuals can harness the potency of meditation even within their bustling lives. The research scrutinized in this report underscores the import of virtual meditation as a comprehensive approach towards attaining holistic wellness.

1.4 Scope and Objectives of Research

The scope of this research chapter encompasses a comprehensive exploration of the emerging paradigm of Metaverse Virtual Meditation, where the convergence of VR, mindfulness practices, and immersive technologies creates a novel domain for personal well-being and mental flourishing. This chapter delves into the conceptual underpinnings of integrating meditation techniques within the expansive realm of the metaverse, shedding light on the transformative potential it holds for individuals seeking holistic wellness in a digitally interconnected world. The primary objectives of this research are twofold: Firstly, to elucidate the multifaceted dimensions of Metaverse Virtual Meditation, ranging from its historical context and theoretical foundations to its practical applications and technological implementations. Secondly, to critically analyze the benefits, challenges, and ethical considerations associated with this emerging fusion of meditation and VR, while also providing insights into its future directions and potential contributions to well-being. By examining the intersections of mindfulness practices, immersive technologies, and cognitive neuroscience, this research aims to provide a comprehensive understanding of how Metaverse Virtual Meditation can positively impact mental health, cognitive function, and overall quality of life. Moreover, it seeks to offer guidance to practitioners, researchers, and developers in designing meaningful, ethically sound, and effective virtual meditation experiences that cater to diverse needs and preferences. Through an in-depth exploration of the subject matter, this chapter aims to contribute to the academic discourse surrounding metaverse technologies, meditation practices, and their harmonious integration for fostering personal growth, stress reduction, and enhanced mindfulness within the context of an increasingly digitized world.

1.5 Key Concepts and Terminology

Metaverse: A virtual shared space, created by the convergence of physical and VR, where users can interact with each other and digital objects in real time. It's often described as the next evolution of the internet, offering immersive and interconnected experiences.

Virtual Meditation: The practice of meditation that takes place within a virtual environment, using technologies like VR or AR to create immersive and engaging meditation experiences.

Immersive Experience: A sensory-rich environment that surrounds a user, providing a strong feeling of presence and engagement. In the context of meditation, it refers to the sensation of being fully absorbed in a virtual environment.

Mindfulness: A mental practice that involves focusing one's awareness on the present moment, typically achieved through meditation techniques. It promotes self-awareness, stress reduction, and emotional regulation.

Guided Meditation: A form of meditation in which a narrator leads the practitioner through a series of visualizations and instructions, aiding relaxation and mental focus.

Biofeedback: The process of monitoring physiological signals (such as heart rate, brainwaves, and breathing) and providing real-time feedback to help individuals gain control over their bodily functions.

Brain-Computer Interface (BCI): Technology that enables direct communication between the brain and external devices, allowing users to control computers or interact with digital environments using their brain activity.

AI-driven Personalization: The use of artificial intelligence to tailor experiences to individual preferences and needs, such as customizing meditation practices based on user behaviour and responses.

Serene and Calming Virtual Spaces: Virtual environments are designed to evoke feelings of tranquillity and relaxation, often featuring soothing visuals, natural elements, and ambient sounds.

Environmental Soundscapes: The auditory landscape of a particular environment, which can greatly influence mood and emotional states. In virtual meditation, carefully crafted soundscapes contribute to the overall experience.

Neuroscientific Studies: Research focused on understanding the brain's structure and function, including how various activities, such as meditation, impact brain activity and cognitive functions.

Cognitive Benefits: Positive effects on cognitive processes such as attention, memory, and problem-solving, which can be enhanced through meditation practices.

Hybrid Meditation: The integration of virtual and physical meditation practices allows individuals to combine the benefits of immersive technology with traditional techniques.

1.6 Chapter Contribution

This chapter makes a significant contribution to the evolving fields of VR, mindfulness, and well-being by illuminating the transformative potential of Metaverse Virtual Meditation. By synthesizing the realms of digital technology and contemplative practices, this contribution facilitates a deeper understanding of how individuals can harness the metaverse to enhance their mental and emotional well-being. The chapter's central contribution lies in its comprehensive examination of the concept, benefits, challenges, and ethical dimensions of Metaverse Virtual Meditation. It serves as a guiding compass for readers navigating the intersection of immersive virtual environments and meditation techniques. Moreover, the chapter underscores the importance of leveraging technological innovations to create serene and immersive meditation spaces, ensuring that these virtual experiences remain authentic and efficacious. By providing insights into the integration of traditional meditation practices with cutting-edge VR and AR technologies, this chapter addresses the gap between ancient wisdom and contemporary digital advancements. It offers a roadmap for practitioners, researchers, and designers to forge new frontiers in the metaverse, promoting stress reduction, focus enhancement, and inclusive well-being practices. Furthermore, the chapter bridges the scientific and experiential realms, drawing from neuroscientific studies and cognitive research to elucidate the cognitive, emotional, and physiological impacts of Metaverse Virtual Meditation. This synthesis not only enriches our understanding but also opens avenues for future studies, ensuring that the potential of this novel fusion is explored comprehensively. In essence, the chapter's contribution lies in fostering a holistic perspective on the integration of Metaverse Virtual Meditation into everyday life, enabling readers to embrace digital tools as catalysts for personal growth, self-awareness, and mental flourishing within the dynamic landscape of the metaverse.

1.7 Chapter Organization

The chapter is organized to comprehensively explore the integration of virtual meditation within the metaverse. It begins by defining the metaverse and its connection to virtual meditation, highlighting the benefits and significance of this fusion. The understanding of virtual meditation encompasses traditional practices, VR and AR meditation, guided mindfulness apps, and their respective benefits. Technological advancements, including immersive audio-visuals, biofeedback, brain-computer interfaces, and AI-driven personalization, are delved into as crucial components. The creation of serene virtual meditation environments is discussed, emphasizing design principles, soundscapes, and user engagement. The chapter then addresses the application of virtual meditation for specific needs, such as stress management, work-life balance, sleep, and healing, while also exploring the combination of virtual and physical practices and the ensuing challenges. Building and scaling virtual meditation platforms involve business models, user experience, monetization, and community building, followed by an exploration of the scientific and cognitive aspects. Ethical considerations regarding data privacy, mental health, and balancing virtual and real-world connections are examined. Lastly, the chapter outlines future trends, including technological advancements, evolving practices, ethical studies, and new modalities, encapsulating a comprehensive exploration of metaverse virtual meditation.

Figure 3. Metaverse meditation
Source: Redirect Notice (n.d.)

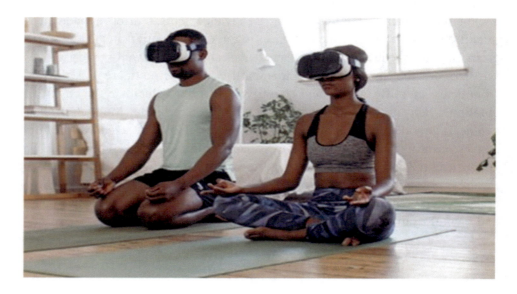

2. UNDERSTANDING VIRTUAL MEDITATION

2.1 Traditional Meditation Practices and Techniques

For centuries, across various cultures, people have utilized age-old meditation practices and methods to improve their mental well-being and spiritual development. These long-standing techniques provide individuals with avenues to foster mindfulness, alleviate stress, and attain a deeper comprehension of both themselves and the world surrounding them.

One widely acknowledged traditional practice is mindfulness meditation, which emphasizes being present in the current moment (Levin, 2023). This technique encourages individuals to observe their thoughts and feelings without passing judgment (Ruan et al., 2023), leading to increased clarity and self-acceptance. An example closely linked to mindfulness is Vipassana, an ancient Indian meditation practice that centres on gaining insight into the nature of reality (McMahan, 2023). Transcendental Meditation (TM), originating from the Vedic tradition, involves repeating specific words to reach a state of deep relaxation and heightened consciousness (Singh & Saxena, 2023). Zen meditation, rooted in Buddhist traditions, places importance on focused breath awareness and detachment from thoughts (Gulick, 2023), resulting in inner tranquillity and equanimity. Within Tibetan Buddhist practices, loving-kindness meditation, or Metta, aims to foster compassion for oneself and others (Slivjak et al., 2023). Yoga Nidra, a yogic technique, induces profound relaxation through guided imagery and body scanning (Robison et al., 2023), facilitating emotional healing and stress reduction. In the Chinese tradition, Qi Gong combines breath regulation, movement, and meditation to balance the body's energy (Liu et al., 2023). Similarly, Tai Chi, another Chinese practice, merges meditation with flowing movements to enhance physical and mental well-being (Park et al., 2023). Numerous traditional meditation methods have demonstrated therapeutic benefits. For instance, Mindfulness-Based Stress Reduction (MBSR), a modification of mindfulness meditation, is widely employed to manage stress-related conditions (Velissaris et al., 2023; Garfin et al., 2023). Mindfulness-Based Cognitive Therapy (MBCT) integrates mindfulness and cognitive therapy, effectively preventing depression relapses (Siwik et al., 2023; Bhattacharya & Hofmann, 2023). In conclusion, time-honoured meditation practices and techniques offer a wide range of approaches to cultivating mindfulness, promoting relaxation, and supporting spiritual growth. Whether through mindfulness, mantra repetition, breath awareness, or body movements, these practices furnish valuable resources for individuals seeking to enhance their mental well-being and embark on a journey of self-discovery. Figure 4 shows the groups of peoples practicing meditation in traditional methods.

2.2 VR Meditation: Overview and Types

VR technology has made notable advancements in various domains, including healthcare and wellness. One of the emerging frontiers is VR meditation, an innovative strategy for augmenting relaxation and mindfulness techniques. VR meditation blends the immersive qualities of VR with the calming methodologies of classical meditation. This document furnishes an overview of VR meditation and delves into its diverse classifications.

VR meditation introduces a fresh avenue for achieving serenity and mental well-being. By utilizing immersive virtual environments, individuals can transcend their immediate physical surroundings and engage with serene, visually captivating landscapes that induce a sense of tranquillity (Harutyunyan, 2023). This technology holds the potential to deepen the meditation practice by offering a focal point and minimizing external disturbances (Pancini et al., 2023). Several categories of VR meditation cater to varying preferences and aspirations. Guided VR Meditation involves following the lead of a virtual instructor, who guides users through mindfulness exercises and breathing methodologies (She et al., 2023). Nature-centric VR Meditation immerses participants in tranquil natural settings, like forests or beaches, harnessing the therapeutic impacts of nature on mental well-being (Pascual et al., 2022). Mindfulness VR Meditation encourages users to remain present within the virtual realm, nurturing awareness of thoughts and sensations without passing judgment (Sun et al., 2023). In contrast, Immersive VR Meditation employs multi-sensory encounters to cultivate a profound feeling of presence, thereby amplifying the meditative state (Schlussel & Frosh, 2023; Haley et al., 2023). Research on the effectiveness of VR meditation is still in progress, but initial findings are promising. Investigations indicate that VR meditation can diminish stress and anxiety levels (King et al., 2023) while enhancing emotional regulation (Pira et al., 2023). However, it's important to acknowledge that individual reactions to VR meditation may differ Figure 3 shows example of metaverse meditation using VR.

In conclusion, VR meditation introduces an inventive approach to mindfulness and relaxation techniques, offering a modern perspective on conventional meditation practices. Its immersive character and assortment of methodologies accommodate diverse preferences, enriching relaxation and mindfulness encounters. The array of its classifications addresses varied inclinations and objectives, granting users a distinctive and immersive channel for engaging in meditation. As this field continues to evolve, further research will furnish a deeper comprehension of its advantages and potential limitations.

Figure 4. Traditional meditation

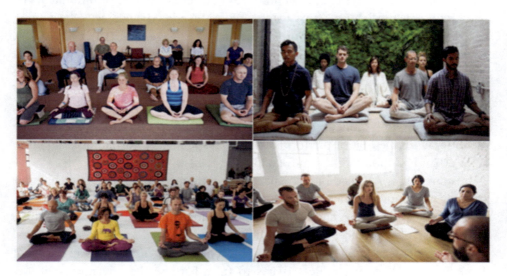

2.3 AR Meditation Experiences

AR has emerged as a promising technological advancement that holds the potential to elevate various dimensions of human encounters. Within this landscape, one promising realm for AR is meditation practices. AR meditation experiences combine conventional mindfulness methodologies with immersive digital components, forming a distinctive fusion that introduces a fresh layer to relaxation and self-awareness.

In AR meditation experiences, AR devices like smart glasses or smartphones overlay digital visuals onto the user's surroundings. This convergence of physical and digital elements empowers users to engage with meditation in innovative ways. Research indicates that such experiences can lead to heightened sensations of tranquillity and reduced stress levels (Eom et al., 2023). The integration of AR in meditation enables users to tailor their surroundings according to their preferences, potentially amplifying focus and engagement (Jo et al., 2023). Visual cues and interactive features within the AR environment can aid in directing breathing rhythms and posture, thereby facilitating a more profound state of meditation (Pal et al., 2023). Furthermore, AR meditation encounters can be adapted to diverse contexts, allowing users to practice mindfulness in their favoured settings, whether indoors or outdoors (Tan et al., 2023). One notable advantage of AR meditation is its accessibility. Users can partake in sessions at their convenience, eliminating the necessity to travel to a specific location. This accessibility has the potential to encourage consistent meditation practices (Lan et al., 2023). Additionally, AR meditation can furnish real-time feedback on a user's advancement, bestowing a sense of achievement and incentive for further engagement (Li et al., 2023). Nevertheless, challenges persist in refining AR meditation experiences. Technical considerations like device limitations and user interface design can impact the efficacy of these encounters (Y. Liu et al., 2023). The seamless integration of digital components with the physical environment, minus disruptive elements, is crucial. Additionally, ethical concerns tied to privacy and data security necessitate attention, as AR meditation platforms accumulate personal information (Randazzo et al., 2023; Hillebrand & Hornuf, 2023).

In summation, AR meditation experiences introduce an innovative avenue for elevating mindfulness practices. The convergence of time-honoured meditation methodologies with AR technology holds the potential to offer adaptable, accessible, and immersive experiences that can culminate in decreased stress and heightened well-being. Yet, meticulous consideration must be devoted to optimizing technical elements and addressing ethical issues to fully harness the advantages of AR meditation. Figure 5 shows benefits of metaverse meditation.

Figure 5. Benefits of metaverse meditation

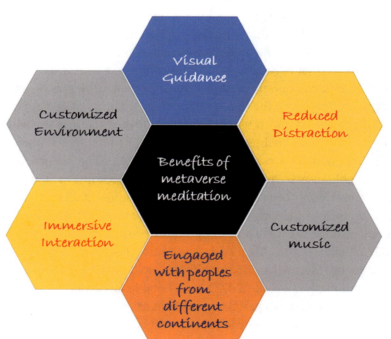

2.4 Guided Meditation and Mindfulness Apps in the Metaverse

The convergence of physical and VR, resulting in a virtual shared space, has introduced innovative possibilities across various domains. A noteworthy area gaining traction is the integration of guided meditation and mindfulness practices within the metaverse environment. This segment delves into the assimilation of guided meditation and mindfulness applications in the metaverse, spotlighting their potential advantages, challenges, and implications for individuals' mental well-being.

Guided meditation and mindfulness applications have garnered considerable popularity due to their capacity to assist individuals in alleviating stress, honing concentration, and enhancing overall mental wellness (Sullivan et al., 2023; Schwartz et al., 2022). These applications provide users with auditory, visual, or text-based guidance through meditation sessions, often focusing on breath awareness, body scans, and mindfulness methods. The accessibility and user-friendly interfaces of these apps have contributed to their widespread adoption. In the metaverse, known for its immersive and interactive characteristics, there exists a distinctive platform for integrating guided meditation and mindfulness practices. Users can fashion avatars, immerse themselves in virtual environments, and connect with others, creating an ideal milieu for nurturing relaxation and self-awareness. Guided meditation sessions within the metaverse can replicate serene landscapes, granting users a taste of calmness and tranquillity (Liedgren et al., 2023). The amalgamation of guided meditation and mindfulness apps within the metaverse yields several benefits. Primarily, the immersive nature of the metaverse amplifies the potential for profound relaxation, enabling users to engage more fully in the meditation experience (Priest, 2023). Secondly, the social dimension of the metaverse enables individuals to engage in collective meditation, cultivating a sense of community and interconnectedness (Covaci et al., 2023). Additionally, the integration of biometric data feedback, such as heart rate variability, within the metaverse can furnish users with real-time insights into their physiological responses during meditation, facilitating more effective stress management (Fernandes & Werner, 2023). The integration of guided meditation and mindfulness applications within the metaverse unveils a promising avenue for augmenting mental well-being. The metaverse's immersive and interactive attributes can provide distinctive meditation encounters, nurturing relaxation, social cohesion, and self-awareness.

3. BENEFITS OF VIRTUAL MEDITATION IN THE METAVERSE

3.1 Stress Reduction and Mental Well-Being

The rise in instances of stress-related disorders and mental health problems in contemporary society has spurred inventive strategies for addressing these issues.

The metaverse, an amalgamation of augmented and VR, has paved the way for fresh methods of tackling mental health concerns. Within this context, metaverse meditation involves the application of mindfulness and relaxation techniques within digital realms.

Metaverse meditation presents a range of potential advantages for mitigating stress and fostering mental wellness. Initially, the immersive quality of VR can establish an atmosphere conducive to relaxation. A study conducted by Gagliardi et al. (2023) suggests that engagement with virtual environments can divert individuals from real-world stressors, thus cultivating a sensation of tranquillity. Secondly, metaverse meditation empowers users to customize their surroundings, constructing tranquil settings that heighten the meditation experience (Wong et al., 2022). This customization aspect empowers users to opt for serene landscapes or calming visuals, thereby contributing to relaxation and stress reduction. The impact of metaverse meditation on neurophysiology is noteworthy. Participating in meditation within virtual settings has been demonstrated to activate brain regions linked to relaxation and stress reduction (Browning et al., 2023). Functional MRI scans have disclosed heightened activity in the prefrontal cortex, which is associated with emotional regulation. Additionally, investigations into heart rate variability (Snodgrass, 2023) suggest that metaverse meditation might foster equilibrium within the autonomic nervous system, fostering a relaxation response.

Another element that plays into stress reduction is social interaction. While metaverse meditation is often viewed as an individual practice, numerous platforms furnish communal spaces for collective meditation experiences (Priest, 2023b). Engaging in meditation alongside others nurtures a sense of inclusion and mutual support, both of which are correlated with enhanced mental well-being (Damaris, 2023; Chen et al., 2023). The metaverse's capacity to transcend geographical constraints enables individuals worldwide to connect and exchange their meditation encounters. Despite the encouraging possibilities linked to metaverse meditation, several factors require consideration. Ethical dilemmas, including potential addiction or detachment from reality, necessitate further exploration (Koohang et al., 2023). It's also important to investigate the long-term impact on mental health and to compare metaverse meditation with conventional approaches. Prospective research could utilize longitudinal studies to gauge the enduring advantages of metaverse meditation.

Metaverse meditation exhibits potential as an inventive strategy for alleviating stress and elevating mental well-being. The immersive atmosphere of virtual settings, options for personalization, neurophysiological effects, social bonding, and inclusiveness all contribute to its prospective benefits. As the metaverse continues to develop, further inquiry is crucial to gain a comprehensive understanding of the lasting consequences of metaverse meditation on mental health.

3.2 Enhanced Focus and Concentration

In today's digital era, maintaining one's focus and concentration has become an increasingly formidable task due to the constant stream of notifications, information overload, and the habit of multitasking. In response to this challenge, innovative solutions are emerging, including the adoption of metaverse meditation as a means to bolster focus and concentration. Metaverse meditation involves the practice of immersive meditation within VR or AR settings. Metaverse meditation provides a distinct platform for individuals to detach from the disruptions of the physical world and fully engage in tranquil virtual environments, which in turn promotes relaxation and heightened focus. Research conducted by Wang et al. (2022) indicates that participating in meditation within VR environments can lead to elevated alpha brainwave activity, which is associated with improved attention and concentration. Furthermore, findings from a study by You and Youn (2023) reveal that the immersive nature of metaverse meditation minimizes external distractions, enabling individuals to channel their attention inward and amplify their levels of concentration.

The immersive aspect of metaverse meditation plays a pivotal role in augmenting focus and concentration. An investigation by Ren (2023) suggests that the multisensory encounter of VR meditation triggers an intensified state of presence, empowering participants to concentrate deeply on their meditation practice. Additionally, according to Mulders (2023), this sense of "presence" in VR environments leads to a state of "flow," where individuals become completely engrossed in their activities, consequently leading to enhanced focus and performance. Metaverse meditation holds the potential to capitalize on the principles of neuroplasticity to enhance cognitive abilities. As highlighted by Ali et al. (2023), the brain's ability to restructure itself in response to novel experiences can be leveraged through focused cognitive training, such as meditation in VR. The research of Sharmin et al. (2023) proposes that consistent metaverse meditation could result in structural modifications within brain regions responsible for attention control, culminating in improved concentration over time. Mindfulness, a central tenet of metaverse meditation, has been correlated with improved regulation of attention. Holley et al. (2022) suggest that practising mindfulness within virtual environments assists individuals in cultivating greater awareness of their thoughts and diversions, empowering them to redirect their focus and uphold concentration more effectively. Furthermore, the study by Loveys et al. (2023) demonstrates that metaverse meditation encourages individuals to adopt an open and non-judgmental stance toward their experiences, thereby further bolstering sustained attention.

In conclusion, metaverse meditation offers a promising avenue for heightening focus and concentration within a digitally saturated world. The immersive qualities of VR surroundings, coupled with the cognitive and neuroplastic advantages of meditation, contribute to enhanced attention control and concentration levels. Through the cultivation of mindfulness and the utilization of immersive experiences, metaverse meditation provides a contemporary solution to the modern challenge of maintaining focus amidst an array of distractions. Figure 6 illustrates the five common types of meditation.

Figure 6. Type of meditation

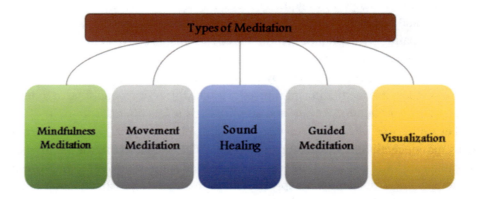

3.3 Accessibility and Inclusivity in Virtual Meditation

Accessibility pertains to the creation and execution of digital environments that cater to the needs of individuals with disabilities, facilitating their full and independent participation. Inclusivity, on the other hand, extends beyond mere accessibility, encompassing a wider spectrum of diversity, including factors such as age, gender, ethnicity, and socio-economic status. Ensuring both accessibility and inclusivity within the context of metaverse meditation is of paramount importance to foster equitable engagement and unlock the maximum potential of this emerging technology.

In crafting an accessible metaverse meditation experience, it's imperative to address visual impairments and hearing disabilities. This involves employing interfaces that are compatible with screen readers and providing audio descriptions for visual elements, enhancing the involvement of individuals with visual impairments (Whiting et al., 2023). Additionally, the inclusion of captions and sign language interpretation for meditation sessions can cater to users who have hearing disabilities (Shannon, 2023). For those with mobility challenges, navigation through virtual environments can pose challenges. By incorporating intuitive controls and adaptable interaction methods, individuals with mobility limitations can be empowered to participate in metaverse meditation effectively (Ponce et al., 2023). Furthermore, the provision of options for seated or reclined meditation postures ensures that individuals with limited mobility can engage comfortably.

Cognitive diversity encompasses a range of cognitive abilities and preferences. To cater to individuals with varying cognitive capacities, designing metaverse meditation experiences with lucid instructions, uncomplicated interfaces, and adjustable meditation durations is essential (Han et al., 2023). Cultural and linguistic diversity also plays a pivotal role in achieving inclusivity. The availability of meditation sessions in multiple languages and the integration of diverse cultural practices can render metaverse meditation more accessible on a global scale (A. Singh et al., 2023). Collaboration with cultural experts can aid in ensuring accurate representation and preventing cultural appropriation. Affordability and access to technology are fundamental aspects of achieving inclusivity. Striving for compatibility with an array of devices, including more affordable options, can extend access to metaverse meditation for individuals with varying levels of technological resources. Furthermore, offering both free or low-cost meditation experiences and premium options can foster accessibility regardless of financial constraints.

In the ever-expanding landscape of the metaverse, the emphasis on accessibility and inclusivity within meditation experiences is pivotal for realizing the full potential of this technology. By thoughtfully addressing concerns related to visual impairments, hearing disabilities, mobility limitations, cognitive diversity, and cultural and linguistic inclusivity, along with affordability and technological access, metaverse meditation can evolve into a space where all individuals can discover tranquillity and personal development. Figure 7 displays a selection of typical meditation benefits.

Figure 7. Benefits of meditation

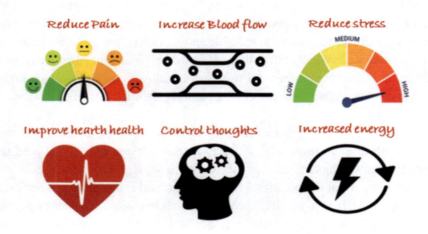

4. TECHNOLOGICAL INNOVATIONS IN VIRTUAL MEDITATION

4.1 Immersive Audio and Visuals for Virtual Meditation

The utilization of immersive audio technologies, such as binaural beats and 3D soundscapes, has garnered attention due to their capacity to manipulate brainwave frequencies and induce meditative states. Binaural beats, a type of auditory illusion, involve presenting slightly divergent frequencies to each ear, resulting in a perceived beat that can synchronize with desired brainwave patterns (Ingendoh et al., 2023). This technique has been linked to heightened relaxation and focus during meditation. Additionally, immersive 3D soundscapes, crafted using methods like ambisonics, envelop the listener within a three-dimensional auditory environment, amplifying the sense of presence and tranquillity (De Engenharia, 2023).

The visual components of virtual meditation significantly contribute to the overall immersive experience. VR headsets provide a canvas for crafting visually captivating meditation settings. These environments span from serene natural landscapes to abstract, soothing scenarios. Research indicates that VR-based meditation can lead to augmented feelings of relaxation and diminished stress (Kaleva & Riches, 2023). Moreover, the integration of biofeedback devices with visual elements enables users to observe real-time shifts in physiological responses, thereby enhancing mindfulness and self-regulation (Jerath et al., 2023). The amalgamation of immersive audio and visual technologies within virtual meditation showcases encouraging outcomes in terms of user engagement and results. A study by Ma et al. (2023) showcased that participants who engaged in virtual meditation sessions featuring immersive elements reported higher levels of relaxation and decreased anxiety in comparison to conventional meditation methods. Another investigation by Seetharaman et al. (2023) unveiled that individuals employing immersive binaural beats reported improved concentration and more profound meditation experiences. Nonetheless, while the application of immersive audio and visual technologies holds significant promise, several considerations demand attention. Individual preferences for audio and visual content can widely differ, thus necessitating personalized options for users. Moreover, ensuring the ethical and responsible utilization of these technologies, without exploiting vulnerable users or supplanting traditional meditation practices, remains pivotal.

In summation, the integration of immersive audio and visual elements within virtual meditation presents a promising avenue for enriching the meditation journey. By harnessing technologies like binaural beats, 3D soundscapes, and VR, individuals can attain deeper states of relaxation and mindfulness. The research underscores the affirmative influence of these technologies on user engagement and overall well-being. Nevertheless, prudent attention must be granted to customization, ethical implementation, and upholding traditional meditation principles. As technology continues its evolution, immersive audio and visual methodologies have the potential to emerge as valuable tools in nurturing mental health and elevating meditation practices.

4.2 Biofeedback and Wearable Devices in VR Meditation

Biofeedback and wearable technologies have garnered significant attention recently as supplementary aids for enhancing meditation encounters, particularly when integrated with VR (VR). Meditation is renowned for its capacity to enhance mental well-being and alleviate stress. The incorporation of biofeedback and wearable devices into VR meditation presents a promising strategy to amplify the advantages of meditation.

Biofeedback entails the measurement of physiological parameters like heart rate, skin conductance, and brainwave activity to furnish individuals with real-time insights into their physiological state (Joshi, 2023; Lucas et al., 2023). Conversely, wearable devices are outfitted with sensors that monitor diverse physiological functions and furnish users with instant input (Mirlou & Beker, 2023). Through the amalgamation of these technologies into VR meditation, participants can promptly and precisely assess their meditation practice, a factor that aids in achieving heightened states of relaxation and concentration (Miller et al., 2023). The convergence of VR meditation, coupled with biofeedback and wearable devices, engenders an immersive and interactive encounter. Users can visualize their physiological responses within the virtual milieu, thus cultivating a more robust connection between the mind and body (Tan et al., 2023). This visual input augments individuals' cognizance of their body's reactions to meditation techniques, empowering them to effectuate real-time modifications for optimizing their practice. Empirical evidence demonstrates that the fusion of biofeedback, wearables, and VR can culminate in enhanced meditation results. A study by Pratviel et al. (2023) underscored that participants who employed biofeedback in tandem with VR meditation reported diminished stress levels and heightened relaxation in comparison to conventional meditation methods. Another study by Gaertner et al. (2023) revealed that participants utilizing wearable devices during VR meditation were adept at sustaining a steady heart rate variability pattern, indicative of enhanced autonomic nervous system regulation. Moreover, wearable devices can chart users' advancement over time and provide tailored recommendations for refining meditation techniques (K. Li et al., 2023). This adaptability assures that users sustain favourable outcomes and sustain engagement in their meditation practice.

To conclude, the convergence of biofeedback and wearable technologies in VR meditation boasts substantial potential for elevating meditation encounters. The instantaneous feedback furnished by these technologies bolsters self-awareness, relaxation, and concentration, all of which contribute to improved mental well-being.

The mounting corpus of research lends support to the efficacy of amalgamating these tools within the VR meditation milieu. As technology progresses, it is plausible that these approaches will become more accessible and customized to individual requisites, ushering in a new epoch of meditation practice.

4.3 Brain-Computer Interface (BCI) for Mindful Interaction

The incorporation of Brain-Computer Interface (BCI) technology into the metaverse has unveiled fresh opportunities for conscious engagement, bridging the domains of neuroscience and VR. BCI facilitates direct communication between the human brain and external devices, such as computers, by converting neural signals into actionable commands. Within the Metaverse, a shared virtual space, the integration of BCI introduces transformative prospects for enhancing user experiences and fostering mindfulness.

BCI technology within the metaverse facilitates real-time interaction by utilizing brainwave patterns to govern virtual elements. Through the interpretation of Electroencephalography (EEG) data, BCI deciphers brain signals connected to intention and attention, enabling users to navigate and manipulate virtual surroundings seamlessly. This shift in interaction mechanisms eliminates the necessity for conventional input tools, nurturing a more immersive and instinctive involvement with the metaverse (Carrión, 2023). The notion of mindfulness, characterized by being fully present and engaged in the present moment, aligns harmoniously with the objectives of exploring the metaverse. BCI-mediated mindful interaction employs mechanisms of neurofeedback to nurture concentrated attention and emotional regulation. Research indicates that BCI-supported mindfulness training can amplify cognitive capabilities and alleviate stress (Mitsea et al., 2023). By weaving mindfulness practices into metaverse encounters, users stand to gain heightened self-awareness and enhanced cognitive mastery (Turdialiev, 2023). BCI's influence on mental health and overall well-being is particularly salient in this context. The metaverse provides a platform for individuals to partake in therapeutic encounters utilizing BCI-driven mindfulness interventions. Studies illustrate the effectiveness of neurofeedback techniques in managing anxiety and depression (Sanku et al., 2023). Through the amalgamation of BCI technology with metaverse environments, users can engage in immersive mindfulness sessions, potentially offering relief from mental health difficulties. Incorporating BCI into the metaverse necessitates paramount attention to ethical aspects encompassing data privacy and user consent. Striking a balance between enhancing user experience and safeguarding personal information holds the utmost importance (Ray, 2023). Moreover, inclusivity concerns must be addressed to ensure that BCI-enhanced metaverse experiences remain accessible to individuals with diverse cognitive abilities.

In summary, the fusion of Brain-Computer Interface technology with the metaverse ushers in a groundbreaking avenue for mindful engagement. By tapping into neural signals, BCI facilitates seamless interaction with virtual environments, in harmony with the principles of mindfulness. This integration bears the potential to nurture cognitive well-being and mental health; nonetheless, a vigilant focus on ethical and accessibility considerations remains imperative

4.4 AI-driven Personalization and Customization of Meditation Experiences

AI advancements have given rise to personalized meditation platforms that cater to the unique requirements of users. These platforms employ AI algorithms to analyze real-time data, evaluating users' emotional states, meditation preferences, and objectives (Anderson et al., 2023). This data guides the AI systems in selecting suitable meditation techniques, durations, and content that align with each user's specific context (Mazlan et al., 2023; Singhal et al., 2020)). Consequently, individuals partake in meditation sessions that harmonize with their present mindset and emotional necessities.

Moreover, AI-driven meditation applications elevate personalization by providing a wide array of meditation styles. These applications leverage natural language processing (NLP) to scrutinize user input and adapt meditation content accordingly (Omranian et al., 2023; Dogra et al., 2022)). For instance, if a user expresses a fondness for guided imagery, subsequent sessions are tailored by the AI system to incorporate more of this element. This personalized approach enhances the engagement and efficacy of the meditation journey. The incorporation of AI-generated ambient sounds further enhances user involvement. AI models generate calming sounds based on individual preferences, cultivating an immersive meditation atmosphere (Tan et al., 2023; Qureshi, 2023). These ambient sounds dynamically shift to match the meditation's theme and the user's emotional state, intensifying the personalized encounter. AI's impact extends beyond individual preferences, extending to group meditation sessions. Algorithms analyze the schedules and time zones of participants, facilitating the arrangement of group meditations at times most conducive for maximum involvement (Ekandjo, 2023; Hamid et al., 2019)). This personalized scheduling nurtures a sense of community among participants while accommodating their routines. In conclusion, AI-powered personalization and customization are revolutionizing meditation encounters. By scrutinizing users' emotional states, preferences, and objectives, AI tailors meditation content to suit individual requirements. NLP-fueled customization and AI-generated ambient sounds enrich the experience, heightening its immersive and engaging nature. Even group meditation sessions benefit from AI's involvement, with algorithms optimizing scheduling for participants' convenience. As AI continues to evolve, the potential for crafting more tailored and effective meditation experiences becomes increasingly promising

5. CREATING IMMERSIVE VIRTUAL MEDITATION ENVIRONMENTS

5.1 Designing Serene and Calming Virtual Spaces

Crafting virtual settings that evoke tranquillity and peacefulness plays a pivotal role in heightening the efficacy of virtual meditation encounters. To augment the effectiveness of these experiences, the architectural layout of virtual domains assumes a pivotal function in evoking feelings of serenity and placidity. Research shows that employing soft and subdued colour schemes can directly impact emotional states (Chauhan & Agarwal, 2023). Within virtual meditation spaces, shades like delicate blues and mild greens cultivate a sense of calmness (J. Li et al., 2023). These colours evoke the essence of nature and expansive skies, infusing a serene atmosphere that fosters relaxation and attentiveness. Integrating natural elements into virtual meditation environments can transport users to soothing outdoor landscapes. The gentle rush of water, rustling leaves, and the melodies of birdsong replicate the tranquillity of nature, establishing a profound connection to the outdoors (Tekin & Gutiérrez, 2023). This immersive encounter with a simulated natural milieu can mitigate stress and kindle a sensation of tranquillity.

A minimalist design approach adopted in virtual meditation spaces serves to eliminate visual chaos, mitigating sensory overload (Krueger, 2022). Clean contours and uncluttered visuals instil a feeling of simplicity and equilibrium. This unembellished aesthetic nurtures a lucid and focused mentality, amplifying the meditation journey. Soft and diffused illumination, akin to natural sunlight, can engender a mild and soothing ambience (Sarasalin, 2023). This lighting pattern emulates the innate rhythms of daylight, fostering relaxation. It sidesteps glaring brightness, establishing a calming setting conducive to meditation. Incorporating ambient sounds such as rain or gentle instrumental melodies can proficiently mask distracting noises and intensify the immersive episode (Crawford, 2023). These sounds produce a tranquil auditory backdrop that complements the visual constituents, cultivating a more profound state of repose. Empowering users to personalize their virtual settings according to their inclinations adds a personalized dimension, nurturing a sense of belonging and ease (Zhang, 2023). This individualization can cultivate a deeper emotional affinity with the virtual environment, enriching the comprehensive meditation journey.

Infusing these design tenets into virtual meditation settings can lead to immersive and impactful episodes that promote relaxation, mindfulness, and emotional well-being. By thoughtfully considering aspects like colour selection, incorporation of natural elements, minimalist aesthetics, lighting techniques, auditory ambience, user engagement, and customization, developers can mould virtual spaces that proffer individuals a serene expedition of self-discovery and inner tranquillity.

Figure 8. BCI technology framework

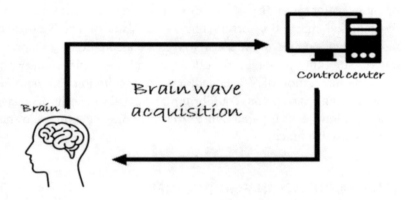

5.2 Interaction and Engagement in VR Meditation

Active involvement holds a pivotal role in the realm of VR meditation experiences, as it empowers users to actively interact with their virtual surroundings. Within the meditation context, interaction entails users' capacity to manipulate both the virtual environment and its constituent objects. VR meditation platforms frequently incorporate interactive functionalities like choosing meditation settings (Zainab et al., 2023), fine-tuning ambient sounds, and engaging with virtual guides. Such interactions foster a sense of control, heightening user engagement by permitting individuals to tailor their meditation sessions to their preferences.

Engagement denotes the degree to which users are captivated and absorbed in the VR meditation encounter. VR's immersive nature holds the potential to amplify engagement compared to conventional meditation approaches (Huang et al., 2023). The feeling of presence and embodiment within a tranquil virtual landscape can seize users' focus and mitigate potential distractions. Additionally, interactive elements like real-time biofeedback during meditation contribute to sustained engagement by offering users tangible insights into their mental state. The interplay between interaction and engagement in the realm of VR meditation brings forth numerous advantages. Firstly, the personalization facilitated by interactive features augments user contentment and adherence to meditation routines (Räsänen et al., 2023). Secondly, heightened engagement heightens the probability of attaining mindfulness and relaxation objectives (Angelos, n.d.). Furthermore, VR meditation's immersive nature might more effectively alleviate anxiety and stress in comparison to conventional approaches (Riches et al., 2023). Nevertheless, ethical concerns linked to potential addiction and overreliance on technology in meditative practices need acknowledgement (Moyer, 2023).

The amalgamation of interaction and engagement in VR meditation presents promising pathways for elevating meditation experiences. By granting users the ability to actively shape their meditation surroundings and cultivate immersive engagement, VR technology stands poised to transform traditional meditation paradigms. While continuous research into its long-term effects is underway, preliminary findings indicate that the integration of VR technology into meditation can yield positive outcomes. Achieving a harmonious equilibrium between the benefits of engagement and the potential drawbacks is paramount as this technology continues to shape the evolution of meditative practices

6. VIRTUAL MEDITATION FOR SPECIFIC NEEDS AND POPULATIONS

6.1 Virtual Meditation for Stress and Anxiety Management

The modern world's rapid pace has led to the widespread prevalence of stress and anxiety, impacting individuals' overall wellness and life quality. Given that conventional methods of addressing these concerns might not always be accessible or effective, virtual meditation has emerged as an encouraging alternative. This section delves into the pivotal role of virtual meditation as a means of managing stress and anxiety. It highlights its advantages, supported by pertinent research.

Virtual meditation encompasses the practice of mindfulness and relaxation techniques through digital platforms, providing individuals with the flexibility to engage in meditation anywhere and at any time. The research underscores the considerable efficacy of virtual meditation in mitigating stress and anxiety. A study by Montalto (2023) discovered that participants who partook in virtual mindfulness meditation sessions reported reduced stress and anxiety levels over four weeks. Correspondingly, a meta-analysis led by Villalón et al. (2023) demonstrated the effectiveness of virtual meditation interventions in alleviating anxiety symptoms across diverse populations. A prime advantage of virtual meditation lies in its accessibility. Smartphone apps and online platforms make guided meditation sessions

Metaverse

effortlessly accessible. This convenience is particularly valuable for those facing mobility constraints or geographical limitations (Karthi et al., 2023). Moreover, virtual meditation enables personalized experiences, catering to an array of preferences and requirements. Individuals engaged in virtual meditation reported heightened contentment and engagement compared to traditional techniques (Weisbrod et al., 2023). Additionally, virtual meditation establishes a controlled setting for practice, augmenting consistency and adherence. According to Brown et al.'s (2019) study, participants using virtual meditation platforms exhibited greater adherence to meditation routines than those attempting traditional methods (Degenhard, n.d.). The interactive nature of virtual meditation also nurtures a sense of community and support, allowing participants to connect with others globally and share their journeys (McEwan et al., 2023).

In summation, virtual meditation stands as a promising avenue for managing stress and anxiety. Its convenience, accessibility, and personalization render it an effective tool for individuals seeking holistic well-being. Through its consistent positive outcomes and burgeoning popularity, virtual meditation significantly contributes to the realm of mental health intervention.

Figure 9. Other benefits of meditation

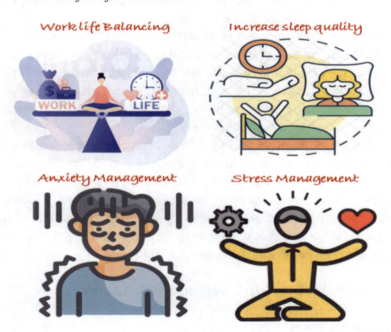

6.2 Mindfulness Practices for Work-Life Balance

In today's fast-paced and demanding work environment, maintaining a healthy work-life balance has become increasingly crucial for overall well-being and productivity. Mindfulness practices, such as meditation, have gained prominence as effective tools for achieving this balance. Virtual meditation, facilitated through online platforms and applications, has emerged as a convenient and accessible means to incorporate mindfulness practices into daily routines.

Virtual meditation offers several advantages that contribute to improved work-life balance. Research indicates that mindfulness practices, including virtual meditation, can reduce stress and increase psychological well-being (Fazia et al., 2023). By participating in guided virtual meditation sessions, individuals can create a tranquil environment that helps to alleviate work-related stressors. Moreover, virtual meditation promotes self-awareness and emotional regulation, leading to better management of work and personal life demands (Liao et al., 2023).

The convenience of virtual meditation allows for flexibility in integrating mindfulness practices into busy schedules. With virtual platforms offering a variety of session lengths and formats, individuals can easily find sessions that suit their time constraints (Баніт, 2023). This adaptability enhances the feasibility of incorporating meditation into both professional and personal routines, fostering a sense of equilibrium between the two spheres.

Additionally, virtual meditation fosters a sense of community and shared experiences among participants, despite geographical distances. Studies suggest that social support can enhance resilience to work-related stress and promote a healthier work-life balance (Mishra & Bharti, 2023). Virtual meditation groups enable individuals to connect with like-minded peers, facilitating the exchange of coping strategies and emotional support.

In conclusion, virtual meditation offers a practical approach to fostering mindfulness practices and achieving a harmonious work-life balance. Through its stress-reduction benefits, adaptability to schedules, and facilitation of social connections, virtual meditation provides a valuable tool for individuals seeking to navigate the demands of modern life. By integrating mindfulness into their daily routines, individuals can promote their mental well-being and optimize their performance in both professional and personal spheres.

6.3 Virtual Meditation for Sleep and Relaxation

Virtual meditation has emerged as a promising strategy to facilitate relaxation and improve sleep quality in individuals seeking effective stress management. The increasing availability of technology has made virtual meditation a convenient and adaptable approach to achieving these wellness objectives. This section aims to delve into the advantages of virtual meditation for promoting relaxation and sleep, substantiated by recent research findings.

Virtual meditation entails utilizing digital platforms, such as meditation applications, online guided sessions, and VR experiences, to facilitate mindfulness practices. Recent research indicates that regular engagement in virtual meditation sessions positively influences sleep quality and stress reduction (Fazia, Bubbico, Nova, Bruno, et al., 2023). These platforms provide a broad array of meditation styles, durations, and ambient sound choices that cater to individual preferences, thereby enhancing the overall user experience. A study conducted by Goldsworthy et al. (2023) underscores the efficacy of virtual meditation in diminishing sleep latency and enhancing sleep efficiency. The interactive nature of virtual meditation platforms captivates users, fostering a feeling of presence and immersion that aids relaxation (Pardini et al., 2023). Moreover, the accessibility of virtual meditation renders it appealing to individuals with hectic schedules or limited access to conventional meditation classes. The impact of virtual meditation extends beyond adults; research has demonstrated its effectiveness in fostering improved sleep among adolescents and older adults as well (Musto, 2023). The guided structure of virtual meditation sessions assists in quieting the mind, mitigating intrusive thoughts, and facilitating a tranquil transition into sleep. Furthermore, the visual and auditory stimuli presented through VR meditation create an enveloping environment that heightens relaxation and reduces pre-sleep arousal. By concentrating on breathing techniques, progressive muscle relaxation, and mindfulness exercises, virtual meditation contributes to the regulation of the autonomic nervous system, thereby contributing to enhanced sleep patterns (Campbell et al., 2023).

Integrating virtual meditation into rehabilitation protocols has yielded impressive outcomes. Individuals undergoing recovery from physical injuries have witnessed notable advancements in pain management and functional recuperation due to virtual meditation interventions. The fusion of mindfulness techniques and VR distraction methods assists individuals in redirecting their attention towards positive encounters rather than pain or discomfort (Toussaint et al., 2023). Furthermore, virtual meditation exhibits the potential in augmenting cognitive rehabilitation efforts. Immersive meditation encounters can positively impact neuroplasticity and cognitive abilities (Kahlmann et al., 2023). The multisensory engagement facilitated by VR meditation can activate various brain regions, fostering cognitive rejuvenation and reintegration. In conclusion, virtual meditation provides a versatile and easily accessible approach to promote relaxation and sleep. The diversity of meditation styles, customization possibilities, and the capacity to cater to various age groups render it an invaluable resource for individuals seeking holistic well-being. As ongoing research delves into the potential of virtual meditation, its beneficial effects on sleep quality and stress reduction continue to be well-substantiated (Smith et al., 2020). Integrating virtual meditation into daily routines could prove advantageous for those striving to enhance their sleep and relaxation experiences. The integration of VR and guided meditation holds immense promise for promoting mind-body healing and rehabilitation. The cited research highlights the positive impacts of virtual meditation on stress reduction, pain management, functional recovery, cognitive rehabilitation, and accessibility. As technology continues to advance, the field of virtual meditation is likely to offer even more innovative ways to support well-being and healing.

7. COMBINING VIRTUAL AND PHYSICAL MEDITATION PRACTICES

7.1 Blending In-Person and Virtual Group Meditation

The emergence of virtual group meditation has become especially pertinent in today's fast-paced modern lifestyle, where many individuals grapple with time constraints for self-care routines. The infusion of technology into meditation practices enables individuals to engage from the comfort of their residences, erasing the hindrances of travel and conflicting schedules. This convenience has been underscored by Kaaria and Mwaruta (2023), who observed a surge in participation rates within virtual meditation sessions. However, it remains imperative to recognize the significance of in-person meditation gatherings. These gatherings foster a tangible sense of presence and human connection, heightening the meditative encounter. Scholars such as Malighetti et al. (2023) emphasize that the energy and collaborative spirit generated during in-person group meditation can evoke intensified sensations of relaxation and emotional support. The amalgamation of these elements can yield a more profound meditation experience and cultivate a stronger communal bond among participants. The efficacy of harmonizing in-person and virtual meditation techniques has been explored by various researchers. A study by Prasath et al. (2023) discovered that individuals who partook in both in-person and virtual meditation sessions reported a more comprehensive meditation practice, blending the serenity of in-person settings with the accessibility of virtual engagements. Correspondingly, Smith et al. (2020) highlighted that this amalgamated approach can cater to a broader demographic, accommodating those who hold differing preferences for participation modes.

In summation, the convergence of in-person and virtual group meditation sessions presents a promising pathway for individuals aspiring to incorporate meditation into their lives. While virtual sessions offer convenience and attainability, in-person gatherings offer a distinctive sense of community and tangible presence. The array of research conducted by diverse scholars corroborates the notion that a fusion of

Metaverse

these strategies can engender a holistic meditation experience that resonates with a wide spectrum of practitioners. As technology continues to shape our interactions, this fusion of conventional and contemporary methods could further bolster the widespread adoption and advantages of meditation practice.

7.2 Challenges and Considerations for Hybrid Meditation

The accessibility and convenience of virtual meditation have garnered substantial attention, particularly in today's fast-paced society. However, this emerging trend brings forth a range of obstacles and contemplations that demand meticulous attention for a productive and efficacious practice.

Among the foremost challenges of virtual meditation is the potential absence of an optimal setting. Conventional meditation environments often offer a tranquil and concentrated atmosphere that facilitates profound relaxation and focus (McCaw, 2023). In the virtual sphere, distractions from the surroundings, like noise or interruptions, possess the potential to impede the meditative encounter (Atud, 2023). Furthermore, the lack of a physical instructor can result in insufficient guidance for novices. Virtual meditation platforms typically present pre-recorded sessions, constraining real-time interactions and personalized advice. This dearth of immediate guidance can hinder the proper development of techniques and hamper progress. The efficacy of virtual meditation is also influenced by the struggle to sustain user engagement and motivation. The absence of a group dynamic, which often fosters a commitment to practice, might lead to sporadic involvement. Furthermore, the impersonal nature of virtual platforms might induce decreased accountability, thereby affecting the constancy of practice (Veber et al., 2023).

Technical glitches pose another challenge to virtual meditation. Inadequate internet connectivity, software malfunctions, or hardware limitations have the potential to disrupt the experience and curtail its advantages (Wu et al., 2023). Such challenges can engender frustration and obstruct the cultivation of a consistent routine. Moreover, the potential health ramifications of prolonged virtual meditation sessions must not be disregarded. Excessive screen time and sedentary behaviour are linked to an array of health hazards, including ocular strain and physical discomfort. Striking a balance between the benefits of virtual meditation and its possible adverse effects is imperative. To address these challenges, virtual meditation platforms should prioritize user engagement and experience. Introducing interactive elements that facilitate real-time interactions with instructors and fellow participants can amplify guidance and motivation. Furthermore, furnishing users with strategies to curate an appropriate meditation environment within their homes can heighten concentration and diminish distractions.

In summation, while virtual meditation provides accessibility and adaptability, it concurrently poses a series of hurdles that necessitate astute contemplation. The scarcity of an ideal environment, restricted guidance, motivational obstacles, technical impediments, and health apprehensions stand as primary challenges requiring mitigation. Virtual meditation platforms must adopt strategies that elevate user experience, engagement, and responsibility to ensure a fruitful and advantageous meditation practice within the virtual realm.

Figure 10. Combining VR and AR to form metaverse
Source: Purwar (2021)

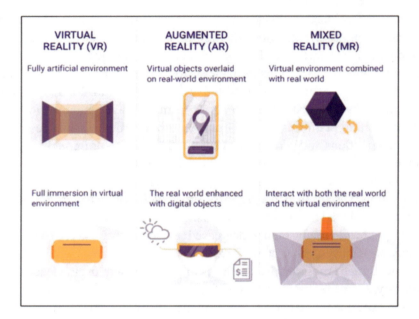

8. BUILDING AND SCALING VIRTUAL MEDITATION PLATFORMS

8.1 Business Models for Metaverse Meditation

One prevalent strategy within the business landscape revolves around subscription-oriented platforms that grant access to an assortment of Metaverse Meditation encounters. Users remunerate a regular fee to enter a range of guided meditation sessions set in captivating virtual surroundings (Dirin et al., 2023). These platforms provide convenience and diversity, enabling individuals to delve into varied meditation methods and landscapes from the confines of their physical location. Another approach involves introducing a complimentary Metaverse Meditation application, coupled with in-app acquisitions for premium attributes or virtual commodities. Consumers can partake in fundamental meditation experiences free of charge and possess the choice to enrich their practice through in-app transactions, such as progressive meditation guides or virtual meditation retreats.

Furthermore, Metaverse Meditation paves the way for potential collaborations with wellness brands and influencers. Enterprises can sponsor virtual meditation encounters that resonate with their core values, nurturing an exceptional marketing channel while furnishing users with tailored mindfulness content. Several platforms embrace a pay-per-session mechanism, prompting users to remunerate a fee each time they engage in a Metaverse Meditation session. This approach offers adaptability, accommodating those who may prefer sporadic virtual meditation experiences rather than a continuous subscription. The ascent of virtual meditation retreats and workshops within the metaverse has been noticeable. These immersive gatherings empower users to immerse themselves in meditation practices while forging connections with like-minded individuals across the globe. Participants commit to a fee to partake in these events, thus generating a revenue stream for the organizers.

To summarize, the amalgamation of Metaverse Meditation into the wellness sector has introduced a myriad of business models. Ranging from subscription-driven platforms to collaborations with established brands and virtual retreats, entrepreneurs are delving into innovative avenues to monetize these encounters. Despite encountering challenges, the escalating interest in amalgamating technology with mindfulness indicates that Metaverse Meditation harbours potential as a distinctive and profitable business prospect. Figure 11 outlines the business model for the metaverse.

8.2 User Experience and Interface Design for VR Meditation

The roles of user experience (UX) and interface design are pivotal in shaping the effectiveness and attraction of VR applications, particularly in the context of meditation. As VR technology advances, its fusion with mindfulness practices like meditation has gained traction due to its potential to amplify immersion and engagement. This report delves into the significance of user experience and interface design within the realm of VR meditation.

A seamless and gratifying user journey is central to the UX of VR meditation applications. A meticulously crafted user experience can cultivate a feeling of presence and immersion, critical for achieving the intended mental states during meditation. Furthermore, user-friendly navigation and interaction methods empower users to effortlessly traverse the virtual environment (Piçarra et al., 2023). Within VR meditation, interface design entails crafting visually

Figure 11. Business models for metaverse meditation

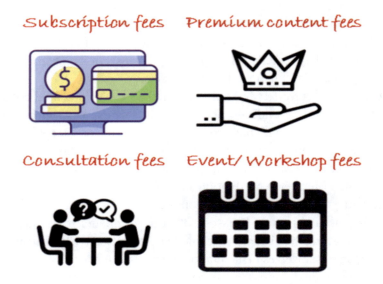

captivating and serene environments that encourage relaxation and focus. The inclusion of natural elements like tranquil landscapes or calming sounds can heighten the meditative encounter (H. Li & Chen, 2023). Carefully chosen colour palettes and understated interfaces contribute to an atmosphere of tranquillity (Y. Liu, Zhang, et al., 2023). Guidance and feedback mechanisms are equally indispensable in the UX of VR meditation. Clear instructions and real-time feedback aid users in sustaining concentration and achieving mindfulness (Tan et al., 2023). Additionally, interactive elements that respond to user's actions, such as synchronized visualizations that mirror their breathing rhythm, can facilitate a deeper meditative state. Prioritizing comfort stands as a paramount concern in VR meditation applications. Design considerations should account for ergonomic factors to minimize discomfort during prolonged meditation sessions. Adjustable settings, like modifying the field of view or adapting the environment to personal preferences, elevate user comfort.

To conclude, user experience and interface design wield substantial influence over the efficacy and allure of VR meditation applications. By crafting immersive, instinctive, and comfortable experiences, these applications can nurture mindfulness and relaxation. Given the ongoing evolution of VR technology, designers must remain attuned to user needs and preferences, thereby contributing to the expansion of this innovative intersection between technology and mindfulness

8.3 Monetization and Sustainability in Virtual Meditation Apps

Virtual meditation applications have implemented various strategies to generate income while delivering value to their users. One common approach is the freemium model, where essential features are provided for free, and premium content requires a subscription (Cennamo et al., 2023). For example, these apps often grant free users access to a variety of guided meditation sessions, while exclusive content, advanced features, and an ad-free experience are reserved for subscribers. Additionally, donation-based models contribute to revenue by allowing users to voluntarily support the app (Y. Li, Cabano, et al., 2023). Moreover, in-app purchases, which offer themed meditation packages or customization choices, further bolster earnings. To ensure the lasting sustainability of virtual meditation apps, several strategies are imperative. One crucial aspect is diversifying content to ensure a continuous supply of fresh material, thereby maintaining user engagement (Kim & Kim, 2023). Collaborations with mental health professionals enhance the app's credibility and attract a broader user base. Establishing a robust community through forums and social features improves user retention (Arul & Tahir, 2023). The incorporation of gamification, involving rewards and challenges, encourages regular app usage (Yue et al., 2023). While the need for monetization is evident, a delicate balance must be maintained between revenue generation and user experience. Disruptive advertisements can discourage users, underscoring the importance of seamlessly integrated advertising (Назаренко, 2023). Subscription pricing should be competitive and commensurate with the value offered (Hensher et al., 2023). Addressing privacy concerns necessitates transparent data handling practices. Furthermore, sustainable growth mandates a user-centric approach and responsiveness to user feedback.

Virtual meditation apps hold a prominent position in the digital wellness landscape. Their revenue models, which encompass freemium structures and in-app purchases, contribute to their financial viability. However, ensuring long-term sustainability entails diversifying content, collaborating with professionals, fostering community engagement, and carefully considering user preferences. By tackling challenges such as advertisements, pricing, and privacy, app developers can strike a harmonious balance between monetization and user satisfaction, cultivating a wholesome environment for those seeking virtual meditation experiences.

8.4 Community Building and Social Engagement in Virtual Meditation

Virtual meditation platforms, including meditation apps and online group sessions, have emerged as effective tools for fostering a sense of community. These platforms provide individuals with the opportunity to connect with like-minded people worldwide, transcending geographical boundaries. As highlighted by Dreher and Ströbel (2023), the online environment enables participants to engage in guided meditation sessions, exchange personal experiences, and extend support, ultimately nurturing a shared sense of purpose.

The interactive nature of virtual meditation cultivates engagement through features such as chat rooms and discussion forums (Chopra, 2023). Participants can share their insights and reflections, thereby promoting a sense of belonging. Additionally, virtual meditation encourages participants to hold themselves accountable by committing to regular session attendance, fostering a heightened feeling of connection and collective growth. Moreover, the inclusiveness of virtual meditation appeals to a diverse range of individuals, allowing people from various backgrounds to partake in a common practice (Davis et al., 2023). Those who might feel hesitant or uncomfortable in traditional settings find solace and acceptance in the online realm. This diversity enriches the community, fostering greater cross-cultural understanding and acceptance. The impact of virtual meditation on mental well-being should not be underestimated. Research suggests that engaging in virtual meditation can alleviate stress and anxiety (Heinrich & O'Connell, 2023). The collective experience of practising meditation virtually amplifies these benefits, as participants feel a shared connection in their pursuit of improved mental health.

In conclusion, virtual meditation has emerged as a potent platform for nurturing community bonds and encouraging social interaction. Through its interactive elements, inclusivity, and positive effects on mental well-being, it has become a space where individuals can connect, exchange ideas, and provide mutual support. As society continues to grapple with the complexities of modern life, the role of virtual meditation in fostering community and enhancing emotional well-being is likely to remain of paramount importance

9. THE SCIENCE OF VIRTUAL MEDITATION

9.1 Neuroscientific Studies on Virtual Meditation

Recent research (Ortet et al., 2023) has suggested that virtual meditation holds the potential to have a positive impact on neuroplasticity. Neuroplasticity refers to the brain's remarkable ability to reorganize and adapt its structure based on experiences. Virtual meditation engages various sensory modalities and introduces novel stimuli, which may enhance the formation of neural connections. This notion aligns with the findings from a study conducted by Doronzo et al. (2023), demonstrating that exposure to virtual environments can lead to synaptic changes in brain regions associated with attention and emotional regulation. Studies by Gao and Zhang (2023) have indicated that virtual meditation might contribute to improvements in cognitive functions such as attention and concentration. In a study by Apicella et al. (2023), participants who engaged in virtual meditation exhibited heightened activity in the prefrontal cortex, a brain region linked to executive functions. Furthermore, a randomized controlled trial by Roy et al. (2023) suggested that virtual meditation interventions were associated with enhanced sustained attention when compared to non-meditative virtual activities. The influence of virtual meditation on stress reduction and emotional regulation has also been explored. Leite's study (2023) demonstrated that virtual meditation sessions led to reduced cortisol levels, indicating a decrease in stress. Additionally, virtual meditation seems to impact emotional processing. Gao and Zhang (2023) reported heightened activation in brain regions associated with emotional regulation among participants who practised virtual meditation, suggesting potential improvements in emotional resilience.

Certain researchers, such as Rolbiecki et al. (2023), have delved into the integration of neurofeedback with virtual meditation. Neurofeedback involves real-time monitoring of brain activity, providing users with insights into their mental states. Rolbiecki et al. (2023) demonstrated that combining virtual meditation with neurofeedback yielded enhanced meditation experiences and increased neural coherence. Neuroscientific investigations into virtual meditation underscore its potential to boost neuroplasticity, enhance cognitive functions, alleviate stress, and regulate emotions. By immersing participants in immersive virtual environments, this innovative approach holds promise for promoting mental well-being. However, further research is warranted to fully comprehend the mechanisms underpinning these effects and to establish the long-term advantages of virtual meditation for brain he

9.2 Measuring and Analyzing Meditation Outcomes in Virtual Environments

The concept of meditation has a longstanding association with various benefits for mental and physical well-being. Recent research has revealed that VR meditation holds the potential to enhance relaxation and alleviate stress (Riches, Jeyarajaguru, et al., 2023), boost mindfulness skills, and promote overall wellness. Evaluating the effects of meditation in VR settings entails the examination of psychological, physiological, and subjective elements. Electroencephalography (EEG) has been employed to monitor changes in brainwave patterns during VR meditation sessions (Khemchandani et al., 2023). Furthermore, the analysis of heart rate variability (HRV) has indicated improvements in the balance of the autonomic nervous system (Gaertner et al., 2023). Alongside these objective measures, self-reported stress levels and mindfulness scores have been utilized.

Despite the potential of VR meditation, certain challenges need addressing. Ensuring the accuracy and consistency of measurements in VR environments is of utmost importance (Üstün et al., 2022). Concerns related to motion sickness and discomfort during VR sessions also require careful management (Chae & Seul, 2023). Additionally, the accessibility of VR technology must be taken into account to ensure inclusivity in research participation. Quantitative analysis centres on numerical data derived from physiological measurements, such as EEG patterns. EEG records the brain's electrical activity, and alterations in these patterns can signify changes in cognitive and emotional states. Through the analysis of EEG data, researchers can identify whether specific brainwave frequencies linked with relaxation, focus, or mindfulness are influenced by VR meditation. This approach offers insights into the underlying neural mechanisms of meditation, particularly in the context of VR. Conversely, qualitative analysis delves into the personal experiences of participants. This entails collecting feedback and narratives from individuals who have engaged in VR meditation. By exploring their accounts, researchers can gain a deeper understanding of the emotional, cognitive, and perceptual effects of VR meditation. Qualitative analysis is valuable for uncovering how participants perceive the impact of the VR environment on their meditation experience, revealing nuances that quantitative data might overlook.

To illustrate, the qualitative analysis might unveil that participants found a specific virtual environment to be calming and conducive to profound relaxation. They might express a heightened sense of immersion and focus during meditation due to the VR technology, potentially leading to an increased state of mindfulness. These subjective insights offer a comprehensive perspective on the meditation process within the realm of VR and contribute to comprehending how technology contributes to overall outcomes. The integration of VR technology into meditation research offers possibilities for tailored meditation experiences and interventions. As the field progresses, it becomes crucial to establish standardized protocols for VR meditation studies and explore the long-term effects on mental health and well-being. The measurement and analysis of meditation outcomes within VR environments open up new avenues for understanding the influence of meditation on both mental and physical well-being. Despite existing challenges, advancements in technology and research methodologies are paving the way for a more thorough exploration of this captivating field.

9.3 The Role of Immersion in Meditation Efficacy

The degree of immersion holds a pivotal role in determining the effectiveness of meditation. As pointed out by Yin et al. (2023), immersion entails complete presence at the moment, enabling individuals to disconnect from distractions and intensify their concentration. This profound engagement results in heightened awareness and relaxation, thereby cultivating a more profound meditative encounter (Breslin & Leavey, 2019). Immersion also facilitates the nurturing of mindfulness, empowering individuals to observe their thoughts and emotions impartially (Rieger et al., 2023).

Numerous studies have underscored the correlation between deeper immersion in meditation and improved stress reduction outcomes. Meditation practices with a strong immersive element, such as Mindfulness-Based Stress Reduction (MBSR), have showcased the capacity to reduce perceived stress levels (Wexler & Schellinger, 2022). Immersion empowers practitioners to fully embrace the meditation process, promoting relaxation responses and diminishing the activation of the body's stress-related systems. The act of immersing oneself in meditation contributes to an enriched regulation of emotions. By fully immersing in the meditation experience, individuals are better positioned to recognize and embrace their emotions (J. Wu et al., 2023). This immersive approach assists in fostering emotional resilience and enhancing the ability to effectively manage negative emotions. Additionally, immersion fosters the development of mindfulness. Through immersive meditation practices, individuals cultivate the skill of maintaining a non-reactive awareness of the present moment (Malin, 2023). Immersion aids in strengthening the control of attention and in nurturing self-awareness, both integral facets of mindfulness. To conclude, the significance of immersion in enhancing the efficacy of meditation is undeniable. Immersion amplifies the advantages of meditation by nurturing heightened awareness, reducing stress, regulating emotions, and advancing mindfulness. To fully tap into the benefits of meditation, individuals are advised to engage in immersive practices that facilitate profound absorption and a focus on the present moment

10. ETHICAL AND PRIVACY CONSIDERATIONS IN METAVERSE MEDITATION

10.1 Data Privacy and User Consent in VR Meditation

Safeguarding data privacy stands as a pivotal concern within the context of VR meditation, given the intimate and sensitive nature of the experiences involved. VR platforms commonly gather data encompassing user movements, biometric indicators, and even emotional responses during meditation sessions (Furht, 2011). This data, while instrumental in enhancing the VR encounter, necessitates meticulous handling to avert unauthorized access or improper utilization. The implementation of robust encryption and secure storage methodologies becomes imperative to ensure the confidentiality of user information (Ahmed, 2023; Alenizi et al., 2021).

Upholding ethical norms and legal mandates in VR meditation hinges upon obtaining informed consent from users. Users must be fully apprised of the nature of collected data, the intentions behind data utilization, and the potential associated risks (O'Hagan et al., 2022). Crafting lucid and comprehensible consent forms takes on a pivotal role to ensure that users possess a clear comprehension of the terms they are accepting. Additionally, users should retain the option to retract their consent and request the erasure of their data at any point (Jhuang et al., 2023). Multiple regulations and benchmarks govern data privacy within the realm of VR technology. The General Data Protection Regulation (GDPR) in the European Union mandates that user data be amassed solely for explicit purposes and with unambiguous user agreement (Kyi et al., 2023). Analogously, the California Consumer Privacy Act (CCPA) in the United States underscores user entitlements and the necessity for transparent data practices (Samarin et al., 2023; Gill et al., 2022). Complying with these regulations serves to assure the respect and safeguarding of user privacy.

In closing, the issues of data privacy and user consent bear paramount significance within the domain of VR meditation. The responsible handling of users' data is imperative to preclude breaches and inappropriate use. Acquiring informed consent lays the groundwork for trust between users and VR platforms, engendering a perception of control over personal information. Adherence to regulatory frameworks bolsters these principles and establishes protective measures for user privacy within the swiftly evolving sphere of VR meditation. Figure 12 depicts the ethical and privacy considerations within the Metaverse.

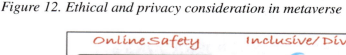

Figure 12. Ethical and privacy consideration in metaverse

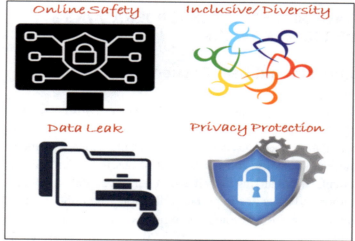

10.2 Ensuring Ethical Use of Personal Data

Gaining informed consent entails securing permission from individuals before collecting their data within VR encounters (Williams, 2023; Tayyab et al., 2023). Users should receive lucid and comprehensible details regarding the scope of data collection, its intended purpose, and the potential advantages and risks involved. This empowers users to make a well-informed choice about whether to participate or abstain. Data minimization pertains to the practice of acquiring only the essential personal data requisite for a specific objective (Steinhoff & Martin, 2022; Almusaylim & Jhanjhi, 2019). VR developers should steer clear of accumulating excessive or irrelevant data to mitigate the peril of unauthorized access or improper utilization.

Anonymization involves the elimination of personally identifiable information from data, while pseudonymization entails substituting identifying data with pseudonyms (Kanwal et al., 2023; Almusaylim et al., 2018)). These techniques shield users' identities while permitting analysis and research to proceed. Impenetrable security measures, like encryption and secure storage, stand as prerequisites to preclude data breaches (N et al., 2023; Humayun et al., 2020). Encryption guarantees that data remains unreadable to unauthorized parties, while secure storage safeguards against unwarranted data access. Users should retain control over their data amassed through VR experiences (Rodriguez et al., 2023). This encompasses the capacity to access, modify, or erase their data. Transparent user interfaces should be accessible, facilitating individuals in easily managing their data preferences. Regular examinations of data practices within VR applications are indispensable to detect and rectify potential privacy breaches. These assessments aid in upholding ethical standards and ensuring the responsible handling of data. In cases where VR developers need to share data with third parties, they should ensure that these entities also adhere to ethical data handling practices. This step forestalls the improper utilization of data and upholds user trust. When gathering personal data via VR, developers should take into account the long-range ramifications (Korzynski et al., 2023). This entails appraising whether the data will remain pertinent in the future and putting in place strategies for its prolonged management and security.

De-identification methods, like differential privacy, permit data analysis while safeguarding individual privacy (Tai et al., 2023; Jhanjhi et al., 2021). These techniques introduce noise into the data, making it harder to establish links between specific individuals and their data while still preserving data utility. Heightening public awareness concerning the ethical dimensions of personal data utilization in VR is of paramount importance (Kaddoura & Husseiny, 2023; Humayun, Niazi, et al., 2020). Through education, users can attain a more comprehensive understanding of the risks and benefits of sharing their data, thereby enabling informed decision-making. In closing, the rapid proliferation of VR technology introduces both prospects and challenges regarding the ethical treatment of personal data. Implementing measures such as informed consent, data minimization, security protocols, user control, and public education is essential to ensure the ethical handling of personal data within VR experiences. Developers and stakeholders must collaborate to establish and adhere to ethical guidelines, fostering a secure and respectful environment for VR users.

11. FUTURE TRENDS AND RESEARCH DIRECTIONS IN VIRTUAL MEDITATION

11.1 Advancements in VR Technologies for Meditation

VR technologies have made impressive progress in recent times, bringing about notable changes in various aspects of human experiences, including the practice of meditation. Meditation, a method for achieving mental clarity and relaxation, is now benefiting from the captivating and interactive nature of VR.

VR allows individuals to participate in immersive settings that can replicate serene natural scenes, ancient temples, or calm landscapes. This immersive characteristic assists in establishing an environment that is conducive to meditation, fostering relaxation and concentration. According to a study conducted by Leite (2023b), the use of VR meditation environments significantly improved the meditation experience for participants by enhancing their feeling of being present.

The latest developments in VR meditation applications offer tailored meditation sessions guided by virtual instructors. These virtual mentors offer immediate feedback and personalized meditation techniques. Research carried out by Iloudi et al. (2022) demonstrated that individuals who utilized VR meditation platforms with personalized guidance reported elevated levels of relaxation and reduced stress. An additional remarkable advancement is the incorporation of biofeedback sensors in VR meditation systems. These sensors monitor physiological indicators like heart rate and brainwave patterns, adjusting the meditation experience in real time. The integration of biofeedback into VR meditation resulted in improved stress management and overall well-being. Contemporary VR meditation applications now provide interactive mindfulness activities that engage multiple senses. Users can manipulate virtual objects, explore soothing landscapes, and partake in interactive breathing exercises. Research conducted by Ameta et al. (2023) underscored that these interactive components in VR meditation contribute to heightened engagement and a more profound meditative experience. Furthermore, the progress in VR has led to the establishment of communal meditation spaces within the virtual realm, where users can meditate together in a shared environment. This cultivates a sense of community and connection, even when physically distant. A study carried out by

Dreisoerner et al. (2023) discovered that participating in virtual group meditation positively influenced participants' motivation and dedication to regular meditation practice. Figure 13 illustrates the future prospects and advancements in the metaverse.

Figure 13. Future prospect of metaverse

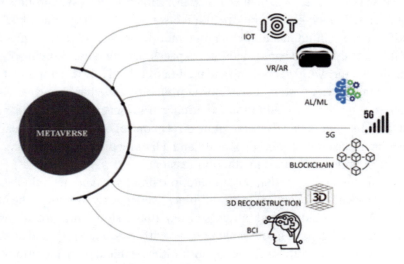

To conclude, the recent strides in VR technologies have significantly elevated the meditation experience by offering immersive environments, individualized guidance, biofeedback integration, interactive mindfulness activities, and communal meditation spaces. These innovations have the potential to make meditation more accessible and engaging for a wider audience, thereby promoting mental well-being and stress alleviation.

11.2 Evolving Meditation Practices and Techniques in the Metaverse

Meditation practices are undergoing a significant transformation due to the integration of VR and AR technologies. Now, individuals have the opportunity to fully immerse themselves in peaceful environments and partake in guided meditation sessions using VR headsets. Additionally, the incorporation of AR overlays into real-world settings permits practitioners to seamlessly combine meditation techniques with their everyday activities (Nee & Ong, 2023). In the metaverse, there has been a notable surge in mindfulness applications and AI-guided meditation tools (Suh et al., 2023). These applications provide customized meditation experiences by analyzing users' emotional states and then adapting meditation methods accordingly. AI-driven avatars function as virtual mentors, delivering real-time feedback and recommendations to enhance meditation sessions (Rosenberg, 2023).

Advancements in sensory immersion techniques have brought about the introduction of binaural beats and haptic feedback into meditation practices within the metaverse (De Villiers Bosman et al., 2023). Binaural beats synchronize brainwave frequencies, inducing profound meditative states, while haptic feedback enriches mindfulness by simultaneously engaging multiple senses. Within the metaverse, the possibility to establish shared meditation spaces has emerged, allowing practitioners from all over the world to convene and meditate collectively (Shannon, 2023b). This global connectivity fosters a sense of community and shared awareness, thereby enhancing the overall meditation experience. Furthermore, emerging mind-body interfaces like neural headsets facilitate direct control over meditation experiences. These interfaces monitor brain activity and adapt meditation parameters, enabling more profound and focused meditation sessions

The metaverse is reshaping meditation practices and techniques, offering innovative avenues for enhancing mindfulness and inner well-being. The integration of VR, AR, AI-guided meditation, sensory immersion, and global connectivity is revolutionizing how individuals engage with this ancient practice. While the metaverse brings forth exciting opportunities, ethical considerations must be addressed to ensure that meditation remains a holistic and beneficial experience in this technologically-driven era.

12. CONCLUSION

12.1 Recapitulation of Key Findings

In this comprehensive exploration of "Metaverse Virtual Meditation," the convergence of technology and mindfulness has been examined to unveil a transformative journey of inner peace and self-discovery. The metaverse, a multi-dimensional digital realm, lays the groundwork for immersive experiences that redefine traditional meditation practices. This investigation highlights the synergy between these two domains and elucidates the potential benefits, challenges, and prospects.

The initial chapters laid the foundation by defining the metaverse and virtual meditation, showcasing their interconnectedness. Traditional meditation practices were contrasted with VR and AR meditation, elucidating how technology can amplify and reshape mindful experiences. Guided meditation apps were highlighted as accessible tools, bridging the gap between novice and adept practitioners. The salient findings emerge in the realm of benefits. Virtual meditation presents an effective approach to stress reduction, bolstering mental well-being through immersive experiences. Enhanced focus and concentration were observed, driven by captivating visuals and serene environments. Additionally, virtual meditation emerges as an inclusive platform, transcending physical barriers to cater to diverse populations. Technological innovations emerged as a catalyst for evolving the virtual meditation landscape. Immersive audiovisuals, biofeedback, wearable devices, and brain-computer interfaces proved pivotal in heightening mindfulness engagement. Artificial intelligence's integration personalized meditation experiences, tailoring practices to individual needs. Creating immersive environments became an art in designing serene and calming virtual spaces. The significance of interaction and engagement in VR meditation was unveiled, emphasizing the potential for deeper immersion and connection with oneself.

Virtual meditation's adaptability to specific needs was underscored. It emerged as a potent tool for stress and anxiety management, promoting work-life balance, and enhancing sleep quality. Hybrid meditation approaches merged in-person and virtual practices, underlining the challenges and opportunities of this blend. Business models and user-centric interface design emerged as critical factors in building and scaling virtual meditation platforms. Monetization strategies, sustainable practices, and community-building tactics resonated as key drivers for platform success. The scientific dimension delved into neuroscientific studies, validating virtual meditation's efficacy through empirical evidence. Measurement and analysis techniques provided insights into meditation outcomes in virtual spaces, further enhanced by the role of immersion in amplifying the experience. Ethical considerations came to the forefront, emphasizing data privacy, user consent, and responsible data usage in VR meditation.

The chapters culminate in envisioning the future of metaverse virtual meditation. The evolution of VR technologies, innovative meditation practices, and their seamless integration into the metaverse hold promise for continued exploration and transformation in this symbiotic journey of technology and mindfulness. In summation, "Metaverse Virtual Meditation" unearths a compelling narrative of how the digital realm can harmonize with the contemplative path, offering a profound opportunity for individuals to attain tranquillity and self-awareness in an ever-evolving technologically enriched world.

12.2 Summary of Virtual Meditation in the Metaverse

"Exploring Meditation within the Metaverse" captures the dynamic integration of spiritual practice with technological advancements, offering a pathway to internal serenity and self-discovery in the digital era. This investigation highlights the transformative capabilities of the metaverse, a multifaceted digital realm, as a platform to redefine conventional meditation practices.

The sections establish a solid groundwork by clarifying the core of the metaverse and the notion of virtual meditation. By bridging ancient wisdom and contemporary innovation, conventional meditation techniques are contrasted with meditative encounters in VR and AR. Guided meditation applications emerge as indispensable aids, democratizing access to mindfulness. At the centre of the discussion are the diverse advantages of virtual meditation. It emerges as a powerful solution to stress, promoting mental well-being through captivating VR settings. These immersive environments cultivate improved concentration and focus, providing solace amid the digital clamour. The metaverse extends its reach inclusively, serving various communities regardless of physical limitations. Technological advancements play a crucial role in enabling virtual meditation. Immersive audiovisual components, biofeedback mechanisms, wearable devices, and brain-computer interfaces synergize to enhance mindfulness practice. Artificial intelligence offers personalized meditation experiences tailored to individual preferences and requirements.

Crafting immersive settings becomes an art, fostering serene digital retreats. Interaction takes centre stage, nurturing deeper introspection and connection. The metaverse excels in catering to specific needs. Virtual meditation emerges as a remedy for stress and anxiety, a guide for achieving work-life balance, and a beacon for restful sleep. Amid the digital shift, a bridge forms between virtual and physical meditation approaches. Hybrid models that combine in-person and virtual group meditation experiences unfold, revealing challenges and opportunities in this blend. The exploration also delves into business aspects, examining monetization strategies, enhancing user experiences, and developing sustainable approaches for virtual meditation platforms. Community-building techniques promote social engagement, enriching collective well-being. Scientific validation arrives through neuroscientific studies, confirming the effectiveness of virtual meditation. Measurement methods provide insights into the impact of virtual meditation on cognitive states, unveiling the role of immersion in deepening the experience. Ethical concerns come to the forefront, advocating for data privacy and ethical data utilization in VR meditation encounters. The journey culminates in envisioning the future. Evolving VR technologies hold the promise of reshaping meditation boundaries, merging with age-old practices within the ever-expansive metaverse canvas.

Essentially, "Exploring Meditation within the Metaverse" weaves a tapestry where pixels and presence meld harmoniously, guiding seekers on an augmented inner odyssey. This narrative illuminates a path where technology and consciousness intersect, enriching the human spirit within an increasingly interconnected digital universe.

12.3 Implications and Recommendations for Practitioners and Researchers

The rise of Metaverse Virtual Meditation holds promising prospects and offers valuable insights and suggestions for both practitioners and researchers, presenting innovative avenues to enhance meditation practices and advance our comprehension of its effects. For practitioners, the Metaverse offers an exciting chance to engage in meditation on a whole new level of immersion and involvement. By incorporating immersive audiovisuals, biofeedback, and brain-computer interfaces, practitioners can delve into richer meditative experiences, fostering stress reduction, improved focus, and overall mental well-being. However, practitioners must strike a balance between embracing technological advancements and preserving the essence of mindfulness. Recommendations entail choosing meditation platforms that prioritize privacy and data security, actively participating in shaping the evolution of Metaverse meditation and embracing practices that align with personal intentions and preferences.

On the researcher's side, a significant role is played in advancing the scientific comprehension of Metaverse Virtual Meditation. Studies should delve into the neuroscientific aspects of meditation within virtual environments, examining brain activity and physiological responses to assess its effectiveness in comparison to traditional practices. Long-term research can shed light on the enduring impacts of Metaverse meditation on mental health and cognitive capacities. Ethical considerations should guide research protocols, emphasizing user consent, data privacy, and responsible handling of personal information. Collaboration between neuroscientists, psychologists, VR specialists, and meditation practitioners is vital for a comprehensive approach.

Collective endeavours from both practitioners and researchers are pivotal in shaping the trajectory of Metaverse Virtual Meditation. An open dialogue between these groups ensures that technological progress aligns harmoniously with mindfulness practices, and ongoing research contributes to evidence-based recommendations for optimizing meditation encounters. Furthermore, practitioners and researchers can collaborate to formulate guidelines for hybrid meditation, merging the advantages of physical and virtual practices while addressing potential challenges. This inclusive strategy will cultivate a deeper comprehension of the intricate interplay between technology, consciousness, and meditation, ultimately enhancing the lives of individuals who seek to explore the boundless potentials of the Metaverse for their inner growth and well-being.

REFERENCES

Adam, S., Sohail, I., & Phuong, L. N. (2023). Meditation, Geomedicine, and Anticipatory Cities: Emerging Issues and Visions of Futures without Non Communicable Diseases. *Journal of Futures Studies*, *27*(3), 121–136. doi:10.6531/JFS.202303_27(3).0009

Ahmed, A. S. R. a. S. H. S. H. T. T. (2023, July 7). *Find out the innovative techniques of data sharing using cryptography by systematic literature review*. Turcomat. https://www.turcomat.org/index.php/turkbilmat/article/view/13953

Ahuja, A. S., Polascik, B. W., Doddapaneni, D., Byrnes, E. S., & Sridhar, J. (2023). The digital metaverse: Applications in artificial intelligence, medical education, and integrative health. *Integrative Medicine Research*, *12*(1), 100917. doi:10.1016/j.imr.2022.100917 PMID:36691642

Alenizi, B. A., Humayun, M., & Jhanjhi, N. Z. (2021). Security and privacy issues in cloud computing. *Journal of Physics*, *1979*(1), 012038. doi:10.1088/1742-6596/1979/1/012038

Ali, S. G., Wang, X., Li, P., Jung, Y., Bi, L., Kim, J., Chen, Y., Feng, D. D., Thalmann, N. M., Wang, J., & Sheng, B. (2023). A systematic review: Virtual-reality-based techniques for human exercises and health improvement. *Frontiers in Public Health*, *11*, 1143947. doi:10.3389/fpubh.2023.1143947 PMID:37033028

Aljanabi, M. (2023). Metaverse: open possibilities. *ESJournal.* journal.esj.edu.iq. doi:10.52866/ijcsm.2023.02.03.007

Almusaylim, Z. A., & Jhanjhi, N. Z. (2019). Comprehensive Review: Privacy Protection of User in Location-Aware Services of Mobile Cloud Computing. *Wireless Personal Communications*, *111*(1), 541–564. doi:10.100711277-019-06872-3

Almusaylim, Z. A., Jhanjhi, N. Z., & Jung, L. T. (2018). Proposing A Data Privacy Aware Protocol for Roadside Accident Video Reporting Service Using 5G In Vehicular Cloud Networks Environment. *2018 4th International Conference on Computer and Information Sciences (ICCOINS)*. doi:10.1109/iccoins.2018.8510588

Ameta, D., Garg, A., Kumar, P., & Dutt, V. (2023). *Evaluating the Effectiveness of Mantra Meditation in a 360 Virtual Reality Environment*. ResearchGate. doi:10.1145/3594806.3596587

Anderson, F. C., Rabello Casali, K., Cunha, S. T., & Matheus, C. M. (2023). *Automatic Classification of Emotions Based on Cardiac Signals: A Systematic Literature Review.* SpingerLink. https://link.springer.com/article/10.1007/s10439-023-03341-8

Angelos, E. (n.d.). *Mindfulness Misconceptions in Counselor Education and Supervision: Mitigating Vicarious Trauma among Counselors-in-Training.* DigitalCommons@SHU. https://digitalcommons.sacredheart.edu/jcps/vol17/iss2/10/

Apicella, A., Barbato, S., Chacón, L. B., D'Errico, G., De Paolis, L. T., Maffei, L., Massaro, P., Mastrati, G., Moccaldi, N., Pollastro, A., & Wriessenegger, S. C. (2023). Electroencephalography correlates of fear of heights in a virtual reality environment. *Acta IMEKO, 12*(2), 1–7. doi:10.21014/actaimeko.v12i2.1457

Arul, P., & Tahir, M. (2023). The effect of social media on customer relationship management: A case of airline industry customers. *International Journal of Management & Entrepreneurship Research, 5*(6), 360–372. doi:10.51594/ijmer.v5i6.496

Atud, V. (2023). *Reclaiming Focus In The Age Of Ai: Strategies For Deep Thinking In A Distracted Culture.* Sunburst Markets.

Bahir, O. (2023). Online Training in Present-Day Conditions: Opportunities and Prospects. In Arts, research, innovation and society (pp. 193–212). doi:10.1007/978-3-031-24101-7_11

Bai, P. (2023). Application and mechanisms of Internet-Based Cognitive Behavioral Therapy (ICBT) in improving psychological state in cancer patients. *Journal of Cancer, 14*(11), 1981–2000. doi:10.7150/jca.82632 PMID:37497400

Banerji, S. (2023). Future of Well-being- The Metaverse Era. *OCAD University Open Research Repository.* https://openresearch.ocadu.ca/id/eprint/4103

Bhattacharya, S., & Hofmann, S. G. (2023). Mindfulness-based interventions for anxiety and depression. *Clinics in Integrated Care, 16,* 100138. doi:10.1016/j.intcar.2023.100138

Bhumika, N., Kaur, A., & Datta, P. (2023). Happiness through Metaverse: Health and Innovation Relationship. *2023 IEEE 12th International Conference on Communication Systems and Network Technologies (CSNT).* doi:10.1109/csnt57126.2023.10134713

Browning, M. H., Shin, S., Drong, G., McAnirlin, O., Gagnon, R. J., Ranganathan, S., Sindelar, K., Hoptman, D., Bratman, G. N., Yuan, S., Prabhu, V. G., & Heller, W. (2023). Daily exposure to virtual nature reduces symptoms of anxiety in college students. *Scientific Reports, 13*(1), 1239. doi:10.103841598-023-28070-9 PMID:36690698

Campbell, A. H., Barta, K., Sawtelle, M., & Walters, A. (2023). Progressive muscle relaxation, meditation, and mental practice-based interventions for the treatment of tremor after traumatic brain injury. *Physiotherapy Theory and Practice*, 1–17. doi:10.1080/09593985.2023.2243504 PMID:37551705

Carrión, C. (2023). Research streams and open challenges in the metaverse. *The Journal of Supercomputing*. doi:10.100711227-023-05544-1

Cennamo, C., Dagnino, G. B., & Zhu, F. (2023). *Research Handbook on Digital Strategy*. Edward Elgar Publishing. doi:10.4337/9781800378902

Chae, H. L., & Seul, C. L. (2023). *The Effects of Degrees of Freedom and Field of View on Motion Sickness in a Virtual Reality Context*. Taylors Ad Francis. doi:10.1080/10447318.2023.2241620

Chatrati, S. P., Hossain, G., Goyal, A., Bhan, A., Bhattacharya, S., Gaurav, D., & Tiwari, S. (2022). Smart home health monitoring system for predicting type 2 diabetes and hypertension. *Journal of King Saud University - Computer and Information Sciences, 34*(3), 862–870. doi:10.1016/j.jksuci.2020.01.010

Chauhan, M., & Agarwal, R. (2023). Impact of screens on how users think. *IEEE Conference P2023 3rd International Conference on Intelligent Technologies (CONIT) Ublication*. IEEE Xplore. 10.1109/CONIT59222.2023.10205565

Chen, Y., He, H., & Yang, Y. (2023). Effects of Social Support on Professional Identity of Secondary Vocational Students major in Preschool Nursery Teacher Program: A Chain Mediating Model of Psychological Adjustment and School Belonging. *Sustainability, 15*(6), 5134. doi:10.3390u15065134

Chopra, R. (2023). *Online Religion*, 521–535. Wiley. doi:10.1002/9781119671619.ch33

Chuanhua, Y. (2023). Using Cognitive Therapy to Explore the Potential Application of Traditional Therapy and Metaverse Therapy from a Cognitive Perspective. *SHS Web of Conferences, 171*, 01030. doi:10.1051hsconf/202317101030

Claisse, C., & Durrant, A. (2023). *'Keeping our Faith Alive': Investigating Buddhism Practice during COVID-19 to Inform Design for the Online Community Practice of Faith*. ACM. doi:10.1145/3544548.3581177

Covaci, A., Alhasan, K., Loonker, M., Farrell, B., Tabbaa, L., Ppali, S., & Ang, C. S. (2023). *No Pie in the (Digital) Sky: Co-Imagining the Food Metaverse*. ACM. doi:10.1145/3544548.3581305

Crawford, T. (2023). *Sonic Urban Exploration: Connections between disused urban environments and electroacoustic music composition*. SES. https://ses.library.usyd.edu.au/handle/2123/31519

Damaris, A. (2023, July 4). *The Effect of Physical Activity on Mental Well-being among College Students*. Cari Journals. https://carijournals.org/journals/index.php/ijars/article/view/1336

Davis, J., Finlay-Jones, A., Bear, N., Prescott, S. L., Silva, D., & Ohan, J. L. (2023). Time-out for well-being: A mixed methods evaluation of attitudes and likelihood to engage in different types of online emotional well-being programmes in the perinatal period. *Women's Health (London, England)*, *19*. doi:10.1177/17455057231184507 PMID:37431205

De Engenharia, F. (2023, July 25). *Instrument Position In Immersive Audio: A Study On Good Practices And Comparison With Stereo Approaches*. https://repositorio-aberto.up.pt/handle/10216/152055

De Villiers Bosman, I., Buruk, O. T., Jørgensen, K., & Hamari, J. (2023). The effect of audio on the experience in virtual reality: A scoping review. *Behaviour & Information Technology*, 1–35. doi:10.1080/0144929X.2022.2158371

Degenhard, S. M. (n.d.). *Mobile phone mindfulness: Effects of app-based meditation intervention on stress and HRV of undergraduate students*. UTC Scholar. https://scholar.utc.edu/mps/vol29/iss1/1/

DeGuzman, K. (2021b). What is Virtual Reality — Games, Movies & Storytelling. *StudioBinder*. https://www.studiobinder.com/blog/what-is-virtual-reality/

Demeco, A., Zola, L., Frizziero, A., Martini, C., Palumbo, A., Foresti, R., Buccino, G., & Cipolla, C. (2023). Immersive Virtual Reality in Post-Stroke Rehabilitation: A Systematic Review. *Sensors (Basel)*, *23*(3), 1712. doi:10.339023031712 PMID:36772757

Dirin, A., Nieminen, M., Laine, T. H., Nieminen, L., & Ghalabani, L. (2023). Emotional contagion in Collaborative Virtual Reality Learning Experiences: An eSports approach. *Education and Information Technologies*. doi:10.100710639-023-11769-7

Dogra, V., Verma, S., Kavita, K., Jhanjhi, N. Z., Ghosh, U., & Le, D. (2022). A comparative analysis of machine learning models for banking news extraction by multiclass classification with imbalanced datasets of financial news: Challenges and solutions. *International Journal of Interactive Multimedia and Artificial Intelligence*, *7*(3), 35. doi:10.9781/ijimai.2022.02.002

Doronzo, F., Nardacchione, G., & Di Muro, E. (2023). Processi neuroplastici associati all'adozione della realtà virtuale: Una revisione sistematica verso un nuovo approccio del trattamento dei disturbi mentali. *IUL Research, 4*(7), 126–147. doi:10.57568/iulresearch.v4i7.411

Dreher, F., & Ströbel, T. (2023). How gamified online loyalty programs enable and facilitate value co-creation: A case study within a sports-related service context. *Journal of Service Theory and Practice, 33*(5), 671–696. doi:10.1108/JSTP-10-2022-0229

Dreisoerner, A., Ferrandina, C., Schulz, A. P., Nater, U. M., & Junker, N. M. (2023). *Using group-based interactive video teleconferencing to make self-compassion more accessible: A randomized controlled trial.* ScienceDirect. doi:10.1016/j.jcbs.2023.08.001

Ekandjo, T. (2023). *Human-ai collaboration in everyday work-life practices: a coregulation perspective.* AIS Electronic Library (AISeL). https://aisel.aisnet.org/ecis2023_rp/213/

Eom, S., Kim, S., Jiang, Y., Chen, R. J., Roghanizad, A. R., Rosenthal, M. Z., Dunn, J., & Gorlatova, M. (2023). Investigation of Thermal Perception and Emotional Response in Augmented Reality using Digital Biomarkers: A Pilot Study. In *2023 IEEE Conference on Virtual Reality and 3D User Interfaces Abstracts and Workshops (VRW).* IEEE. 10.1109/VRW58643.2023.00042

Fazia, T., Bubbico, F., Nova, A., Bruno, S., Iozzi, D., Calgan, B., Caimi, G., Terzaghi, M., Manni, R., & Bernardinelli, L. (2023). Beneficial Effects of an Online Mindfulness-Based Intervention on Sleep Quality in Italian Poor Sleepers during the COVID-19 Pandemic: A Randomized Trial. *International Journal of Environmental Research and Public Health, 20*(3), 2724. doi:10.3390/ijerph20032724 PMID:36768089

Fazia, T., Bubbico, F., Nova, A., Buizza, C., Cela, H., Iozzi, D., Calgan, B., Maggi, F., Floris, V., Sutti, I., Bruno, S., Ghilardi, A., & Bernardinelli, L. (2023). Improving stress management, anxiety, and mental well-being in medical students through an online Mindfulness-Based Intervention: A randomized study. *Scientific Reports, 13*(1), 8214. doi:10.103841598-023-35483-z PMID:37217666

Fernandes, F. A., & Werner, C. M. L. (2023). A Scoping review of the metaverse for Software Engineering Education: Overview, Challenges, and opportunities. *Presence (Cambridge, Mass.),* 1–40. doi:10.1162/pres_a_00371

Furht, B. (2011). *Handbook of Augmented Reality.* Springer Science & Business Media. doi:10.1007/978-1-4614-0064-6

Gaertner, R. J., Kossmann, K. E., Benz, A., Bentele, U. U., Meier, M., Denk, B., Klink, E. S. C., Dimitroff, S. J., & Pruessner, J. C. (2023). Relaxing effects of virtual environments on the autonomic nervous system indicated by heart rate variability: A systematic review. *Journal of Environmental Psychology*, *88*, 102035. doi:10.1016/j.jenvp.2023.102035

Gagliardi, E., Bernardini, G., Quagliarini, E., Schumacher, M., & Calvaresi, D. (2023). Characterization and future perspectives of Virtual Reality Evacuation Drills for safe built environments: A Systematic Literature Review. *Safety Science*, *163*, 106141. doi:10.1016/j.ssci.2023.106141

Gao, Q., & Zhang, L. (2023). Brief mindfulness meditation intervention improves attentional control of athletes in virtual reality shooting competition: Evidence from fNIRS and eye tracking. *Psychology of Sport and Exercise*, 102477. doi:10.1016/j.psychsport.2023.102477 PMID:37665918

Garfin, D. R., Amador, A., Osorio, J., Ruivivar, K. S., Torres, A., & Nyamathi, A. (2023). Adaptation of a mindfulness-based intervention for trauma-exposed, unhoused women with substance use disorder. *Psychological Trauma: Theory, Research, Practice, and Policy*. doi:10.1037/tra0001486 PMID:37307346

Gill, S. H., Razzaq, M. A., Ahmad, M., Almansour, F. M., Haq, I. U., Jhanjhi, N. Z., Alam, M. Z., & Masud, M. (2022). Security and privacy aspects of cloud Computing: A Smart Campus case study. *Intelligent Automation and Soft Computing*, *31*(1), 117–128. doi:10.32604/iasc.2022.016597

Goldsworthy, A., Chawla, J., Birta, J., Baumanna, O., & Gough, S. (2023). Use of extended reality in sleep health, medicine, and research: A scoping review. *Sleep (Basel)*, zsad201. doi:10.1093leep/zsad201 PMID:37498981

Gulick, W. (2023). Polanyi, zen and non-linguistic knowledge. In Comparative philosophy of religion (pp. 91–106). doi:10.1007/978-3-031-18013-2_7

Haley, A. C., Thorpe, D., Pelletier, A., Yarosh, S., & Keefe, D. F. (2023). Inward VR: Toward a qualitative method for investigating interoceptive awareness in VR. *IEEE Transactions on Visualization and Computer Graphics*, *29*(5), 2557–2566. doi:10.1109/TVCG.2023.3247074 PMID:37027715

Hamid, B., Jhanjhi, N. Z., Humayun, M., Khan, A. F., & Alsayat, A. (2019). Cyber Security Issues and Challenges for Smart Cities: A survey. *2019 13th International Conference on Mathematics, Actuarial Science, Computer Science and Statistics (MACS)*. 10.1109/macs48846.2019.9024768

Han, E., Miller, M. R., DeVeaux, C., Jun, H., Nowak, K. L., Hancock, J. T., Ram, N., & Bailenson, J. N. (2023). People, places, and time: A large-scale, longitudinal study of transformed avatars and environmental context in group interaction in the metaverse. *Journal of Computer-Mediated Communication*, *28*(2), zmac031. doi:10.1093/jcmc/zmac031

Harutyunyan, M. (2023). Exploring the Rich Tapestry of Gardens and Parks: A Journey through History, Education, and Artistic Expressions. *Harutyunyan | Indonesian Journal of Multidiciplinary Research*. doi:10.17509/ijomr.v3i2.60561

Hasapeehko, A. (2023). *Marketing determinants of consumer behaviour change in the food market*. SUM DU. https://essuir.sumdu.edu.ua/handle/123456789/92038

Heinrich, D., & O'Connell, K. A. (2023). The effects of mindfulness meditation on nursing students' stress and anxiety levels. *Nursing Education Perspectives*. doi:10.1097/01.NEP.0000000000001159 PMID:37404039

Hensher, D. A., Mulley, C., & Nelson, J. D. (2023). What is an ideal (Utopian) mobility as a service (MaaS) framework? A communication note. *Transportation Research Part A, Policy and Practice*, *172*, 103675. doi:10.1016/j.tra.2023.103675

Hillebrand, K., Hornuf, L., Müller, B., & Vrankar, D. (2023). The social dilemma of big data: Donating personal data to promote social welfare. *Information and Organization*, *33*(1), 100452. doi:10.1016/j.infoandorg.2023.100452

Holley, R., Moldow, E., Chaudhary, S., Gaumond, G., Hacker, R. L., Kahn, P., Boeldt, D., & Hubley, S. (2022). A qualitative study of virtual reality and mindfulness for substance use disorders. *Journal of Technology in Behavioral Science*, *8*(1), 36–46. doi:10.100741347-022-00284-0

Hopkins, J. L., & Bardoel, A. (2023). The future is hybrid: How organisations are designing and supporting sustainable hybrid work models in Post-Pandemic Australia. *Sustainability*, *15*(4), 3086. doi:10.3390u15043086

Huang, H., Li, Y., & Cai, S. (2023). Best Practices for Integrating 360 VR Videos into Psychology Teaching. *2023 9th International Conference on Virtual Reality (ICVR)*. 10.1109/icvr57957.2023.10169358

Humayun, M., Jhanjhi, N. Z., Alruwaili, M., Amalathas, S. S., Balasubramanian, V., & Selvaraj, B. (2020). Privacy protection and energy optimization for 5G-Aided industrial internet of things. *IEEE Access : Practical Innovations, Open Solutions*, *8*, 183665–183677. doi:10.1109/ACCESS.2020.3028764

Humayun, M., Niazi, M., Jhanjhi, N. Z., Alshayeb, M., & Mahmood, S. (2020). Cyber Security Threats and Vulnerabilities: A Systematic Mapping study. *Arabian Journal for Science and Engineering*, *45*(4), 3171–3189. doi:10.100713369-019-04319-2

Iloudi, M., Lindner, P., Ali, L., Wallström, S., Thunström, A. O., Ioannou, M., Anving, N., Johansson, V., Hamilton, W., Falk, Ö., & Steingrimsson, S. (2022). Physical Versus Virtual Reality-based Calm Rooms for Psychiatric Inpatients: A Quasi-randomized Trial (Preprint). *Journal of Medical Internet Research*. doi:10.2196/42365

Ingendoh, R. M., Posny, E. S., & Heine, A. (2023). Binaural beats to entrain the brain? A systematic review of the effects of binaural beat stimulation on brain oscillatory activity, and the implications for psychological research and intervention. *PLoS One*, *18*(5), e0286023. doi:10.1371/journal.pone.0286023 PMID:37205669

Jerath, R., Syam, M., & Ahmed, S. Z. (2023). *The Future of Stress Management: Integration Smartwatches and HRV Technology*. doi:10.20944/preprints202307.1283.v2

Jhanjhi, N. Z., Humayun, M., & Almuayqil, S. N. (2021). Cyber security and privacy issues in industrial internet of things. *Computer Systems Science and Engineering*, *37*(3), 361–380. doi:10.32604/csse.2021.015206

Jhuang, Y., Yan, Y., & Horng, G. (2023). GDPR Personal Privacy Security Mechanism for smart home system. *Electronics (Basel)*, *12*(4), 831. doi:10.3390/electronics12040831

Jin, N., Wu, Y., Park, J., Qin, Z., & Li, Z. (2023). Brain-Metaverse Interaction for Anxiety Regulation. *2023 9th International Conference on Virtual Reality (ICVR)*. 10.1109/icvr57957.2023.10169785

Jo, H. (2023). Tourism in the digital frontier: a study on user continuance intention in the metaverse. *Springer Link*. https://link.springer.com/article/10.1007/s40558-023-00257-w

Jo, H., Seidel, L., Pahud, M., Sinclair, M., & Bianchi, A. (2023). *FlowAR: How Different Augmented Reality Visualizations of Online Fitness Videos Support Flow for At-Home Yoga Exercises*. ACM. doi:10.1145/3544548.3580897

Joshi, J. (2023, August 5). *PhysioKit: open-source, low-cost physiological computing toolkit for single and multi-user studies*. https://arxiv.org/abs/2308.02756

Kaaria, A. G., & Mwaruta, S. S. (2023). Mental Health Ingenuities and the Role of computer Technology on Employees' Mental Health: A Systematic review. *East African Journal of Health & Science*, *6*(1), 219–231. doi:10.37284/eajhs.6.1.1268

Kaddoura, S., & Husseiny, F. A. (2023). The rising trend of Metaverse in education: Challenges, opportunities, and ethical considerations. *PeerJ*, *9*, e1252. doi:10.7717/peerj-cs.1252 PMID:37346578

Kahlmann, V., Moor, C. C., Van Helmondt, S. J., Mostard, R. L. M., Van Der Lee, M., Grutters, J. C., Wijsenbeek, M., & Veltkamp, M. (2023). Online mindfulness-based cognitive therapy for fatigue in patients with sarcoidosis (TIRED): A randomised controlled trial. *The Lancet. Respiratory Medicine*, *11*(3), 265–272. doi:10.1016/S2213-2600(22)00387-3 PMID:36427515

Kaleva, I., & Riches, S. (2023). Stepping inside the whispers and tingles: Multisensory virtual reality for enhanced relaxation and wellbeing. *Frontiers in Digital Health*, *5*, 1212586. doi:10.3389/fdgth.2023.1212586 PMID:37534028

Kanwal, N., Janssen, E. M., & Engan, K. (2023). *Balancing privacy and progress in artificial intelligence: Anonymization in histopathology for biomedical research and education.* Cornell University. doi:10.48550/arxiv.2307.09426

Karthi, M., Alsager, M., Metha, R., & Nash, N. F. (2023). Digital Solution: Breaking the barriers to address stigma of mental health. In *IEEE EUROCON 2023 - 20th International Conference on Smart Technologies*. IEEE. 10.1109/EUROCON56442.2023.10198879

Khemchandani, V., Goswani, K., Teotia, M. P., Chandra, S., & Wadalkar, N. M. (2023). Virtual Reality Based Attention Simulator using EEG Signals. In *2023 2nd Edition of IEEE Delhi Section Flagship Conference (DELCON)*. IEEE. 10.1109/delcon57910.2023.10127358

Kim, D. Y., & Kim, S. Y. (2023). Investigating the effect of customer-generated content on performance in online platform-based experience goods market. *Journal of Retailing and Consumer Services*, *74*, 103409. doi:10.1016/j.jretconser.2023.103409

King, J., Halversen, A., Richards, O., John, K. K., & Strong, B. (2023). Anxiety and physiological responses to virtual reality and audio meditation in racial and ethnic minorities. *Journal of Technology in Behavioral Science*. doi:10.1007/s41347-023-00330-5

Koohang, A., Nord, J. H., Ooi, K., Tan, G. W., Al-Emran, M., Aw, E. C., Baabdullah, A. M., Buhalis, D., Cham, T., Dennis, C., Dutot, V., Dwivedi, Y. K., Hughes, L., Mogaji, E., Pandey, N., Phau, I., Raman, R., Sharma, A., Sigala, M., & Wong, L. (2023). Shaping the Metaverse into Reality: A Holistic Multidisciplinary Understanding of Opportunities, Challenges, and Avenues for Future Investigation. *Journal of Computer Information Systems*, *63*(3), 735–765. doi:10.1080/08874417.2023.2165197

Korzynski, P., Koźmiński, A. K., & Baczyńska, A. (2023). Navigating leadership challenges with technology: Uncovering the potential of ChatGPT, virtual reality, human capital management systems, robotic process automation, and social media. *Przedsiębiorczość Międzynarodowa, 9*(2), 7–18. doi:10.15678/IER.2023.0902.01

Krueger, J. (2022). *Affordances and spatial agency in psychopathology*. Taylors and Francis Online. doi:10.1080/09515089.2023.2243975

Kyi, L., Shivakumar, S. A., Santos, C., Roesner, F., Zufall, F., & Biega, A. J. (2023). *Investigating Deceptive Design in GDPR's Legitimate Interest*. ACM. doi:10.1145/3544548.3580637

Lan, L., Sikov, J., Lejeune, J., Ji, C., Brown, H., Bullock, K., & Spencer, A. E. (2023). A Systematic Review of using Virtual and Augmented Reality for the Diagnosis and Treatment of Psychotic Disorders. *Current Treatment Options in Psychiatry, 10*(2), 87–107. doi:10.100740501-023-00287-5 PMID:37360960

Leite, R. (2023). *The effects of Virtual Reality-Based Mindfulness Meditation on cognition*. STARS. https://stars.library.ucf.edu/honorstheses/1376/

Leite, R. (2023b). *The effects of Virtual Reality-Based Mindfulness Meditation on cognition* [Undergraduate Thesis]. University of Central Florida.

Levin, J. (2023). Being in the present moment: Toward an epidemiology of mindfulness. *Mindfulness*. doi:10.100712671-023-02179-4

Li, H., & Chen, H. (2023). Research on immersive virtual reality healing design based on the Five senses Theory. In Communications in computer and information science (pp. 99–106). doi:10.1007/978-3-031-35992-7_14

Li, J., Kwon, N., Pham, H., Shim, R., & Leshed, G. (2023). *Co-designing Magic Machines for Everyday Mindfulness with Practitioners*. ACM. doi:10.1145/3563657.3595976

Li, K., De Oliveira Cardoso, C., Moctezuma-Ramirez, A., Elgalad, A., & Perin, E. C. (2023). (Preprint). Heart Rate Variability Measurement through a Wearable Device. *Another Breakthrough for Personal Health Monitoring*. doi:10.20944/preprints202308.0732.v1

Li, Y., Cabano, F., & Li, P. (2023). How to attract low prosocial funders in crowdfunding? Matching among funders, project descriptions, and platform types. *Information & Management, 103840*(7), 103840. doi:10.1016/j.im.2023.103840

Li, Y., Ch'ng, E., & Cobb, S. (2023). Factors influencing engagement in hybrid virtual and augmented reality. *ACM Transactions on Computer-Human Interaction*, *30*(4), 1–27. doi:10.1145/3589952

Liao, Y., Huang, T., Lin, S., Wu, C., Chang, K., Hsieh, S., Lin, S., Goh, J. O. S., & Yang, C. (2023). Mediating role of resilience in the relationships of physical activity and mindful self-awareness with peace of mind among college students. *Scientific Reports*, *13*(1), 10386. doi:10.103841598-023-37416-2 PMID:37369802

Liedgren, J., Desmet, P., & Gaggioli, A. (2023). Liminal design: A conceptual framework and three-step approach for developing technology that delivers transcendence and deeper experiences. *Frontiers in Psychology*, *14*, 1043170. doi:10.3389/fpsyg.2023.1043170 PMID:36844338

Liu, H., Liu, S., Li, X., & Bing-Quan, L. (2023). Efficacy of Baduanjin for treatment of fatigue: A systematic review and meta-analysis of randomized controlled trials. *Medicine*, *102*(32), e34707. doi:10.1097/MD.0000000000034707 PMID:37565842

Liu, Y., Bitter, J. L., & Spierling, U. (2023). Evaluating interaction challenges of Head-Mounted Device-Based augmented reality applications for First-Time users at museums and exhibitions. In Lecture Notes in Computer Science (pp. 150–163). doi:10.1007/978-3-031-34732-0_11

Liu, Y., Zhang, Y., Zhang, X., Han, F., & Zhao, Y. (2023). A geographical perspective on the formation of urban nightlife landscape. *Humanities & Social Sciences Communications*, *10*(1), 483. doi:10.105741599-023-01964-9

Loveys, K., Sagar, M., Antoni, M., & Broadbent, E. (2023). *The impact of virtual humans on psychosomatic medicine*. Psychosomatic Medicine. doi:10.1097/PSY.0000000000001227

Lucas, I., Solé-Morata, N., Baenas, I., Rosinska, M., Fernández-Aranda, F., & Jiménez-Murcia, S. (2023). Biofeedback interventions for impulsivity-related processes in addictive disorders. *Current Addiction Reports*, *10*(3), 543–552. doi:10.100740429-023-00499-y

Ma, J., Zhao, D., Xu, N., & Yang, J. (2023). The effectiveness of immersive virtual reality (VR) based mindfulness training on improvement mental-health in adults: A narrative systematic review. *Explore (New York, N.Y.)*, *19*(3), 310–318. doi:10.1016/j.explore.2022.08.001 PMID:36002363

Malighetti, C., Bernardelli, L., Pancini, E., Riva, G., & Villani, D. (2023). Promoting Emotional and Psychological Well-Being During COVID-19 Pandemic: A Self-Help Virtual Reality intervention for university students. *Cyberpsychology, Behavior, and Social Networking*, *26*(4), 309–317. doi:10.1089/cyber.2022.0246 PMID:36940285

Malin, Y. (2023). Others In Mind: A Systematic Review and Meta-Analysis of the Relationship between Mindfulness and Prosociality. *Mindfulness*, *14*(7), 1582–1605. doi:10.100712671-023-02150-3

Mazlan, I., Abdullah, N., & Ahmad, N. (2023). Exploring the impact of hybrid recommender systems on personalized mental health recommendations. *International Journal of Advanced Computer Science and Applications*, *14*(6). doi:10.14569/IJACSA.2023.0140699

McCaw, C. T. (2023). Contemplative practices and teacher professional becoming. *Educational Review*, 1–29. doi:10.1080/00131911.2023.2215467

McEwan, K., Krogh, K. S., Dunlop, K., Khan, M., & Krogh, A. (2023). Virtual Forest Bathing Programming as Experienced by Disabled Adults with Mobility Impairments and/or Low Energy: A Qualitative Study. *Forests*, *14*(5), 1033. doi:10.3390/f14051033

McMahan, D. L. (2023). *Rethinking meditation: Buddhist Practice in the Ancient and Modern Worlds*. Academic Press.

Miller, N., Stepanova, E. R., Desnoyers-Stewart, J., Adhikari, A., Kitson, A., Pennefather, P. P., Quesnel, D., Brauns, K., Friedl-Werner, A., Stahn, A., & Riecke, B. E. (2023). *Awedyssey: Design Tensions in Eliciting Self-transcendent Emotions in Virtual Reality to Support Mental Well-being and Connection*. ACM. doi:10.1145/3563657.3595998

Mirlou, F., & Beker, L. (2023). Wearable Electrochemical Sensors for Healthcare Monitoring: A review of current developments and future Prospects. *IEEE Transactions on Molecular, Biological, and Multi-Scale Communications*, *1*(3), 364–373. doi:10.1109/TMBMC.2023.3304240

Mishra, N., & Bharti, T. (2023). Exploring the nexus of social support, work–life balance and life satisfaction in hybrid work scenario in learning organizations. *The Learning Organization*. doi:10.1108/TLO-08-2022-0099

Mitsea, E., Drigas, A., & Skianis, C. (2023). Brain-computer interfaces in digital mindfulness training for metacognitive, emotional and attention regulation skills: A literature review. *Research. Social Development*, *12*(3), e2512340247. doi:10.33448/rsd-v12i3.40247

Montalto, J. (2023). The Effects Of Mindfulness On Stress Reduction And Academic Performance In Students Studying Health Sciences. *DUNE: DigitalUNE*. https://dune.une.edu/na_capstones/51/

Moyer, M. A. (2023). *Engaging Technologies of the Self with Youth: A Critical Contemplative Pedagogy Action Research Project*. https://etd.ohiolink.edu/acprod/odb_etd/etd/r/1501/10?clear=10&p10_accession_num=miami1689338623782483

Mulders, M. (2023). Learning about Victims of Holocaust in Virtual Reality: The Main, Mediating and Moderating Effects of Technology, Instructional Method, Flow, Presence, and Prior Knowledge. *Multimodal Technologies and Interaction*, *7*(3), 28. doi:10.3390/mti7030028

Musto, S. (2023). Exploring the uses of yoga nidra: An integrative review. *Nursing and Scholarship*. https://sigmapubs.onlinelibrary.wiley.com/doi/abs/10.1111/jnu.12927

N, S., M, S., G, K., & R, R. (2023). *Securing the Cloud: An empirical study on best practices for ensuring data privacy and protection*. doi:10.31033/ijemr.13.2.6

Nagarajan, G. (2023, July 15). *The Role Of The Metaverse In Digital Marketing*. Universidad De Granada. https://digibug.ugr.es/handle/10481/84077

Nee, A. Y. C., & Ong, S. K. (2023). *Springer Handbook of Augmented Reality*. Springer Nature. doi:10.1007/978-3-030-67822-7

O'Hagan, J., Saeghe, P., Gugenheimer, J., Medeiros, D., Marky, K., Khamis, M., & McGill, M. (2022). Privacy-Enhancing technology and everyday augmented reality. *Proceedings of the ACM on Interactive, Mobile, Wearable and Ubiquitous Technologies, 6*(4), 1–35. 10.1145/3569501

Omranian, S., Zolnoori, M., Huang, M., Campos-Castillo, C., & McRoy, S. (2023). Predicting patient satisfaction with medications for treating opioid use Disorder: Case study Applying natural language processing to reviews of methadone and Buprenorphine/Naloxone on Health-Related Social media. *JMIR Infodemiology*, *3*, e37207. doi:10.2196/37207 PMID:37113381

Ortet, C. P., Vairinhos, M., Veloso, A. I., & Costa, L. V. (2023). Virtual Reality Hippotherapy Simulator: A model proposal for Senior citizens. In Lecture Notes in Computer Science (pp. 592–609). doi:10.1007/978-3-031-34866-2_42

Pal, R., Adhikari, D., Heyat, M. B. B., Ullah, I., & You, Z. (2023). Yoga meets intelligent Internet of Things: Recent challenges and future directions. *Bioengineering (Basel, Switzerland)*, *10*(4), 459. doi:10.3390/bioengineering10040459 PMID:37106646

Pancini, E., Di Natale, A. F., & Villani, D. (2023). *Breathing in virtual Reality for Promoting Mental Health: A scoping review. Research Square*. Research Square. doi:10.21203/rs.3.rs-3230685/v1

Pardini, S., Gabrielli, S., Olivetto, S., Fusina, F., Dianti, M., Forti, S., Lancini, C., & Novara, C. (2023). Personalized, naturalistic virtual reality scenarios coupled with Web-Based progressive muscle relaxation training for the general population: Protocol for a Proof-of-Principle randomized controlled trial. *JMIR Research Protocols*, *12*, e44183. doi:10.2196/44183 PMID:37067881

Park, M., Song, R., Ju, K., Shin, J. C., Seo, J., Fan, X., Gao, X., Ryu, A., & Li, Y. (2023). Effects of Tai Chi and Qigong on cognitive and physical functions in older adults: Systematic review, meta-analysis, and meta-regression of randomized clinical trials. *BMC Geriatrics*, *23*(1), 352. doi:10.118612877-023-04070-2 PMID:37280512

Pascual, K. J., Fredman, A., Naum, A., Patil, C., & Sikka, N. (2022). Should mindfulness for health care workers go virtual? A Mindfulness-Based intervention using virtual reality and heart rate variability in the emergency department. *AAOHN Journal*, *71*(4), 188–194. doi:10.1177/21650799221123258 PMID:36377263

Piçarra, M., Rodrigues, A., & Guerreiro, J. (2023). *Evaluating Accessible Navigation for Blind People in Virtual Environments*. ACM. doi:10.1145/3544549.3585813

Pira, G. L., Aquilini, B., Davoli, A., Grandi, S., & Ruini, C. (2023). The Use of Virtual Reality Interventions to Promote Positive Mental Health: Systematic Literature review. *JMIR Mental Health*, *10*, e44998. doi:10.2196/44998 PMID:37410520

Ponce, P., Peffer, T., Garduno, J. I. M., Eicker, U., Molina, A., McDaniel, T., Mimo, E. D. M., Menon, R. P., Kaspar, K., & Hussain, S. (2023). Smart communities and cities as a unified concept. In Studies in big data (pp. 125–168). doi:10.1007/978-3-031-32828-2_5

Prasath, P. R., Xiong, Y., & Zhang, Q. (2023). A practical guide to planning, implementing, and evaluating the mindfulness-based well-being group for international students. *The Journal of Humanistic Counseling*, johc.12200. doi:10.1002/johc.12200

Pratviel, Y., Bouny, P., & Deschodt-Arsac, V. (2023). *Immersion in a relaxing virtual reality environment is associated with similar effects on stress and anxiety as heart rate variability biofeedback*. Research Square. doi:10.21203/rs.3.rs-3221200/v1

Priest, S. (2023). Predicting the future of experiential and adventurous learning in the metaverse. *Journal of Adventure Education and Outdoor Learning*, 1–14. doi:10.1080/14729679.2023.2220835

Purwar, S. (2021, December 8). Designing User Experience for Virtual Reality (VR) applications. *Medium.* https://uxplanet.org/designing-user-experience-for-virtual-reality-vr-applications-fc8e4faadd96

Qureshi, I. (2023, July 10). *Can Music And Artificial Intelligence Influence Customer Behavior In-Store?* RC. https://rc.library.uta.edu/uta-ir/handle/10106/31524

Randazzo, G., Reitano, G., Carletti, F., Iafrate, M., Betto, G., Novara, G., Moro, F. D., & Zattoni, F. (2023). Urology: A trip into metaverse. *World Journal of Urology, 41*(10), 2647–2657. doi:10.100700345-023-04560-3 PMID:37552265

Räsänen, P., Muotka, J., & Lappalainen, R. (2023). Examining coaches' asynchronous written feedback in two blended ACT-based interventions for enhancing university students' wellbeing and reducing psychological distress: A randomized study. *Journal of Contextual Behavioral Science, 29*, 98–108. doi:10.1016/j.jcbs.2023.06.006

Ray, P. P. (2023). ChatGPT: A comprehensive review on background, applications, key challenges, bias, ethics, limitations and future scope. *Internet of Things and Cyber-physical Systems, 3*, 121–154. doi:10.1016/j.iotcps.2023.04.003

Redirect notice. (n.d.). https://www.google.com/url?sa=i&url=https%3A%2F%2Fwww.shutterstock.com%2Fvideo%2Fsearch%2Fvr-meditation&psig=AOvVaw1lDxksdO4j_cUe7TWIDomo&ust=1692327355095000&source=images&cd=vfe&opi=89978449&ved=0CBIQjhxqFwoTCPDmqenY4oADFQAAAAAdAAAAABBg

Ren, C. (2023). *Question the nature of reality through virtual reality Portals of Perception - ProQuest.* New York University Tandon School of Engineering.

Riches, S., Jeyarajaguru, P., Taylor, L., Fialho, C., Little, J. R., Ahmed, L., O'Brien, A., Van Driel, C., Veling, W., & Valmaggia, L. (2023). Virtual reality relaxation for people with mental health conditions: A systematic review. *Social Psychiatry and Psychiatric Epidemiology, 58*(7), 989–1007. doi:10.100700127-022-02417-5 PMID:36658261

Riches, S., Taylor, L., Jeyarajaguru, P., Veling, W., & Valmaggia, L. (2023). Virtual reality and immersive technologies to promote workplace wellbeing: A systematic review. *Journal of Mental Health (Abingdon, England),* 1–21. doi:10.1080/09638237.2023.2182428 PMID:36919828

Richter, S., & Richter, A. (2023). What is novel about the Metaverse? *International Journal of Information Management, 73*, 102684. doi:10.1016/j.ijinfomgt.2023.102684

Rieger, K. L., Hack, T. F., Duff, M. A., Campbell-Enns, H., & West, C. H. (2023). Integrating mindfulness and the expressive arts for meaning making in cancer care: A grounded theory of the processes, facilitators, and challenges. *Supportive Care in Cancer*, *31*(8), 475. doi:10.100700520-023-07909-x PMID:37466723

Robison, J., Walter, T., Godsey, J. A., & Robinson, J. (2023). Chairside yoga therapy alleviates symptoms in patients concurrently receiving outpatient cancer infusions: A Promising Feasibility study. *Journal of Holistic Nursing*. doi:10.1177/08980101231170482 PMID:37128683

Rodriguez, S. D., Rivu, R., Mäkelä, V., & Alt, F. (2023). *Challenges in Virtual Reality Studies: Ethics and Internal and External Validity*. ACM. doi:10.1145/3582700.3582716

Rolbiecki, A. J., Govindarajan, A., & Froeliger, B. (2023). Immersive virtual reality and neurofeedback for the management of cancer symptoms during treatment. *Supportive Care in Cancer*, *31*(8), 493. doi:10.100700520-023-07957-3 PMID:37493785

Rosenberg, L. (2023). The Metaverse and Conversational AI as a Threat Vector for Targeted Influence. In *2023 IEEE 13th Annual Computing and Communication Workshop and Conference (CCWC)*. IEEE. 10.1109/ccwc57344.2023.10099167

Roy, B. L., Martin-Krumm, C., & Trousselard, M. (2023). Mindfulness for adaptation to analog and new technologies emergence for long-term space missions. *Frontiers in Space Technologies*, *4*. doi:10.3389/frspt.2023.1109556

Ruan, H., Pocock, I., & Ruan, H. (2023). "You just have to stick with the practice": A Long-Term weekly mindfulness group at the VA. *Group*, *47*(1–2), 91–114. doi:10.1353/grp.2023.0008

Samarin, N., Kothari, S., Siyed, Z., Bjorkman, O., Yuan, R., Wijesekera, P., Alomar, N., Fischer, J., Hoofnagle, C. J., & Egelman, S. (2023). *Lessons in VCR Repair: Compliance of Android App Developers with the California Consumer Privacy Act (CCPA)*. Cornell University. doi:10.48550/arxiv.2304.00944

Sanku, B. S., Li, Y. J., & He, J. (2023). A Survey of VR-Based Neurofeedback Systems in Physiological Computing for Depression Treatment. *2023 9th International Conference on Virtual Reality (ICVR)*. 10.1109/icvr57957.2023.10169583

Sarasalin, P. (2023). Atmosphere of Place: A case study of a contemporary tropical home. *The International Journal of Design in Society*, *17*(1), 45–78. doi:10.18848/2325-1328/CGP/v17i01/45-78

Schlussel, H., & Frosh, P. (2023). The taste of video: Facebook videos as multi-sensory experiences. *Convergence*, *29*(4), 980–996. doi:10.1177/13548565231179958

Schwartz, K., Ganster, F. M., & Tran, U. S. (2022). Mindfulness-Based Mobile Applications and their Impact on Well-Being in Non-Clinical Populations: A Systematic Review of Randomized Controlled Trials (Preprint). *Journal of Medical Internet Research*. doi:10.2196/44638 PMID:37540550

Seetharaman, R., Avhad, S., & Rane, J. (2023). *Exploring the healing power of singing bowls: An overview of key findings and potential benefits*. Elsevier. doi:10.1016/j.explore.2023.07.007

Shafiq, D. A., Jhanjhi, N. Z., & Abdullah, A. (2021). Machine Learning Approaches for Load Balancing in Cloud Computing Services. *2021 National Computing Colleges Conference (NCCC)*. 10.1109/NCCC49330.2021.9428825

Shannon, L. (2023). *Interconnected realities: How the Metaverse Will Transform Our Relationship with Technology Forever*. John Wiley & Sons.

Sharmin, S. (2023, July 25). *Insights into Cognitive Engagement: Comparing the Effectiveness of Game-Based and Video-Based Learning*. https://arxiv.org/abs/2307.13637

She, Y., Wang, Q., Liu, F., Lin, L., Yang, B., & Hu, B. (2023). An interaction design model for virtual reality mindfulness meditation using imagery-based transformation and positive feedback. *Computer Animation and Virtual Worlds*, *34*(3-4), e2184. doi:10.1002/cav.2184

Singh, A., Sharma, S., Singh, A., Unanoglu, M., & Taneja, S. (2023). *Cultural marketing and metaverse for consumer engagement*. IGI Global. doi:10.4018/978-1-6684-8312-1

Singh, K., & Saxena, G. (2023). *Religious and spiritual practices in India: A Positive Psychological Perspective*. Springer Nature. doi:10.1007/978-981-99-2397-7

Singhal, V., Jain, S. P., Anand, D., Singh, A., Verma, S., Kavita, Rodrigues, J. J. P. C., Jhanjhi, N. Z., Ghosh, U., Jo, O., & Iwendi, C. (2020). Artificial Intelligence Enabled Road Vehicle-Train Collision Risk Assessment Framework for Unmanned railway level crossings. *IEEE Access : Practical Innovations, Open Solutions*, *8*, 113790–113806. doi:10.1109/ACCESS.2020.3002416

Siwik, C., Adler, S. R., Moran, P. J., Kuyken, W., Segal, Z. V., Felder, J. N., Eisendrath, S. J., & Hecht, F. M. (2023). Preventing Depression Relapse: A Qualitative Study on the Need for Additional Structured Support Following Mindfulness-Based Cognitive Therapy. *UCSF*, *12*. doi:10.1177/27536130221144247 PMID:37077178

Slivjak, E., Kirk, A., & Arch, J. J. (2023). The Psychophysiology of Self-Compassion. In Springer eBooks (pp. 291–307). Springer. doi:10.1007/978-3-031-22348-8_17

Snodgrass, J. G. (2023). *The Avatar faculty: Ecstatic Transformations in Religion and Video Games*. Univ of California Press.

Soni, L., & Kaur, A. (2023). Strategies for Implementing Metaverse in Education. In *2023 International Conference on Disruptive Technologies (ICDT)*. IEEE. 10.1109/ICDT57929.2023.10150886

Steinhoff, L., & Martin, K. D. (2022). Putting Data Privacy Regulation into Action: The Differential Capabilities of Service Frontline Interfaces. *Journal of Service Research*, *26*(3), 330–350. doi:10.1177/10946705221141925

Stockly, K. J., & Wildman, W. J. (2022). Interpreting the rapidly changing landscape of spirit tech. *Religion, Brain & Behavior*, *13*(1), 109–118. doi:10.1080/2153599X.2022.2091010

Suh, I. H., McKinney, T., & Siu, K. (2023). Current Perspective of Metaverse Application in Medical Education, Research and Patient Care. *MDPI*, *2*(2), 115–128. doi:10.3390/virtualworlds2020007

Sullivan, M., Huberty, J., Chung, Y., & Stecher, C. (2023). Mindfulness meditation app Abandonment during the COVID-19 Pandemic: An observational study. *Mindfulness*, *14*(6), 1504–1521. doi:10.100712671-023-02125-4 PMID:37362188

Sun, T., Jin, T., Huang, Y., Meng, L., Yun, W., Jiang, Z., & Fu, X. (2023). Restoring Dunhuang Murals: Crafting Cultural Heritage Preservation Knowledge into Immersive Virtual Reality Experience Design. *International Journal of Human-Computer Interaction*, 1–22. doi:10.1080/10447318.2023.2232976

Tai, B., Tsou, Y., Li, S., Huang, Y., Tsai, P., & Tsai, Y. (2023). User-Driven Synthetic Dataset Generation with Quantifiable Differential Privacy. *IEEE Transactions on Services Computing*, *16*(5), 1–14. doi:10.1109/TSC.2023.3287239

Tan, F. F., Ram, A., Haigh, C., & Zhao, S. (2023). *Mindful Moments: Exploring On-the-go Mindfulness Practice On Smart-glasses*. ACM. doi:10.1145/3563657.3596030

Tayyab, M., Marjani, M., Jhanjhi, N. Z., Hashem, I. T., Usmani, R. S. A., & Qamar, F. (2023). A comprehensive review on deep learning algorithms: Security and privacy issues. *Computers & Security*, *131*, 103297. doi:10.1016/j.cose.2023.103297

Tekin, B. H., & Gutiérrez, R. U. (2023). Human-centred health-care environments: A new framework for biophilic design. *Frontiers in Medical Technology*, *5*, 1219897. doi:10.3389/fmedt.2023.1219897 PMID:37560462

Toussaint, L., Huynh, K., Kohls, N., Sirois, F. M., Alberts, H., Hirsch, J. K., Hanshans, C., Nguyen, Q., Van Der Zee-Neuen, A., & Offenbaecher, M. (2023). Expectations regarding Gastein Healing Gallery treatment and their connection to Health-Related quality of life. *International Journal of Environmental Research and Public Health*, *20*(7), 5426. doi:10.3390/ijerph20075426 PMID:37048040

Turdialiev, M. (2023). *Legal discussion of metaverse Law*. doi:10.59022/ijcl.36

Uddin, M., Manickam, S., Ullah, H., Obaidat, M., & Dandoush, A. (2023). Unveiling the metaverse: Exploring emerging trends, multifaceted perspectives, and future challenges. *IEEE Access : Practical Innovations, Open Solutions*, *1*, 87087–87103. doi:10.1109/ACCESS.2023.3281303

Üstün, A., Yılmaz, R., & Yılmaz, F. G. K. (2022). Educational UTAUT-based virtual reality acceptance scale: A validity and reliability study. *Virtual Reality (Waltham Cross)*, *27*(2), 1063–1076. doi:10.100710055-022-00717-4

Veber, M., Pesek, I., & Aberšek, B. (2023). Assessment of supporting visual learning technologies in the Immersive VET Cyber-Physical Learning Model. *Education in Science*, *13*(6), 608. doi:10.3390/educsci13060608

Velissaris, S. L., Davis, M., Fisher, F., Gluyas, C., & Stout, J. C. (2023). A pilot evaluation of an 8-week mindfulness-based stress reduction program for people with pre-symptomatic Huntington's disease. *Journal of Community Genetics*, *14*(4), 395–405. doi:10.100712687-023-00651-1 PMID:37458974

Villalón, F., Moreno, M. I. B., Rivera, R. M., & Venegas, W. G. JVC, N., Soto-Mota, A., & Pemjean, A. (2023). Brief Online Mindfulness- and Compassion-Based Inter-Care Program for Students during COVID-19 Pandemic: A randomized controlled trial. *Mindfulness*. doi:10.100712671-023-02159-8

Wang, Y., Weng, T., Tsai, I. F., Kao, J., & Chang, Y. J. (2022). Effects of virtual reality on creativity performance and perceived immersion: A study of brain waves. *British Journal of Educational Technology*, *54*(2), 581–602. doi:10.1111/bjet.13264

Weisbrod, A. V., Bohman, L., & Ramdial, K. J. (2023). From theory to practice: A novel meditation program at a global corporation. *Current Psychology (New Brunswick, N.J.)*. doi:10.100712144-023-04516-1 PMID:37359588

Wexler, T. M., & Schellinger, J. (2022). Mindfulness-Based Stress Reduction for Nurses: An Integrative Review. *Journal of Holistic Nursing*. doi:10.1177/08980101221079472 PMID:35213264

Whiting, A., Sharma, Y., Grewal, M. K., Ghulam, Z., Sajid, W., Dewan, N., Peladeau-Pigeon, M., & Dutta, T. (2023). Virtual Accessible Bilingual conference planning: The Parks Accessibility Conference. *International Journal of Environmental Research and Public Health*, *20*(3), 2302. doi:10.3390/ijerph20032302 PMID:36767670

Williams, R. (2023). Think piece: Ethics for the virtual researcher. *Practice*, *5*(1), 1–7. doi:10.1080/25783858.2023.2179893

Wong, I. A., Lu, M. V., Lin, S. K., & Lin, Z. (2022). The transformative virtual experience paradigm: The case of Airbnb's online experience. *International Journal of Contemporary Hospitality Management*. doi:10.1108/ijchm-12-2021-1554

Wu, J., Tang, J., & Agyeiwaah, E. (2023). 'I had more time to listen to my inner voice': Zen meditation tourism for Generation Z. *Tourist Studies*. doi:10.1177/14687976231189833

Wu, Y. C., Maymon, C., Paden, J., & Liu, W. (2023). Launching your VR Neuroscience Laboratory. In Current topics in behavioral neurosciences. doi:10.1007/7854_2023_420

Yin, C., Huang, Y., Kim, D., & Kim, K. (2023). The Effect of Esports Content Attributes on Viewing Flow and Well-Being: A focus on the moderating effect of esports involvement. *Sustainability*, *15*(16), 12207. doi:10.3390u151612207

You, Y., & Youn, C. T. (2023). Research on the happiness experience structure of elderly people in metaverse. *Han'gug Di'jain Munhwa Haghoeji*, *29*(2), 339–353. doi:10.18208/ksdc.2023.29.2.339

Yue, Y., Yi, S., Nan, X., Leo, Y.-H. L., Shigyo, K., Liwenhan, X., Wicaksana, J., & Cheng, K.-T. (2023). FoodWise: Food Waste Reduction and Behavior Change on Campus with Data Visualization and Gamification. In *Proceedings of the 6th ACM SIGCAS/SIGCHI Conference on Computing and Sustainable Societies*. ACM. 10.1145/3588001.3609364

Zainab, H. E., Bawany, N. Z., Rehman, W., & Imran, J. (2023). Design and development of virtual reality exposure therapy systems: Requirements, challenges and solutions. *Multimedia Tools and Applications*. doi:10.100711042-023-15756-5

Zaman, N., Gaur, L., & Humayun, M. (2022). *Approaches and applications of deep learning in virtual medical care*. IGI Global. doi:10.4018/978-1-7998-8929-8

Zhang, J. (2023). *Exploring gender expression and identity in virtual reality : The interplay of avatars, role-adoption, and social interaction in VRChat*. DIVA. https://www.diva-portal.org/smash/record.jsf?pid=diva2%3A1765332&dswid=-4051

Zhi, L. J., Heng, T. M., & Taojun, X. (2023). Evaluating the impact of digital economy collaborations in ASEAN. In Routledge eBooks (pp. 8–27). doi:10.4324/9781003308751-2

Chapter 4
A Combined Survey on Machine Learning for Cognitive Radio Deployed on Secure WBAN Environments

M. V. Karthikeyan
St. Joseph's Institute of Technology, India

Tephillah Sophia
https://orcid.org/0000-0002-6554-4813
St. Joseph's Institute of Technology, India

M. Senthil Murugan
St. Joseph's Institute of Technology, India

D. Suresh
St. Joseph's Institute of Technology, India

M. Samayaraj Murali Kishanlal
St. Joseph's Institute of Technology, India

T. Siva
St. Joseph's Institute of Technology, India

ABSTRACT

Wireless body area network (WBAN) security and cognitive radio networks (CRNs) are two separate topics in the field of wireless communication, but they can be related in some ways. WBANs are wireless networks that are designed to operate on or around the human body, typically for medical or healthcare applications. These networks often involve small, low-power devices that can monitor vital signs, track movement, or even deliver medication. Security is a critical concern in WBANs, as they often deal with sensitive personal information and may be vulnerable to various types of attacks. Some of the security challenges in WBANs include confidentiality, integrity, availability, privacy, and authentication. CRNs are wireless networks that allow devices to dynamically adapt to their environment by changing their transmission and reception parameters. This technology can improve the efficiency and reliability of wireless communication, but it also introduces security challenges, an attacker may try to manipulate the cognitive radio's sensing mechanism or jam the spectrum to disrupt the network. potential connections between WBAN security and CRNs. For instance, cognitive radios can be used to enhance the security of WBANs by providing more secure communication channels or detecting and mitigating attacks. Some of the security mechanisms developed for WBANs, such as secure authentication and encryption protocols, can be applied to CRNs to improve their security posture. WBAN security and CRNs are distinct topics, there is potential for these technologies to complement each other and enhance the overall security of wireless networks. the relationship between WBAN and CRN's is the specific objective is the primarily centered around spectrum management, interference mitigation, and secure spectrum sharing. By intelligently adapting to the wireless environment and optimizing spectrum usage, CR can enhance the security and reliability of WBAN communication in healthcare and other contexts where WBANs are deployed.

DOI: 10.4018/978-1-6684-9823-1.ch004

1. INTRODUCTION WBAN

The new inventions in health care devices have led to a considerable increase in the human life span. Miniaturized bio-sensing elements and dedicated wireless communication bands have led to the development of a new arena called Wireless Body Area Networks (WBANs) (IEEE 802.11.6). WBAN was first introduced by Zimmerman T.G (1996), and was initially known as Wireless Personal Area Networks (WPAN) in which the node has a transmission range of three meters. Body Area Networks (BAN) plays a significant role in medical, non-medical, military and emergency services. According to the World Health Organization (WHO) survey, cardiovascular diseases affected an estimated 17.5 million people in 2012, representing 31 percent of all global sicknesses. All over the world, 180 million people are currently affected by diabetes and around the year 2030, it is expected to be 360 million. A rapid rise in Neuro-degenerative diseases such as Alzheimer's and Parkinson's is threatening millions more. In India, there is a significant growth in the population of aged people and the expenses spent on caretakers are getting increased. The author [1] mentioned the need for an inexpensive monitoring device and a secure communication system for monitoring at the doctor's end.

Devices like wearable ECG, Electromyography (EMG), Electroencephalography (EEG), Blood Pressure (BP), Oxygen Saturation (SpO2) and temperature monitor the subject and collect the data. The developments of WBAN technology made it practical to sense and communicate various medical and non-medical signal applications as shown in Figure 1.

Figure 1. WBAN applications

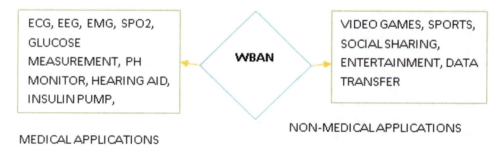

This vital information is communicated through an open wireless channel to the doctor's programming device on demand or on a daily basis. The communication of these signals are made through dedicated frequencies like Wireless Medical Telemetry Services (WMTS), unlicensed Industrial Scientific and Medical (ISM)

Band, Ultra-Wide Band and Medical Implanted Communication services (MICS) band for bio-medical signal transmission [2] . The WMTS is urged by Federal Communication Commission (FCC) only eight medical devices operate on the 14 MHz band and only authorized persons are allowed to operate this medical frequency. A licensed MICS band used to communicate between sensors which operate in a frequency range of 402 – 405MHz. Thus, a more collusion free radio network is provided, but still, the data transmitted is kept open in the transmission medium [3]. This Body area Node (BN) or Implantable Medical Devices (IMDs) are kept invasive to the human body, thus making a miniature structure. The BN consists of a wireless module, a small processor and a miniature battery. Therefore, it became mandatory to design a Light Weight (LW) operating system with an LW security algorithm to protect the data and device from an attacker. The IMD placed in the human body is connected to another reliable node or to an IMD programmer through a wireless telemetry interface. The wireless communication between devices is not an authenticated channel and unencrypted information is transmitted. The wireless module has simple password protection, and once it is cracked, it's possible to wirelessly re-configure the software protocol (that is intended for a lifesaving purpose) or alter the transmitted signal. This PV has more valuable information when hacked during communication and can mislead to false treatment leading to life-threatening situations. The various wireless telemetry interface security threats are analyzed. And also security attacks with special emphasis are given for the security issues of data privacy and device authentication during communication.

1.2 WBAN Architecture

Each IMD is an electronic device, implanted in the human body to monitor and/or collect the PV forwards to it. The Body area Network Coordinator (BNC) or simply called as a programmer is an external device which has the ability to access data in the IMD and program it wirelessly. Both the devices are currently standard medical devices and most IMDs have the capability of measuring the ECG signal [4]. The architecture of WBAN with various communication levels shown in Figure 2 [5].

The general WBAN communication level is detailed below:

i) Tire 1 / Level 1: This forms the basic transmission structure of the WBAN communication with a three-meter range. The BN kept invasive is in direct contact with the human body at the lower level, and senses the PV from the human. The BN that measures the PV is communicated to the BNC. The authentication of the device and the privacy of the data between the communicating nodes are focused. The BNC can be an external programming device within less than one meter to configure the IMD.

Figure 2. Architecture of WBAN

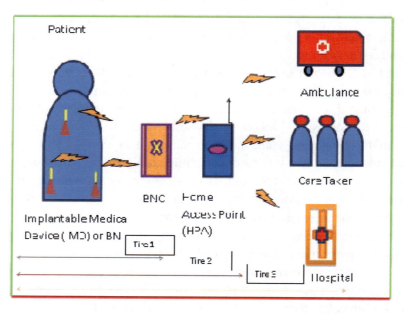

ii) Tire 2 / Level 2: The BNC collects the data but does not have any resource constraint like computation complexity, memory and energy consumption because it is kept outside the human body. Then it forwards the aggregated data to the Home Access Point (HAP).

iii) Tire 3/ Level 3: The data collected in the HAP is transmitted over a secure channel for long distance to a Hospital, caretaker and to an ambulatory service during emergencies.

The work is concentrated in level 1 WBAN device security, since it is necessary to refer various threats arising in it a satisfactory security solutions is needed. The working scenario is shown with IMD and programmer in Figure 3. A LW security solution is developed for data privacy and device authentication between the devices. The IMD in WBAN is a combination of the following sub-systems; a sensing element, a radio transceiver, an Analog to Digital Converter (ADC), memory to store the sensed information, patients' identity, microprocessor to compile the application specific programmer and battery to manage the overall device power requirement. Only authorized medical staff should be able to adjust the IMD settings and access the data stored in the IMD. Current commercialized IMD have limited resources for applying security measures and are placed in the market without any preventive method against security threats. In fact, the possibilities for a hacker to break into a

ML for Cognitive Radio Deployed on Secure WBAN Environments

Figure 3. Proposed system model with IMD and programmer in WBAN

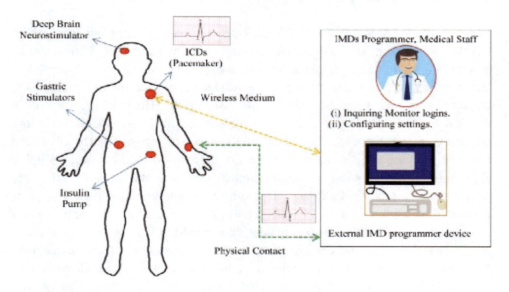

device to obtain sensitive health-related data and alter the device settings intentionally to malfunction have been reported.

The proposed system consists of two components – an Implantable Cardioverter Defibrillator (ICD) and an external programmer. The ICD is a medical device which is implanted in the patient's body to continuously monitor the patient's health. Hereafter, the ICD or any other re-configurable device is represented as IMD. An external ECG sensor placed on the patient's wrist is connected to the programmer and measures the ECG signal. The IMDs are surgically implanted systems and wireless communication with an external programmer should be established to access the IMD configuration. The IMDs such as Implantable Cardioverter Defibrillators (ICDs) and Implantable drug delivery pumps sense the disorders and treat patients with therapies. Then a doctor uses a programmer device to communicate and diagnose the problem. In some situations when a change in the IMD setting is needed, by connecting the programming device the IMD can be reconfigured to act according to the patient's current medical condition; all these actions will be done through the wireless module of the IMD. However, IMDs wirelessly communicate with programmers, use Radio Frequency (RF) through the MICS band, and have greater communication ranges and higher data rates. The IMDs have a battery that can last for up to eight years for Neuro-stimulators and ten years for pacemakers. The exact period is dependent on the patient's abnormal physiological conditions over time, and more energy will be consumed by the IMD to react and apply therapy.

1.3 WBAN Security

Wireless Body Area Networks (WBANs) have been a game-changer in the healthcare industry, but they also present new security challenges. With sensitive patient information being transmitted wirelessly, it's crucial to ensure the privacy and confidentiality of this data. Device producers, regulatory agencies (FDA, Department of Homeland Security), trade associations (Heart Rhythm Society), medical professionals, IT security experts, and, last but not least, patients (including advocacy groups) work together to ensure the cybersecurity of CIEDs. Given the resource limitations on computation and the necessity to address cryptographic algorithms, the cybersecurity elements must be taken into account during the device's design process. Following this, a thorough and unbiased review of post-implant threat analysis and accurate reporting of cyberattack incidents should be conducted. When it's feasible, patient data should always be encrypted using asymmetrical encryption techniques. On the basis of the values of secrecy, integrity, authenticity, accountability, and reliability, strict data transfer procedures should be adhered to.One of the biggest concerns is unauthorized access or interception of data by malicious individuals. This is where encryption techniques come into play. By encrypting the data, it becomes unreadable for anyone who doesn't have a decryption key, making it virtually impossible to be intercepted.Another concern is ensuring that only authorized devices are connected to the WBAN network. One solution to this problem is using authentication protocols that require devices to provide credentials before being granted access.In addition to these measures, physical security of devices must also be considered. Lost or stolen devices can compromise patient data integrity and confidentiality. Having strict policies in place for device use and storage can help mitigate these risks.While WBANs offer many benefits in healthcare settings, it's important that their security isn't compromised. Implementing robust security measures can help ensure both efficiency and safety when using wireless technology in healthcare applications

1.4 Biomedical Device Security With Secret Key Generation

Machine learning has become a valuable tool in biomedical research, but the increasing use of connected medical devices also raises concerns about security. To address this issue, biomedical device manufacturers are looking into adopting strong security practices [6]. One approach to securing connected devices involves authenticating each device using secret identification codes. This can be done through challenge-response protocols to ensure that the device is genuine, and the use of secret key generation can strengthen security measures. By implementing these security measures, patients can have more peace of mind knowing that their medical devices are secure and trustworthy.

Biomedical device manufacturers are taking strong security measures to ensure the security and authenticity of their devices. This includes the adoption of secret identification codes and secret key generation to prevent counterfeit devices from being introduced to the market. For wireless medical devices, cryptographic techniques such as encryption, authentication, and secure key storage are necessary to protect communications and accesses. [7] In addition, multi-party quantum key agreement protocols have been proposed as a secure method for secret key generation in biomedical device security. These measures are crucial in ensuring the safety and privacy of patients as well as the integrity of biomedical research. Machine learning has been proposed as a method for generating secret keys to ensure the security and authenticity of medical devices. This approach involves using machine learning algorithms to generate a private key, which can then be used for encrypting and decrypting sensitive patient data. In addition to this, healthcare security solutions that utilize machine learning have been developed to enhance the quality and performance of the Internet of Medical Things (IoMT). These solutions analyze the data collected from medical devices using edge computing to detect and prevent security breaches. Such measures are crucial in protecting the privacy and safety of patients and maintaining the integrity of biomedical research.

The proposed model [8] by the author is an ECG signal based one-time secret key generation with a lightweight Secure Force (SF) Algorithm. In this model the patient ECG signals monitored for a predetermined amount of time, over it eight different values are calculated and the least significant values are extracted to create the 8-bit secret key. This one time key is securely shared with the external device. The main advantage is the key is generated with the highly random bits, thus it will be unique and reputation impossible. This entire module is implemented in a raspberry pi3 stand-alone module.

1.5 Biomedical Device Security With Secret Key Agreement

Machine learning has become an important tool in biomedical research, used for tasks such as drug discovery, disease diagnosis, and personalized treatment recommendations. [6] However, the increasing use of connected medical devices raises concerns about security. Biomedical device manufacturers are adopting strong security practices such as secret identification codes and secret key generation to ensure that the devices are genuine and secure. [7] Multi-party quantum key agreement protocols have been proposed to set up a secure secret key between two users in biomedical device security. [8]

Machine learning has proven to be a valuable tool in the field of biomedical research, helping researchers with tasks such as drug discovery and disease diagnosis. [6] Biomedical device manufacturers are aware of the importance of security and are adopting strong security practices, including secret identification codes and secret key generation, to ensure the devices are genuine and secure. [7] In the case of wireless medical devices, cryptographic techniques such as encryption, authentication, and secure key storage are necessary to protect communications and accesses. [8] Multi-party quantum key agreement protocols have been proposed for secure secret key generation in biomedical device security.

Machine learning has been proposed as a method for generating secret keys and enhancing the quality and performance of the Internet of Medical Things (IoMT) healthcare security solutions. One such approach is to use machine learning algorithms to aggregate secret keys generated by different devices in a secure and efficient manner. This method can improve the security of medical devices, while also reducing the computational overhead. The key aggregation process involves combining the individual secret keys generated by multiple devices into a single shared key. Machine learning algorithms can be used to analyze the individual keys and determine the optimal way to combine them [9]. This approach can improve the overall security of the IoMT system, as it reduces the risk of individual keys being compromised.

Machine learning algorithms can also be used to generate secret keys from biometric data, such as fingerprints or facial recognition. This approach can provide an additional layer of security, as biometric data is unique to each individual and difficult to replicate. Overall, machine learning-based secret key aggregation is a promising approach for enhancing the security of medical devices in the IoMT system. By adopting strong security practices, biomedical device manufacturers can protect the privacy and safety of patients, while maintaining the integrity of biomedical research.

The secret key must be securely shared with the implanted pacemaker and the external device for data extraction and for remote programming. In this proposed work [7], the Implanted Medical Device (IMD) and the external ECG machine must be synchronized first, then both the devices sense the monitor the ECG signal. In the next stage the IMD generate a random number with Pseudo Random Number Generation; this is hidden in the ECG signal. In the next stage, with reference as QRS points from the ECG signal, with the Flower Pollination Algorithm (FPA) which is a Light weight Algorithm generates the chaff points. All the three values, ECG signal, chaff points and the secret key are transmitted to the external ECG programming machine. At the same time the external ECG machine also measures the ECG signal in a time synchronized manner, based on the ECG signal QRS reference points with FPA the chaff points are generated. During the last stage both the received signal from IMD is subtracted with the locally generated signal, both the ECG signal and chaff point get cancelled, the left out data is the secret key. Thus securely the secret key is agreed with both the devices and now the IMD shared its secret key with the external device and starts its communication [8]. This entire module is implemented in a raspberry pi 3 stand-alone module.

The use of IMDs facilitates the remote monitoring of the health of a patient [9]. The IMDs specially improve the quality of life of elderly people, who other has problem to move easily. A doctor can provide them remote consultation on the basis of their health data, which is collected by the help of IMDs. However, wireless communication raises serious threats in the IMD deployment. In this paper, we proposed a remote user authentication scheme through which a user (a doctor) and a controller node can mutually authenticate each other and establish a session key for their future secure communication [9]. Apart from that the pairwise key establishment between a controller node and its IMDs is also provided in the proposed scheme for the secure communication between them. The computation and communication costs of the proposed scheme are comparable with the existing related schemes. In addition, the proposed scheme also provides better security and more functionality features, such as password and biometric update phase, dynamic controller node and IMD addition phases, as compared to other existing related schemes.

In 6G-enabled devices there is lot of convenience which includes the flexibility and speed, which can be well deployed in various industrial applications and significantly useful in medical related areas, which the possibility various passive and active attacks due to the insecure channel communication between entities. In the proposed work [10] IMD(Implantable Medicinal Device) application present three-factor remote client validation convention for implantable therapeutic gadgets correspondence condition, the proposed plan, in that the client (for instance, a patient) their body is set in with (IMDs), such as insulin, siphon and pacemaker. All these IMDs screen the patient's wellbeing. IMDs have its very own functionalities and offer administrations to the patient based on their side effects. IMDs likewise have remote correspondence include (for instance, Bluetooth innovation) utilizing through which the they can transfer the patient's verified information to the close-by controller hub. Gathers detected data safely from IMD. Assume there is a client (for instance, a specialist) User needs to get to the ongoing information from a specific hub for observing and analysis of the patient remotely. In this situation, we require verification among User and hubs. After common verification among User and hubs, they set up a session key for the further secure correspondence.

Machine learning is being increasingly utilized in the healthcare industry to improve the security of biomedical devices and protect patient privacy. One of the applications is the generation of secret keys and the aggregation of keys using machine learning techniques. By using machine learning, the quality and performance of the

Internet of Medical Things (IoMT) is enhanced. Additionally, machine learning-based secret key aggregation is a promising approach for improving the security of medical devices in the IoMT system. This approach addresses challenges such as statistical heterogeneity, data partitioning, and fragmentation [9]. The use of cryptographic techniques such as encryption and authentication, along with the generation of secret identification codes, is also being implemented to ensure authenticity and protect patient privacy. Wireless Body Area Networks (WBANs) and Machine Learning (ML) are two important areas of research in the field of healthcare technology. WBANs refer to a network of wearable or implantable devices that can monitor various physiological parameters of a person such as heart rate, blood pressure, body temperature, and so on. ML, on the other hand, is a subset of Artificial Intelligence that uses algorithms to analyze data, identify patterns, and make predictions. The combination of WBANs and ML can have numerous applications in healthcare. For example, ML algorithms can be trained on data collected from WBANs to predict the onset of certain medical conditions such as heart disease, diabetes, or epilepsy. Additionally, ML can be used to analyze data from WBANs to identify trends and patterns that can help healthcare providers make more informed decisions about a patient's care.[10-11] However, there are also challenges associated with the use of WBANs and ML in healthcare. One major challenge is the need to ensure the security and privacy of the data collected from WBANs. Additionally, there is a need for more research to develop robust ML algorithms that can accurately analyze the complex and heterogeneous data collected from WBANs. Overall, the combination of WBANs and ML has the potential to revolutionize healthcare by providing real-time monitoring and analysis of a patient's physiological parameters, leading to better diagnosis, treatment, and management of medical conditions.

To address cyber security issues related to CIEDs, it is crucial that all parties, including medical device manufacturers, federal regulatory agencies, doctors, and patient advocacy groups, unite on a common platform. Security should be taken into account from the design stage to the implementation and post-marketing survey stages. The lack of transparency and persistent denial on the part of medical makers about the security issues brought up by independent auditors and cyber security firms is a concern in post marketing surveillance. Federal agencies, particularly the FDA, should play a crucial role as the gatekeeper of such dialogues and should keep an eye on businesses to ensure that security concerns are addressed quickly. It will improve patient communication and enhance adherence to firmware and other security updates proposed by manufacturers if physicians are involved in the dialogue to create a better awareness on their part of such security risks. Security is a critical concern when it comes to Wireless Body Area Networks (WBANs) and Machine Learning (ML). WBANs typically involve the transmission of sensitive medical data over wireless networks, which make them vulnerable to various security threats such as eavesdropping, data tampering, and unauthorized access.ML algorithms can also be vulnerable to security threats such as adversarial attacks, where an attacker intentionally modifies the input data to deceive the ML algorithm and cause it to produce incorrect results. To address these security concerns, various techniques can be employed. For example, encryption can be used to secure the transmission of data over wireless networks. Access control mechanisms can also be implemented to ensure that only authorized users have access to the data collected from WBANs. In addition, ML algorithms can be designed to be more robust to security threats. For example, techniques such as anomaly detection and outlier analysis can be used to detect and mitigate adversarial attacks. Overall, security is an important consideration when it comes to WBANs and ML. By employing appropriate security measures, the potential benefits of WBANs and ML can be realized while minimizing the risks associated with security threats.

2. WBAN AND COGNITIVE RADIO (CR) NETWORKS

Wireless Body Area Networks (WBANs) have revolutionized the healthcare industry by enabling continuous, non-invasive monitoring of patients in real-time. However, with this new technology comes new challenges, especially when it comes to security. That's where Cognitive Radio Networks come into play! In this blog post, we'll explore how WBANs and Cognitive Radio Networks work together to ensure both efficiency and safety in the world of wireless healthcare. So grab a cup of coffee and let's dive in!

2.1 WBAN Usage Cognitive Radio Networks

Wireless Body Area Networks (WBANs) have been around for quite some time now and they are a promising technology that can revolutionize healthcare. WBANs are low-power, wireless devices used to monitor the vital signs of humans such as heart rate, blood pressure, temperature, and more. They enable real-time monitoring of patients which is crucial in emergency situations.Cognitive Radio Networks (CRNs), on the other hand, are intelligent radio networks that dynamically allocate spectrum bands to different radio devices based on their requirements. With CRNs in place alongside WBANs, there is now an opportunity to improve not only the functionality of WBANs but also its security.The usage of cognitive radio networks in WBANs allows for improved network reliability and better efficiency utilization of scarce bandwidth resources by enabling dynamic channel allocation algorithms based on network conditions. This ensures optimal use of available frequencies while reducing interference between different medical sensors operating within the same room or vicinity.Moreover, this combination enables secure communication between different medical sensors and health care providers by utilizing advanced encryption techniques such as LightWeight Cryptography (LWC). Using Cognitive Radio Networks with Wireless Body Area Networks can significantly improve healthcare services while maintaining security standards.

2.2 Cognitive Radio Networks

Cognitive radio networks have emerged as a promising solution for efficient utilization of wireless spectrum resources. With the increasing demand for wireless communication and the limited availability of frequency bands, cognitive radio networks are becoming more important than ever before.By combining WBANs with cognitive radio technologies, we can achieve better security and reliability in healthcare applications. The ability to sense the environment and adapt to changing network conditions makes it possible to create dynamic networks that can adjust their parameters on-the-fly.As technology continues to evolve at an unprecedented pace, there will be many challenges ahead in terms of designing secure and efficient wireless communication systems. However, by leveraging the power of cognitive radio networks together with WBANs, we can address these challenges and pave the way towards a brighter future for wireless communications.CRN defines the new paradigm for sharing the unused and used spectrum effectively in the proliferation environment. The intelligent device formulates the dynamic behavior of the spectrum and its availability to the unlicensed user to maximize the utilization efficiency.

In [12], have given a contempary survey on the utility of ML for CR applications. Spectrum sensing is one of the basic and important task of CRN, [13] have specified the ML framework for spectrum sensing. In [14], the deep convolution neural network has been proposed. The NN is trained with power spectrum of the input signal with different types of modulation schemes such as BPSK, QPSK and QAM. Another Deep learning algorithm model is specified in [15] for checking the status of the PU, where the energy measurement in each frequency band is taken in matrix form to train the algorithm. The Reinforcement Learning algorithm decreases the overhead by the above method by selecting only few CR's for updating the energy levels. Another task of the CR is the spectrum allocation. Two strategies are proposed, namely Wide Band Predictive Sensing (WBPS) and Q-learning enabled WBPS (QWBPS) in [16]. This technique enables the prediction of various traffic of radio access technologies.

With regard to cooperative spectrum sensing, orthogonal and non-orthogonal multiple access techniques are used to increase the spectrum utility. In [17], different ML algorithms such as K-means, SVM, KNN and back propagation are trained with the energy measured from the CR's over some time slots and tested with the same. For

Heterogeneous CRN with more mobile CR, the spectrum availability can be affected by shadowing, fading etc. The authors in [18] have specified a Bayesian ML model in which the spatial temporal correlation in spectrum sensing results collected by the mobile CR's are exploited in order to provide the correct sensing results in case of above mentioned demerits. Spectrum auction or leasing is also one of the techniques to utilize the spectrum. ML have also proved their efficiency in the domain. In [19] authors have specified KNN to provide the spectrum to genuine CR's. The KNN classifies the CR's based on the geographical locations, thereby differentiating the virtual and real buyers of spectrum. Ml's also have aided in spectrum prediction of CR. In spectrum prediction, the CR predicts the channel with high probability to become vacant during the next time slot. The authors in [20-22] have specified four different MLs such as recurrent NN, SVM for different traffics. The SVM with linear kernel proved to predict the best among the comparison. In [23], the LSTM model is proposed based on the real world occupancy of spectrum through the analysis of time –frequency correlation. This model was specified in order to overcome the long time dependencies of the spectrum sensing results. The model uses the history of spectrum availability in the form of spectral temporal correlation.

To predict over multiple slots with respect to time, the authors in [24-25] have proposed a deep learning based approach. Initially the samples are collected using the short and long frequency data using deep learning. Further the data from these frequencies are processed by residual networks. Without the prior knowledge of the traffic of primary user, using multilayer perceptron model the predictions are made in [26], thus enabling the implementation in real time scenarios.

The authors in [27-28], in order to learn temporal features from spectral data and to take advantage of other environmental activity statistics like energy, distance, and duty cycle duration for the improvement of sensing performance, the authors propose a hybrid combination of long short-term memory (LSTM) and extreme learning machines (ELM). Security is highly essential in CRN due to the wireless communication between the SU's and PU's. Recent studies have implemented ML algorithms to identify MU's as they provide a way of learning a system without being programmed explicitly [29-30].ML takes the advantage of eliminating need for redesign of the system, maximizes the resource utilization and increases the life span of the network. The rigid approaches proposed in literature cannot combat to the time varying attacks in wireless environment. ML forms a solution to these adaptable behaviors as it learns from the input applied. Also scaling the network to large number of user increases the probability of MU's, which makes its identification difficult. ML handles the difficulty of identification at ease as it can handle large and complex datasets.

Recently ML has found its application in in securing of CRN. The proficiency of ML in distinguishing MU's from honest SU's depends on the better selection of features, training methodology and evaluation procedures [31-32] Many supervised and unsupervised learning methods have been proposed in literature. The analytics provide the description of SVDD algorithm. But the detection of MU's by the formation of the hemisphere is not defined clearly .However, the probabilities of detection and false alarm are highly dependent on the number of attackers and if this number is higher than 20, the probability of detection decreases to 50 percent and the probability of false alarm increases to 100 percent. In [33] the authors have investigated a defense against byzantine attack using supervised ML's- Neural Network, SVM, Naïve Bayes and Ensemble Classifiers. The ML's are considered under two categories i) training and test data draw from the same data set and ii) separate data sets for training and testing. The FC records the sensing results and applies majority voting rule. The frequency of occurrence of the binary output regarding sensing is considered as the types of events and is grouped as dibits and the data set is built. NN, NB, SVM and Ensemble average are the ML's chosen for training. NN and ensemble have proved their consistency in good performance. A comparison of non ML methods with ML methods has proved the robustness of the ML's. A detailed analysis on the design of Neural Network model has also been presented. The validation of the chosen ML's have also been performed for further justification of the optimal model for detecting the MU's. The results are considered for always yes, always no, random yes and random no types of SSDF attackers. The selfish and alternator types of SSDF attackers are not addressed.

The authors in [34] have presented a boosted tree algorithm (BTA) using Adaboost. The method identifies four different SSDF attackers by increasing the weight of weak classifiers. Sensing energies from the SU's are used as feature vectors to the classifier and the classifier categorizes the input energy into either the presence or absence of the PU signal. To avoid biased predictions using individual classifiers, BTA-Ensemble of classifiers has been used [35]. The ensemble classifiers prove the detection accuracy at higher value. The simulations have proven the results. Also global decisions using soft decision schemes have been performed. Comparison of the proposed BTA with other types of ML algorithms for choice of the optimal model is not presented. The author in [36] has suggested the SVM based ML to combat the PUE attack by classifying whether the primary user is genuine or not. The Renyi entropy is given as the input to the SVM. The method proves its uniqueness in low SNR environments. Gaussian Minimum Shift Keying and OFDM are the modulations performed for the SVM to learn the environment. OFDM had a threshold near to lower SNR range. Using the energy detector, the SNR and the Renyi entropy the SVM learns the environment. The SVM plots the hyper plane and classifies the PU whether it is genuine or not. SVM uses the SNR and entropy of the input signal to plot the hyper plane with maximal margin. The results have also proved that the solution increased the detection probability and detects MU's for PUEA in mobile CRN's. Finally the SDR test bed is implemented to prove the practicality of the proposed algorithm.

The authors in [37] have proposed a SETM algorithm to secure the CRN against spectrum sensing data falsification attack. Also the authors have exploited the use of different types of MLs in implementation of SETM algorithm when the number of Secondary users is increased. The logistic regression algorithm has proved to be the best out of SVM, NN, Decision Tree and Bayesian model for a network with 70 SU's.

On the whole ML's have acquired a rapid growth in different applications of CRN. ML's outperform when the scalability of the network increases. Also the choice of training data and number of data used to train the system increases the reliability of ML in different applications.

ML in CRN is also used for spectrum sensing. The energy statistics is utilized as a feature to train the classifiers and assess the status of various frequency channels in order to carry out spectrum sensing. There are two steps in this process: The first distinguishes between the two classes using k-means clustering, an unsupervised machine-learning technique. Additionally, the elements in the data base are labeled. In the second phase, this dataset is used to train a number of supervised machine learning classifiers, which must learn to categorise each channel using these attributes. The probabilities of detection, miss-detection, false alarm, and accuracy are the attributes to assess the effectiveness of the machine learning-based spectrum sensing systems. The possibility of claiming that the main user signal is present when it is truly there is referred to as the probability of detection. The ratio of the number of times the primary user signal is declared present to the total number of times the primary user is present is used to determine this. The probability of missing a principal user signal when one is present is referred to as the probability of miss-detection. It is calculated as the ratio of the number of times the primary user is truly active to the number of times it is detected as inactive. The likelihood that the approach may mistakenly detect the primary user's presence when they are not using it is known as the probability of false alarm. This is determined by dividing the total number of times the primary user has been declared active by the number of times it has been inactive. Another popular statistic in classification issues is classification accuracy. It relates to the likelihood of both recognizing the PU as active when it is actually inactive and detecting it as inactive when it is truly active.

The authors in [38] have developed a machine learning-based approach for spectrum sensing in this study. Using machine learning classifiers, this model performs spectrum sensing to estimate the availability of frequency channels. A large-scale comprehensive dataset is produced and utilized to train, validate, and test various machine learning approaches. In terms of probabilities of detection, false alarm, and miss-detection as well as accuracy, a performance comparison between random forest and the other classifiers such as support vector machines with different classifiers, logistic regression, K-nearest neighbours, and Naive Bayes. For every performance review, random forest yields the best results, with an accuracy rate of up to 99.65%.

The authors in [39, 40] have employed the K-means method in the first stage to determine the primary user's current state. The new input data is collected into one of the classes defined by the K-means method in the first stage using a support vector machine or a classifier of a similar type in the second step. The second group of methods rely on supervised machine learning techniques to train For instance, the authors of [41] utilized supervised machine-learning classifiers such as Nave Bayes, K- closest neighbour, support vector machine, and decision tree in a single step. n models in a single step while presuming that the sensing classes are well-known. The majority of these earlier machine learning models lacked feature selection, which is essential in the context of machine learning theory since it enables the selection of the most pertinent features, which in turn enables the classifiers to have high accuracy.[42-43]

3. COMPARING DIFFERENT MACHINE LEARNING TECHNIQUES APPLIED TO CRNS IN THE CONTEXT OF WBAN SECURITY

Applying machine learning techniques to Cognitive Radio Networks (CRNs) in the context of Wireless Body Area Network (WBAN) security can significantly enhance the security and performance of such networks. Here's a comparison of various machine learning techniques in this context:

3.1. Anomaly Detection

Support vector Machine (SVM):
Pros: SVMs are effective at identifying outliers and anomalies in the network traffic, making them suitable for detecting unusual or suspicious activities in a WBAN.
Cons: They may struggle with high-dimensional data and require careful selection of hyperparameters.
Random Forerst:
Pros: Random Forests can handle high-dimensional data and provide feature importance rankings, which can be helpful in understanding which features are critical for detecting anomalies.
Cons: They may overfit on small datasets.
Neural Networks
Pros: Deep learning models, such as autoencoders, can capture complex patterns in data and are effective at anomaly detection.

Cons: They require a large amount of labeled data for training, which can be a limitation in some cases.

Comparison: All three techniques can be effective for anomaly detection in WBANs. SVMs and Random Forests may be more suitable for smaller datasets, while neural networks excel with larger datasets and complex patterns.

3.2. Intrusion Detection

Decision Trees:

Pros: Decision trees are interpretable and can be used to build rule-based intrusion detection systems.

Cons: They can be prone to overfitting and might not capture complex attack patterns effectively.

K-Nearest Neighbors (KNN):

Pros: KNN can be used for both anomaly detection and classification-based intrusion detection. It's simple to implement.

Cons: It can be sensitive to the choice of the "k" parameter and the distance metric.

Deep Learning (e.g., Convolutional Neural Networks):

Pros: Deep learning models can automatically learn features from data, making them suitable for capturing complex attack patterns.

Cons: They require a substantial amount of labeled data and computational resources for training

Comparison: Decision trees and KNN can be useful for simple intrusion detection tasks in WBANs, while deep learning models can excel when dealing with more sophisticated and evolving attacks

3.3. Resource Management

Reinforcement Learning:

Pros: Reinforcement learning can be used to optimize spectrum allocation in CRNs dynamically, improving resource utilization and reducing interference.

Cons: RL models can be computationally expensive to train and might require extensive fine-tuning.

Q-Learning:

Pros: Q-learning can be used for channel selection in CRNs to minimize interference and maximize throughput.

Cons: It may require a substantial amount of time to converge, and the Q-table can become large for complex CRN scenarios.

Comparison: Reinforcement learning techniques, such as Q-learning or deep reinforcement learning, can be powerful for optimizing resource management in CRNs, including spectrum allocation and interference mitigation.

In conclusion, the choice of machine learning technique for enhancing WBAN security within CRNs depends on the specific security objectives and the available data. Anomaly detection and intrusion detection methods can help identify and respond to security threats, while resource management techniques can optimize the network's performance and resilience. The suitability of each technique also depends on factors like dataset size, computational resources, and the complexity of the problem at hand.[39-40]

4. CONCLUSION

Wireless Body Area Networks (WBANs) and Cognitive Radio (CR) are two distinct technologies in the field of wireless communication, but they can be related in terms of security considerations and potential interactions. Tailored Security Objectives: The security objectives of a WBAN within a CRN should be aligned with the specific use case and application. Different healthcare scenarios may have varying security priorities. For example, ensuring patient data privacy might be the top concern in some cases, while in others, it could be interference mitigation or device authentication. Customized Security Measures: Depending on the objectives, different security measures and techniques may be more appropriate. For instance, if the primary concern is data privacy, encryption and access control mechanisms may take precedence. In contrast, if interference mitigation is crucial, spectrum management and interference detection methods become more critical. Resource Constraints: WBANs typically operate in resource-constrained environments, which can influence the choice of security mechanisms. The network's energy efficiency, processing power, and bandwidth limitations must be considered when implementing security solutions. Adaptability and Flexibility: CRNs are known for their adaptability to dynamic environments. Security solutions within CRNs should be flexible and capable of adjusting to changes in the network conditions and security threats. Cognitive radios can assist in adapting security measures to evolving situations. Interplay of Machine Learning: Machine learning techniques can play a significant role in enhancing WBAN security within CRNs. The choice of machine learning algorithms should also be tailored to the specific security objectives, whether it's anomaly detection, intrusion detection, or resource optimization. In, conclusion, WBAN security within

CRNs is not a one-size-fits-all approach. It requires a careful assessment of the unique security requirements and objectives of the specific use case. By tailoring security measures to these objectives and considering the constraints and opportunities presented by CR technology, organizations can create robust and effective security solutions for their WBAN deployments.

REFERENCES

Agarwal, A., Dubey, S., Khan, M. A., Gangopadhyay, R., & Debnath, S. (2016). Learning based primary user activity prediction in cognitive radio networks for efficient dynamic spectrum access. *Proc. International Conference on Signal Processing and Communications (SPCOM),* (pp. 1–5). IEEE. 10.1109/SPCOM.2016.7746632

Arjoune, Y., & Kaabouch, N. (2019). On Spectrum Sensing, a Machine Learning Method for Cognitive Radio Systems. *2019 IEEE International Conference on Electro Information Technology (EIT),* (pp. 333-338). IEEE. 10.1109/EIT.2019.8834099

Bourouis, A., Feham, M., & Bouchachia, A. (2011). Ubiquitous Mobile Health Monitoring System for Elderly (UMHMSE). *International Journal of Computer Science and Information Technologies*, *3*(3), 74–82. doi:10.5121/ijcsit.2011.3306

Chaudhary, M., Gaur, L., Chakrabarti, A., & Jhanjhi, N. Z. (2023). Unravelling the Barriers of Human Resource Analytics: Multi-Criteria Decision-Making Approach. *Journal of Survey in Fisheries Sciences*, 306-321.

Crosby, G., Ghosh, T., Murimi, R., & Chin, C. (2012). Wireless Body Area Networks for Healthcare: A Survey. *International Journal of Ad hoc, Sensor & Ubiquitous Computing, 3.*

Karthikeyan, M. V. (2019ECG-Signal Based Secret Key Generation (ESKG) Scheme for WBAN and Hardware Implementation. *J. Martin Leo Manickam, Wireless Personal Communications, Springer, 106*(4), 2037–2052. doi:10.100711277-018-5924-x

Gul, N., Khan, M. S., Kim, S. M., Kim, J., Elahi, A., & Khalil, Z. (2020). Boosted trees algorithm as reliable spectrum sensing scheme in the presence of malicious users. *Electronics (Basel)*, *9*(6), 1–23. doi:10.3390/electronics9061038

Karthikeyan, M. V. & Manickam, M. (2017). A 128-Bit Secret Key Generation Using Unique Ecg Bio-Signal for Medical Data Cryptography in Lightweight Wireless Body Area Networks. *Journal of Pakistan journal of Biotechnology, 14*(2), 257-264.

Karthikeyan, M. V. & Manickam, M. (2017). A novel fast chaff point generation method using bio-inspired flower pollination algorithm for fuzzy vault systems with physiological signal for wireless body area sensor networks. *Artificial Intelligent Techniques for Bio-Medical Signal Processing.* Biomedical Research.

Karthikeyan, M. V. & Manickam, M. (2017). An enhanced flower pollination algorithm based chaff point generation method with hardware implementation in WBAN. *International Journal of Communication Systems.* Wiley. . doi:10.1002/dac.4447

Karthikeyan, M. V. & Manickam, M. (2017). Efficient Bio-Signal Feature Based Secure Secret Key Generation Scheme a Simplified Model for Wireless Body Area Network (EFSKG Scheme). *Journal of Medical Imaging and Health Informatics, American Scientific Publishers, 8*(5). . doi:10.1166/jmihi.2018.2415

Karthikeyan, M. V. & Manickam, M. (2017). Security Issues in Wireless Body Area Networks: In Bio-signal Input Fuzzy Security. *Research Journal of Pharmaceutical, Biological and Chemical Sciences,. 7*(6), 1755-1773.

Karthikeyan, M. V. & Manickam, M. (2017). Secret Key Generation Of 128-Bits Using Patient ECG Signal and Secret Transmission For IMDs Authentication. *International Journal of Pure and Applied Mathematics.*

Karthikeyan, M. V. (2021). Raspberry Pi implemented with MATLAB simulation and communication of Physiological Signal based fast Chaff point (RPSC) generation algorithm for WBAN systems. *Biomedical Engineering/Biomedizinische Technik, 66*(2). . doi:10.1515/bmt-2019-0336

Khalfi, B., Zaid, A., & Hamdaoui, B. (2017). When Machine Learning Meets Compressive Sampling for Wideband Spectrum Sensing. *Wireless Communications and Mobile Computing Conference,* (pp. 1120-1125). IEEE. 10.1109/IWCMC.2017.7986442

Li, H., Ding, X., Yang, Y., Huang, X., & Zhang, G. (2019). Spectrum occupancy prediction for internet of things via long short-term memory. *Proc. IEEE International Conference on Consumer Electronics - Taiwan (ICCE-TW).* IEEE. 10.1109/ICCE-TW46550.2019.8991968

Liu, H., Zhu, X., & Fujii, T. (2019). Ensemble deep learning based cooperative spectrum sensing with semi-soft stacking fusion center. In *Proceedings of the 2019 IEEE Wireless Communications and Networking Conference (WCNC),* Marrakesh, Morocco. 10.1109/WCNC.2019.8885866

Lu, Y., Zhu, P., Wang, D., & Fattouche, M. (2016). Machine Learning Techniques with Probability Vector for Cooperative Spectrum Sensing in Cognitive Radio Networks. *IEEE Wireless Communications and Networking Conference*, (pp. 1-6). IEEE. 10.1109/WCNC.2016.7564840

Madushan, K., Kae, T., Choi, W., Saquib, N., & Hossain, E. (2013). Machine Learning Techniques for Cooperative Spectrum Sensing in Cognitive Radio Networks. *IEEE Journal on Selected Areas in Communications*, *31*(11), 2209–2221. doi:10.1109/JSAC.2013.131120

Mohanakurup, V., Baghela, V. S., Kumar, S., Srivastava, P. K., Doohan, N. V., Soni, M., & Awal, H. (2022). 5G Cognitive Radio Networks Using Reliable Hybrid Deep Learning Based on Spectrum Sensing. Wireless Communications and Mobile Computing. doi:10.1155/2022/1830497

Mohanavalli, S.S. & Anand, S. (2011). International Journal of Ad hoc [IJASUC]. *Sensor & Ubiquitous Computing*, *2*(1), 60–69. doi:10.5121/ijasuc.2011.2106

Munivel, K. V., Samraj, T., Kandasamy, V., & Chilamkurti, N. (2020). Improving the Lifetime of an Out-Patient Implanted Medical Device Using a Novel Flower Pollination-Based Optimization Algorithm in WBAN Systems. M. V. Karthikeyan, Advances in Mathematical Methods for Machine Learning Algorithms for Computer Aided Diagnostic Systems. mathematics. *Mathematics*, *8*(12), 2189. doi:10.3390/math8122189

Muñoz, E. C., Luis, F. P. M., & Jorge, E. O. T. (2020). Detection of Malicious Primary User Emulation Based on a Support Vector Machine for a Mobile Cognitive Radio Network Using Software-Defined Radio. *Electronics, MDPI*, *9*, 1–17.

Santosh, K. C., Gaur, L., Santosh, K. C., & Gaur, L. (2021). *AI in Sustainable Public Healthcare. Artificial Intelligence and Machine Learning in Public Healthcare: Opportunities and Societal Impact*, (pp. 33-40). IGI Global.

Santosh, K. C., Gaur, L., Santosh, K. C., & Gaur, L. (2021). Case Studies—AI for Infectious Disease. *Artificial Intelligence and Machine Learning in Public Healthcare: Opportunities and Societal Impact,* (pp. 55-63). IGI Global.

Sarikhani, R., & Keynia, F. (2020, July). Cooperative spectrum sensing meets machine learning: Deep reinforcement learning approach. *IEEE Communications Letters*, *24*(7), 1459–1462. doi:10.1109/LCOMM.2020.2984430

Sarmah, R., Taggu, A., & Marchang, N. (2020). Detecting Byzantine attack in cognitive radio networks using machine learning. *Wireless Networks*, *26*(8), 5939–5950. doi:10.100711276-020-02398-w

Shalev-Shwartz, S., Livni, R., & Shamir, O. (2014). On the computational efficiency of training neural networks. *Proceedings of the 27th International Conference on Neural Information Processing Systems*, (pp. 855-863). IEEE.

Shawel, B. S., Woldegebreal, D. H., & Pollin, S. (2019). Convolutional lstmbased long-term spectrum prediction for dynamic spectrum access. *Proceedings of the ... European Signal Processing Conference (EUSIPCO). EUSIPCO (Conference)*, (Sep), 1–5.

Shi, Y., Erpek, T., Sagduyu, Y. E., & Li, J. H. (2018). Spectrum Data Poisoning with Adversarial Deep Learning. *MILCOM IEEE Military Communications Conference*, Los Angeles, CA. 10.1109/MILCOM.2018.8599832

Tephillah, S., & Martin Leo Manickam, J. (2020). An SETM Algorithm for Combating SSDF Attack in Cognitive Radio Networks. Wireless Communications and Mobile Computing. doi:10.1155/2020/9047809

Karthikeyan, M. V. & Manickam, M. (2017). Three Tire Proxy Re-Encryption Secret Key (PRESK) Generation for Secure Transmission of Biosignals in Wireless Body Area Sensor Networks. *Journal of Chemical and Pharmaceutical Sciences*.

Tian, J., Cheng, P., Chen, Z., Li, M., Hu, H., Li, Y., & Vucetic, B. (2019). A machine learning-enabled spectrum sensing method for ofdm systems. *IEEE Trans. Veh. Technol., 68*(11).

Timcenko, V., & Gajin, S. (2017). Ensemble classifiers for supervised anomaly based network intrusion detection. *Proceedings of the 13th IEEE International Conference on Intelligent Computer Communication and Processing (ICCP)*, Cluj-Napoca, Romania. 10.1109/ICCP.2017.8116977

Tumuluru, V. K., Wang, P., & Niyato, D. (2010). A neural network based spectrum prediction scheme for cognitive radio. *Proc. IEEE International Conference on Communications*. IEEE. 10.1109/ICC.2010.5502348

Ullah, S., & Khan, P. (2009). NiamatUllah, Shahnaz Saleem, Henry Higgins, Kyung Sup Kwak. *International Journal of Communications, Network and Systems Sciences*, 797–803. doi:10.4236/ijcns.2009.28093

Umar R. & Sheikh, A. (2012). A Comparative Study of Spectrum Awareness Techniques for Cognitive Radio Oriented Wireless Networks. *Physical Communication*.

Upadhye, A. (2021). A survey on machine learning algorithms for applications in cognitive radio networks. *2021 IEEE International Conference on Electronics, Computing and Communication Technologies (CONECCT)*. IEEE. 10.1109/CONECCT52877.2021.9622610

Xu, Y., Cheng, P., Chen, Z., Li, Y., & Vucetic, B. (2018, November). Mobile collaborative spectrum sensing for heterogeneous networks: A bayesian machine learning approach. *IEEE Transactions on Signal Processing*, 66(21), 5634–5647. doi:10.1109/TSP.2018.2870379

Yu, L., Chen, J., Zhang, Y., Zhou, H., & Sun, J. (2018, September). Deep spectrum prediction in high frequency communication based on temporal-spectral residual network. *China Communications*, 15(9), 25–34. doi:10.1109/CC.2018.8456449

Zhang, H., Poon, C., & Zhang, Y. (2011). *ISNR Communication and Networking*.

Zhao F., & Tang, Q. (2018). A knn learning algorithm for collusion-resistant spectrum auction in small cell networks. *IEEE Access, 6*, 796–4.

Zheng, S., Chen, S., Qi, P., Zhou, H., & Yang, X. (2020, February). Spectrum sensing based on deep learning classification for cognitive radios. *China Communications*, 17(2), 138–148. doi:10.23919/JCC.2020.02.012

Chapter 5
A Metaverse-Based Approach to Rehabilitation Healthcare

V. Vivekitha
https://orcid.org/0000-0002-0573-4164
Sri Ramakrishna Engineering College, India

S. Caroline Vinnetia
Bannari Amman Institute of Technology, India

R. Sri Roshini
Dr. N.G.P. Institute of Technology, India

ABSTRACT

Rehabilitative healthcare is focused on restoring physical and cognitive abilities in individuals following injuries or diseases and has largely relied on traditional methods such as physical therapy and medical interventions over time. However, the metaverse, a collaborative virtual environment, has opened new possibilities for the field of rehabilitation. In comparison to traditional rehabilitation, this technology provides increased accessibility and convenience by allowing individuals to participate in therapy from the comfort of their own homes. The immersive and engaging nature of virtual reality (VR) and augmented reality (AR) technologies increases patient motivation and compliance with therapy regimens. Through the integration of telemedicine, wearable technologies, and artificial intelligence, rehabilitation can become more sophisticated and personalized. The use of these technologies can enable the acquisition, analysis, and tracking of patient data, as well as providing real-time feedback for the improvement of treatment regimens and outcomes.

DOI: 10.4018/978-1-6684-9823-1.ch005

1. INTRODUCTION

As virtual reality technology continues to advance, more and more people are exploring the concept of a metaverse- a shared virtual realm that transcends physical limitations (Aung & Al-Jumaily, 2017; Cho et al., 2023). The word itself merges "universe" with "meta", which has Greek origins implying transcendence beyond usual limits. Within this space, users can engage with one another synchronously, co-create projects, and potentially even conduct commerce. There is virtually no limit to applications for such an immersive digital platform- it has already been proposed as an innovative solution for rehabilitation therapies.

In healthcare, rehabilitation is essential because it aids in patients' recovery from ailments, accidents, or impairments (Beristain-Colorado et al., 2020). It seeks to restore their quality of life and ability to carry out everyday tasks by enhancing their physical, mental, and emotional functions. The need for remote and virtual therapy has increased as a result of the COVID-19 epidemic, and the metaverse may offer a solution to the problems of isolation and restricted access to conventional rehabilitation facilities (Beristain-Colorado et al., 2020). It can enhance therapy methods by adding the metaverse into rehabilitation courses. The metaverse could offer a secure and regulated environment for patients to exercise the skills they need to recover from physical or mental health issues because it can imitate a variety of real-world settings and environments. Although it is still in its infancy, the metaverse has the potential to fundamentally alter how we communicate and use technology. Additionally, using the metaverse for rehabilitation may allow for distant therapy.

Virtual rehabilitation programmes can help patients who are unable to travel to physical therapy appointments due to distance or mobility concerns (Jee, 2023). This can greatly increase access to medical treatment, particularly for people who live in rural or distant places. To sum up, the metaverse has the potential to completely transform the healthcare sector, especially in the area of rehabilitation. It can improve patient experience, enable remote rehabilitation, and ultimately raise the standard of healthcare services by offering immersive virtual environments. It also holds the potential to serve as a substantial repository of data and insights, thus contributing significantly to the continuous advancement of medical knowledge and the delivery of personalized care. By seamlessly integrating telemedicine, wearable devices, and artificial intelligence within the metaverse, healthcare providers are enabled to access real-time data pertaining to patient progress, vital signs, and rehabilitation performance (Gaur et al., 2023). This data-driven approach empowers healthcare professionals to precisely tailor treatment regimens, thereby optimizing therapeutic outcomes and permitting the flexibility to adapt strategies as warranted.

Furthermore, the metaverse affords unique opportunities for innovative forms of therapy and holistic well-being (Moon et al., 2023). Beyond conventional physical therapy, the immersive and dynamic nature of the metaverse enables the creation of inventive, gamified rehabilitation exercises, rendering the process of recovery engaging and enjoyable for patients. They are granted the ability to partake in activities that simulate their daily routines, whether it be navigating lifelike cityscapes or engaging in virtual shopping experiences. This immersive approach serves to fortify physical and cognitive abilities within a context that feels both familiar and relatable. In addition to its therapeutic aspects, the social dimension of the metaverse fosters a sense of community among patients undergoing rehabilitation. The provision of peer support and shared experiences within virtual environments can be profoundly motivating and therapeutic. It serves as a countermeasure against the feelings of isolation and depression that can often accompany physical or mental health challenges, thus contributing to an overall sense of emotional well-being (Shao et al., 2023).

In summation, the metaverse significance in healthcare, particularly within the realm of rehabilitation, transcends immediate advantages in terms of accessibility and engagement. It emerges as a multifaceted instrument capable of facilitating data-driven, personalized care, pioneering innovative therapeutic methodologies, and nurturing supportive virtual communities. As the metaverse continues its evolution, it stands poised to redefine the parameters of healthcare and elevate the quality of life for a multitude of individuals embarking on their path to recovery and well-being. Embracing this transformative paradigm is imperative for healthcare systems and professionals as they endeavor to meet the evolving needs of patients in an ever-changing digital landscape.

2. THEORETICAL BACKGROUND OF METAVERSE-BASED REHABILITATION HEALTHCARE

For several decades ago, the idea of using virtual worlds for rehabilitation has been around. Computer-based programmes were first the main technique utilized to enhance cognitive and physical function. These programmes tended to be brief and uncomplicated, giving exercises like those used in basic physical rehabilitation and memory and attention training. However, there has been a shift recently towards more immersive and interactive settings that provide a stronger sense of presence and participation. The development of virtual reality (VR) and related technologies, which enabled the production of extremely lifelike and adaptable virtual environments, has had a huge impact on this change. The techniques for rehabilitation that have been used in the past are covered in this chapter.

2.1 History and Evolution of Rehabilitation Healthcare

For individuals who have been injured, ill, or disabled, rehabilitation healthcare is essential for regaining and improving their functional abilities and quality of life. Due to developments in technology, medicine, and a better understanding of human physiology, the area of rehabilitation has seen major changes throughout history. Early types of rehabilitation have been used by many civilizations throughout history to help people with disabilities heal and reintegrate (Hall, 2007; Coulter, 1947). Prosthetics constructed of leather and wood were utilized in ancient Egypt to help amputees regain their movement and function. Orthopaedics became a specialized field during the Industrial Revolution, and musculoskeletal disorders-focused hospitals and clinics were established. Significant advances in medical knowledge and the creation of specialized facilities for the treatment of people with disabilities are to blame for the development of modern rehabilitation. Rehab healthcare had significant changes in the 19th and 20th centuries that influenced the industry. The evolution of rehabilitation was significantly aided by the establishment of orthopedics as a distinct medical specialty. Orthopaedics concentrated on diagnosing and treating musculoskeletal diseases, giving rehabilitation techniques a strong foundation.

In order to cater exclusively to people with disabilities, orthopaedic hospitals and clinics were built with the belief that focused interventions and therapies could improve recovery. These developments had a significant impact on people with disabilities' psychological wellbeing and social integration in addition to improving their physical skills (Cooper et al., 2006). The acceptance of the value of interdisciplinary cooperation was another factor in the development of contemporary rehabilitation. To deliver comprehensive and patient-centered care, medical experts such as doctors, physiotherapists, occupational therapists, psychologists, and social workers started collaborating in multidisciplinary teams. This method recognized the intricate interplay between a person's physical, psychological, and social components in their recovery and emphasized the significance of taking care of all aspects of rehabilitation. The development and history of rehabilitation medicine show the remarkable strides made in regaining the independence, functionality, and quality of life for people with disabilities. Rehabilitation has seen considerable changes as a result of the transition from traditional treatment methods to the use of cutting-edge technology and interdisciplinary cooperation over time.

2.2 Theoretical Framework of Rehabilitation Healthcare in the Metaverse

Recently, the idea of the metaverse has attracted a lot of attention because it holds the potential to fundamentally alter how we connect, operate at work, and enjoy ourselves in virtual spaces. A collaborative virtual environment known as the metaverse allows people to interact in real time with one another and computer-generated settings. A wide variety of immersive technologies, virtual worlds, augmented reality, social media platforms, and online gaming are all included in this ecosystem, which is both rich and linked. This article explores the metaverse ecosystem, its core elements, and the potential for transformation it holds for various facets of our life. The ecology of the metaverse is made up of a number of essential parts that work together to create a dynamic and engaging virtual world.

The ability of the metaverse to seamlessly integrate the virtual and real worlds is one of its intrinsic qualities. Figure 1 exhibits the fundamental idea of the metaverse, which employs augmented and virtual reality, a technology that enhances users' vision and interaction with the real world by superimposing digital information concerning it. The development of rehabilitation healthcare in the metaverse is greatly influenced by theoretical frameworks (Calabrò et al., 2022). A framework in the metaverse is made up of ideas, rules, and standards that influence the virtual world. It places a strong emphasis on user-centricity, paying particular attention to trust, identification, and privacy rights. There many principles which is used as a basic framework some of them include ecological systems theory, social cognitive theory, self-determination theory, Cognitive load theory etc. By incorporating these theoretical foundations, rehabilitation professionals can design immersive and effective interventions that promote engagement, motivation, and positive outcomes in the metaverse. These theories also inform the evaluation and research efforts to measure the impact and effectiveness of virtual interventions in enhancing rehabilitation outcomes.

Figure 1. Components of metaverse

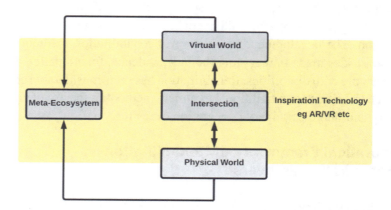

In the metaverse, the scientific foundations of rehabilitation healthcare provide beneficial insights to establish effective virtual therapies. These frameworks guide the understanding of the underlying principles and processes involved in rehabilitation, allowing for the creation of immersive and impactful experiences. In this regard, some key theoretical foundations are very relevant. The ecological systems theory emphasizes the dynamic interaction of individuals with their surroundings. According to this idea, while constructing treatments in the metaverse, the virtual environment, social interactions, and personal characteristics should all be considered. By understanding how these components interact, rehabilitation practitioners can create virtual environments that increase engagement, learning, and positive outcomes. According to the social cognitive theory, social interactions, observational learning, and self-efficacy all impact behaviour change. Incorporating social components into the metaverse, such as virtual support groups or shared rehabilitation experiences, can enhance motivation, self-belief, and healthy habit adoption. By allowing people to express themselves, social cognitive theory can help to promote good rehabilitation outcomes. The self-determination theory focuses on autonomy, competence, and relatedness as key factors in fostering intrinsic motivation and well-being (Ibanez Valdes et al., 2023).

In the metaverse, virtual rehabilitation interventions should offer choices, opportunities for mastery, and social connections. By addressing these psychological needs, self-determination theory supports active engagement and meaningful outcomes in rehabilitation. Lastly, cognitive load theory explores how cognitive demands impact learning and problem-solving. In the metaverse, designing virtual interventions that optimize cognitive load is crucial. Clear instructions, scaffolding learning experiences, and gradually increasing task complexity can enhance learning and skill acquisition. By incorporating these theoretical foundations into the design and implementation of virtual interventions, rehabilitation professionals can create immersive and effective experiences in the metaverse. These theories inform the development of interventions that promote engagement, motivation, and positive outcomes. Additionally, they guide the evaluation and research efforts to assess the impact and effectiveness of virtual rehabilitation interventions. As technology advances and our understanding of the metaverse evolve, continued exploration and integration of theoretical frameworks will contribute to further advancements in rehabilitation healthcare.

2.3 Differences Between Traditional and Metaverse-Based Rehabilitation Healthcare

Traditional rehabilitation refers to the conventional approach of providing medical, therapeutic, and supportive care to individuals who have suffered from injury, illness, or disability. It involves the use of physical settings like hospitals, clinics, and rehabilitation centers, where a team of healthcare professionals delivers hands-on treatment and therapies to enhance patients' functional abilities, mobility, and overall well-being. The execution of rehabilitation services is very different between conventional rehabilitation healthcare and rehabilitation healthcare based in the metaverse. Traditional rehabilitation takes place in real-world locations like hospitals and clinics, whereas metaverse-based rehabilitation happens in virtual settings with the use of virtual reality (VR) or augmented reality (AR) technologies (Desai et al., 2019).

The ease of access and convenience they provide is one important difference. Travelling to physical sites is a need in traditional rehabilitation, which can be difficult for people with mobility impairments or those who live in distant areas. In contrast, patients can attend therapy sessions and exercises using VR/AR devices or internet platforms from the comfort of their homes with metaverse-based rehabilitation (Dionísio Corrêa et al., 2012). Additionally, interactions and responses take in several forms. In traditional rehabilitation, medical staff can speak with patients face-to-face, lend a hand, and give quick feedback on exercises and motions. Patients engage in virtual interactions while receiving feedback from haptic feedback, motion tracking devices, visual and aural cues, and guided exercises in metaverse-based therapy. Healthcare practitioners are less visible physically, though. In all strategies, customization and agility are essential. Traditional rehabilitation enables medical personnel to tailor care regimens based on patients' needs and development (Elor and Kurniawan, 2019).

Metaverse-based rehabilitation also offers personalization by tailoring virtual exercises and activities to specific requirements, and the programs can dynamically adapt based on real-time data and patient feedback. One significant advantage of metaverse-based rehabilitation is the immersive and engaging experience it provides. Virtual environments can simulate real-world scenarios and gamify rehabilitation exercises, enhancing patient motivation and adherence to therapy programs. In contrast, traditional rehabilitation may rely more on conventional exercises and therapy techniques without the same level of immersive experiences (Liu et al., 2020).

Collaborative and social interaction opportunities differ as well. Traditional rehabilitation often involves face-to-face interactions between patients and healthcare professionals, as well as group therapy sessions for peer support and learning. Through virtual environments, metaverse-based rehabilitation provides similar collaborative and social networks, allowing patients to connect with peers, participate in group activities, and receive support from healthcare experts and online communities. Both approaches have advantages and disadvantages, and a comprehensive rehabilitation program may use parts from both to improve patient outcomes (Feng et al., 2019).

3. METAVERSE-BASED APPROACHES TO REHABILITATION HEALTHCARE

Metaverse-based approaches to rehabilitative healthcare hold significant possibilities for enhancing patient outcomes and transforming rehabilitation service delivery. Virtual exercises and simulations have the potential to enhance therapy by improving mobility, strength and coordination. To ensure the metaverse becomes a platform it is crucial to incorporate the following technologies.

3.1 Virtual Reality for Rehabilitation

Virtual reality (VR) is an emerging technological innovation that engenders a simulated environment, thereby affording users an immersive and interactive experience. Within the realm of healthcare, VR has emerged as a promising therapeutic tool, chiefly owing to its inherent capability to furnish patients with immersive and captivating experiences. Within this simulated milieu, patients are able to engage in physical exercise and participate in therapeutic activities. Significantly, VR augments the rehabilitation process by bestowing upon patients a profound sense of presence and personal agency, thereby serving as a potent motivational catalyst for active engagement in their recuperative journey. Figure 2 shows how a virtual reality system operates by establishing a connection between the user and the virtual environment via an input/output loop.

Figure 2. VR architecture for rehabilitation

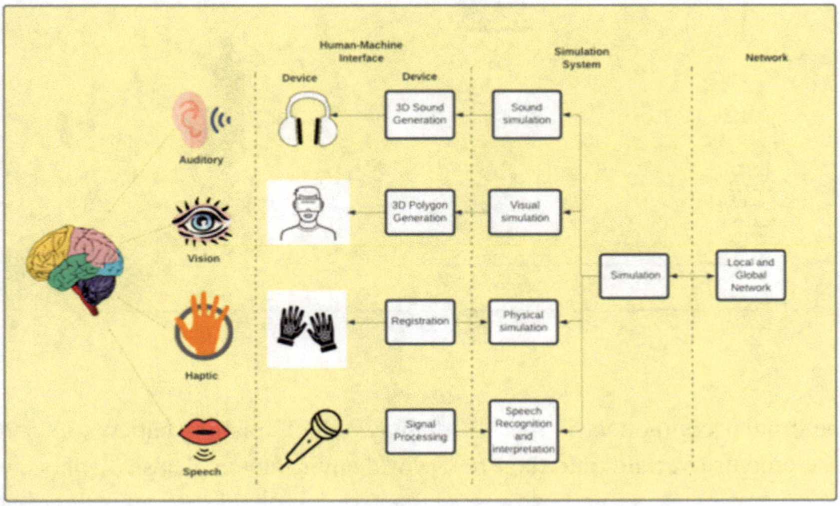

Users can engage with virtual objects and perform actions relevant to their rehabilitation goals via controllers, gestures, or voice commands. Because VR is immersive and engaging, patients can get immediate visual and aural feedback that helps them better understand their actions and performances. They can change and develop as a result of the real-time feedback, which encourages a more successful rehabilitation process. Additionally, patients can practise functional motions, enhance balance and coordination, and concentrate on specific rehabilitation objectives in a secure and controlled setting with VR. VR presents a singular chance for patients to engage in rehabilitation exercises that mimic real-life circumstances by bridging the gap between the physical and virtual worlds.

3.2 Augmented Reality for Rehabilitation

Augmented Reality (AR) is a technology that enriches the real-world environment by overlaying virtual content onto it. For improved perception and interaction with the environment, AR mixes computer-generated images, audio, and other sensory inputs. VR and AR each have particular applications. Through the use of AR, patients can interact with virtual content while staying aware of their physical environment. On the other hand, VR creates completely immersive virtual settings that mimic real-life situations. AR systems comprise several key components that play important roles in facilitating the rehabilitation process as shown in the figure 3.

Figure 3. Components of AR system for rehabilitation

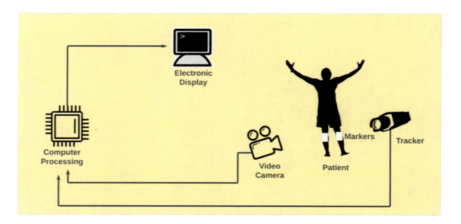

One crucial component is the AR display, which enables patients to perceive virtual elements overlaid onto their real-world environment. These displays, which can take forms of wearable headsets, glasses, or handheld devices, allow patients to see both their physical surroundings and the virtual content at the same time. The quality of the display, encompassing aspects such as resolution and clarity, holds paramount significance for the effective visualization of virtual objects and cues. Additionally, a pivotal component within this context is the tracking system, responsible for both gathering and monitoring the patient's movements, as well as the ambient environment. This system meticulously records the patient's actions and subsequently correlates them with the virtual elements through the utilization of an array of sensors, cameras, or cutting-edge motion capture technology. Precise and unfaltering tracking capabilities facilitate the provision of real-time feedback and guidance during rehabilitation exercises, with a strong emphasis on maintaining proper form and technique.

Augmented Reality (AR) rehabilitation systems leverage dedicated software or applications to create virtual content, fostering patient involvement within this digital environment. This specialized software is meticulously designed for rehabilitation objectives, offering an array of tailored workouts, activities, and simulations, finely tuned to individual requirements. It is imperative that this software is not only user-friendly but also intuitive, ensuring a fluid and captivating experience for patients. Furthermore, a pivotal facet enabling patients to interact with the virtual environment is the input mechanism. Possibilities range from handheld controllers to voice commands and gesture recognition programs, exemplifying the diverse means through which patients can engage with the virtual world.

The input technique needs to be flexible and open-ended so that patients with different physical capabilities and restrictions can use it to interact with the virtual information. Systems for augmented reality (AR) provide feedback mechanisms to improve the rehabilitation experience. Patients are given real-time information through these systems, which helps them comprehend their performance and progress. In order to give patients quick feedback during workouts so they may change their movements and improve their technique, auditory input, haptic feedback (such as vibrations or tactile sensations), and visual cues are frequently used. An AR display, tracking system, software or application, input method, and feedback mechanisms make up an AR system in rehabilitation. Together, these elements provide an immersive and interactive rehabilitation environment that enables patients to perform customized exercises, get immediate feedback, and track their development. Rehabilitation professionals can improve therapy results, inspire patients, and provide dynamic and entertaining rehabilitation experiences by implementing AR technology.

3.3 Gamification for Rehabilitation

Gamification is the process of integrating aspects of game design into therapy to increase patient motivation, engagement and adherence. It turns mundane exercises into exciting and engaging experiences. These elements include points and scoring systems to track progress and provide a sense of accomplishment. Levels and progression mechanics offer a clear sense of advancement, unlocking new challenges and activities. Setting specific goals and challenges adds structure and purpose to rehabilitation, motivating active participation. Rewards and incentives, such as virtual badges or trophies, reinforce positive behavior and acknowledge achievements.

Feedback and progress tracking enable timely evaluation and identification of areas for improvement. Avatars and customization options personalize the experience, allowing patients to reflect their progress visually. Competition elements, like leaderboards, and social interaction through multiplayer modes or online communities foster engagement and peer support. Storytelling and narrative elements create an immersive experience, giving context and meaning to the rehabilitation journey. Customization of these components is important to meet individual patient needs and goals. The Gamification elements are shown in the figure 4.

Figure 4. Classification of gamification elements

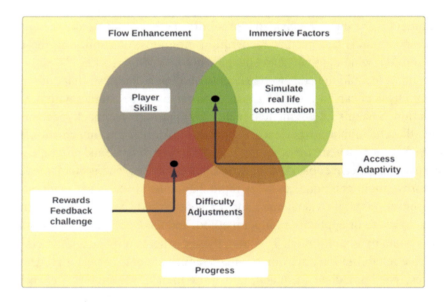

Overall, Gamification in rehabilitation offers a motivating and rewarding therapeutic approach, leading to improved patient outcomes and increased participation. Telemedicine, also known as Telehealth, has emerged as a valuable approach in the field of rehabilitation, enabling remote delivery of healthcare services through technology and telecommunications. It encompasses various components specifically designed for rehabilitation purposes.

4. INTEGRATION WITH ARTIFICIAL INTELLIGENCE AND MACHINE LEARNING

There is a huge potential for metaverse adapted rehabilitation therapy. With technology progress, we may be able to anticipate more sophisticated and Immersive Virtual Environments which can deliver a more personalized and real rehabilitation experience (Kaswan et al., 2021). Future development of metaverse based rehabilitation is identified as follows:

Advanced Virtual Reality (VR) and Augmented Reality (AR) Technologies: Patients will be able to use more realistic and natural methods of interaction with virtual environments as advanced VR and Augmented Reality technology matures, which can improve the effectiveness of rehabilitation.

Wearable technology and sensors: Wearable technology and sensors enable real time monitoring and feedback of the patient's mobility, heart rate, and other physiological data. This can allow the patient to alter his or her exercise and movement so as to result in better recovery.

Artificial Intelligence (AI): Individualized advice and support can be given to patients by AI powered Virtual Assistants on the basis of their specific needs and capabilities. In order to provide more accurate and personalized treatment regimens, AI can also look at the data from patients (Gaur et al., 2023).

Multi-user virtual environments: Virtual environments, facilitated by the inclusion of multiple users, have the potential to cultivate a more congenial and supportive atmosphere for interactions between patients and their healthcare providers. This increased social dimension enhances the overall experience.

Looking ahead, the prospects for metaverse-based rehabilitation seem promising. While there are undoubtedly challenges and ethical considerations to navigate, the potential advantages of this technology could bring about a paradigm shift in our approach to healthcare and rehabilitation. The integration of Artificial Intelligence (AI) and Machine Learning (ML) stands as a transformative force in metaverse-based rehabilitation, promising personalized and adaptive treatment regimens, real-time monitoring, and data-driven insights that have the potential to revolutionize the field. The incorporation of sensors and wearable devices for gathering data on patients' movements, biometrics, and relevant metrics holds immense potential for integrating AI and ML into metaverse-based therapy. This data can subsequently undergo analysis through machine learning algorithms to unveil intricate patterns and trends, which in turn can be harnessed to craft bespoke treatment plans tailored to individual needs(Mahbub et al., 2022). For instance, machine learning techniques can be employed to scrutinize sensor data obtained from a patient's devices, effectively pinpointing areas where they may be encountering balance or movement-related challenges. With this knowledge, healthcare providers can create individualized workouts or activities that address these identified areas of concern, hence improving the efficacy of rehabilitation and therapy.

AI and machine learning can play a critical role in providing real-time feedback and support to patients during rehabilitation sessions. The use of an AI-powered virtual assistant, for example, can give patients with step-by-step instructions and advice during their workouts. It may vary the difficulty level dynamically based on the patient's performance and even recommend alternative activities when necessary. Furthermore, AI and ML can be used to build predictive models that anticipate patient outcomes by taking into account a variety of parameters such as age, medical history, and numerous data points. Physicians can then use these insights to fine-tune and adapt rehabilitation regimens to meet the specific needs of each patient, increasing the likelihood of successful outcomes.

4.1 Block Chain and Crypto Currency in Metaverse-Based Rehabilitation

A metaverse-based rehabilitation system has the potential to significantly benefit from the use of blockchain and crypto currencies. The term "metaverse" describes a virtual reality environment where users can communicate with one another and digital items in a made-up setting (Laver et al., 2017). Including crypto currency and blockchain technology in such a system can have the following advantages:

Security and Transparency: The use of blockchain technology guarantees the security and immutability of data and transactions. A metaverse-based rehabilitation system may safely store and distribute sensitive patient data, treatment records, and progress reports by using blockchain. This increases openness and fosters trust among those involved in the recovery process.

Decentralization: Crypto currencies run on decentralized networks, which mean that no single entity has control over them. This decentralization can be used to spread ownership and decision-making power in a metaverse rehabilitation system. For instance, people can exert more control over their own health information and treatment regimens, while healthcare professionals can contribute their knowledge by joining a decentralized network (Gaur et al., 2021).

Tokenization of Assets: In the metaverse, there are many different assets and services that can be tokenized using crypto currencies. This can involve tokenizing certain therapy sessions, virtual medical tools, or even customized avatars in the context of rehabilitation. Tokens can be utilized to speed up transactions and reward participation, resulting in a more engaging and immersive rehab experience.

Smart Contracts: Self-executing contracts with established terms and conditions are known as smart contracts. Smart contracts can be used in a metaverse-based rehabilitation system to automate a number of procedures. For instance, a smart contract may be set up to compensate a virtual therapist when certain rehabilitation objectives are met. By doing this, administrative costs are cut and it is made sure that everyone engaged abides by the conditions.

Economic Incentives: In the metaverse, crypto currencies can be used to create financial incentives that promote participation and cooperation. Patients who meet their rehabilitation objectives may receive tokens as compensation, which can then be used elsewhere in the metaverse ecosystem. This incentive system can increase engagement in the rehabilitation process overall, motivation, and adherence to treatment regimens.

It's vital to remember, too, that integrating blockchain and crypto currency into a metaverse-based rehabilitation system has its own set of difficulties. Scalability, energy use, regulatory issues, and user adoption are some of these difficulties. To successfully integrate blockchain and crypto currencies into the rehabilitation process, there must be meticulous planning, a strong technological foundation, and consideration of the ethical aspects.

4.2 Ethical Considerations in Metaverse-Based Rehabilitation

To ensure the safety and privacy of participants, it is essential to take into account several ethical aspects when creating a metaverse-based rehabilitation system. Here a few important moral points to remember.

Privacy and Data Protection: Solutions for patient rehabilitation based in the metaverse capture and store private patient information. To safeguard against unauthorized access, security breaches, and exploitation of this data, it is crucial to develop strong privacy protocols. To protect people's privacy, it's crucial to have clear data usage policies, informed consent processes, and secure data storage.

Inclusivity and Accessibility: Metaverse platforms ought to be inclusive and easy to use for people with special needs or disabilities. Diverse demographics, including those with visual impairments, hearing impairments, or mobility restrictions, should be taken into account. Accessible technologies, adaptable user interfaces, and different communication channels can improve the rehabilitation process.

Informed Consent and Autonomy: Participants in a metaverse-based rehabilitation system ought to be free to choose whether or not to take part. They should have the choice to provide or withhold consent after being given enough information about the system's purpose, risks, and advantages. To ensure that participants fully comprehend the metaverse environment and its ramifications, it is important to give concise and accessible explanations.

Ethical Use of AI and Algorithms: A metaverse-based rehabilitation system can use AI algorithms and machine learning models to personalize care and improve results. However, it is crucial to guarantee that these algorithms are open, impartial, and fair. To sustain ethical standards, it is essential to avoid discriminatory practices, constantly audit algorithms for biases, and provide justifications for algorithmic conclusions.

Informed User Interface Design: The user's physical and mental wellness should come first in the metaverse interface design. It should refrain from preying on people's psychological weak points or addictive tendencies. A good balance between virtual and real-world activities can be maintained with the use of notifications, time restrictions, and features that promote breaks and self-care.

Ethical Content and Interactions: The interactions and content within the metaverse ecosystem should follow moral standards. A safe and encouraging rehabilitation environment must be maintained by making sure that there is no damaging, offensive, or discriminating information. Mechanisms for moderation and reporting should be in place to deal with any problems right away.

Continuous Evaluation and Improvement: The metaverse-based rehabilitation system needs to be monitored and evaluated frequently in order to spot any emergent ethical issues and deal with them. To continue to enhance and uphold ethical standards, it is important to take into account participant, healthcare provider, and ethical expert feedback. If a metaverse-based rehabilitation system takes these moral issues into account, it can work to give participants access to a secure, welcoming, and empowered environment that will promote their general well-being and recovery success.

5. METAVERSE BASED REHABILITATION PROGRAM IN PRACTISE

5.1 Stroke Rehabilitation

Stroke rehabilitation is the process of regaining function and enhancing quality of life after a stroke. A stroke happens when the blood flow to the brain is disrupted, either by a blood vessel rupture or an arterial obstruction. This disruption can cause a variety of physical, cognitive, and emotional issues. Stroke rehabilitation can often start immediately following a stroke, frequently while the patient is still in the hospital, with the goal of assisting the patient in regaining as much independence and function as possible. A multidisciplinary team of medical specialists, including psychologists, occupational therapists, speech therapists, and physical therapists, is involved in rehabilitation. Medication, assistive devices, and adjustments to lifestyles may also be included. Medications can be provided to treat symptoms like pain or sadness while also lowering the risk of future strokes. Mobility devices, such as wheelchairs or braces, may be offered to help with movement. In summary, stroke rehabilitation is a difficult procedure that necessitates a customized strategy to meet the specific demands of each patient. Many stroke patients can restore function and independence with the correct combination of therapies and care, improving their overall quality of life.

Traditional techniques to stroke recovery, on the other hand, have limits. Patients are frequently required to physically attend therapy sessions at medical institutions, which can be difficult for individuals with restricted mobility or who live in remote places. Furthermore, reproducing real-world circumstances in clinical settings lacks realism, making it difficult for stroke patients to practice daily chores in context-appropriate settings. Furthermore, by reducing options for peer support and emotional connection among stroke patients, these traditional strategies may unintentionally promote to social isolation. For addressing these issues, a metaverse-based approach to stroke therapy has emerged as a promising answer. This method allows patients to engage in therapy sessions regardless of their geographical location. This is especially advantageous for people living in rural or isolated locations since it expands their access to rehabilitation programs. Furthermore, virtual worlds within the metaverse provide deep realism, closely mimicking real-life scenarios and allowing stroke survivors to practice daily activities in a secure and realistic setting, increasing skill development and speeding up the rehabilitation process (Ventura et al.,2022).

Apart from physical benefits, the metaverse-based approach boosts social support. Stroke survivors can connect with peers, healthcare experts, and support groups through Metaverse virtual communities, which promote social engagement and emotional well-being. This efficiently tackles the social isolation issue that can emerge with traditional rehabilitation procedures. Finally, the metaverse-based approach to stroke therapy is a possible alternative to standard approaches. It provides a viable path for stroke survivors to engage in rehabilitation and improve their quality of life by providing remote accessibility, immersive realism, and greater social support through virtual environments and communities.

5.2 Occupational Therapy

The main objective of occupational therapy practitioners is to assist clients in learning or reacquiring the skills required to engage in their everyday employment, sometimes known as their "occupations." Occupational therapists help patients who have physical, emotional, or cognitive difficulties that make it difficult for them to operate normally in daily life. The primary objective of occupational therapy is to help patients attain the best level of independence and functionality achievable by addressing the underlying issues that impede their capacity to perform daily activities.

Occupational therapists operate in a variety of settings, including hospitals, educational institutions, rehabilitation centers, and community facilities, and serve a wide spectrum of clients, from infants to the elderly. Occupational therapy has a wide scope, encompassing many aspects of human functioning. It comprises assisting people in developing their fine motor abilities, which include tasks like holding and manipulating objects with precision, as seen in handwriting, typing, and proficient tool use. Furthermore, occupational therapy plays a critical role in addressing foundational activities of daily living (ADLs) such as bathing, dressing, personal grooming, and gaining meal consumption autonomy. Occupational therapists engage closely with their patients to support skill development, ultimately increasing their capacity to participate in meaningful and independent activities. Instrumental Activities of Daily Living (IADLs): These entail more sophisticated responsibilities such as medication management, housekeeping, and meal preparation. Sensory processing refers to the ability to process and respond to sensory input such as touch, hearing, and sight. Memory, attention, problem-solving, and decision-making ability are examples of cognitive capabilities.

Occupational therapy, in its entirety, is a comprehensive approach that focuses on enhancing a person's overall quality of life by treating physical, emotional, and cognitive issues that limit their ability to engage in activities of daily living. The potential applications of the metaverse in occupational therapy have not yet been fully investigated as the idea is still relatively new and spreading quickly. There are some possible uses for the metaverse in occupational therapy strategies, nevertheless. For instance, occupational therapy is already using virtual reality (VR) technology to simulate real-world environments and activities to help patients hone and develop their skills. The metaverse might offer even more choices for creating realistic, interactive virtual environments that are catered to a person's preferences and needs. A simpler and more inclusive platform for occupational therapy services may be offered by the metaverse.

Patients who have limited mobility, live in remote areas, or have difficulty attending in-person sessions may be able to participate in virtual sessions via the metaverse. The metaverse may also aid in social involvement and community building, which are important aspects of occupational therapy. Patients could engage with people who have similar experiences and interests by joining virtual support groups, recreational activities, and educational initiatives. However, it is critical to underline that the use of metaverse technology in occupational therapy would need to be properly researched and tailored to individual patients' needs and preferences. The metaverse-based approach to occupational therapy offers several advantages for stroke rehabilitation. It provides highly customizable virtual environments tailored to individual rehabilitation requirements, allowing for personalized and targeted therapy sessions. These virtual environments closely replicate real-life situations, enabling stroke survivors to practice daily activities safely and realistically. This facilitates skill development and motor skill recovery. Additionally, the metaverse-based approach allows for remote participation, improving accessibility to essential care regardless of geographical location. It also offers enhanced social support through virtual communities within the metaverse, addressing social isolation and promoting emotional well-being . Overall, the metaverse-based approach overcomes existing approaches' shortcomings and offers a viable option for stroke recovery in occupational therapy.

5.3 Cognitive Rehabilitation

Cognitive rehabilitation is a series of interventions aimed to assist people with cognitive impairments, which are frequently caused by disorders such as brain injuries, strokes, or neurodegenerative diseases, in restoring cognitive functioning and the capacity to conduct daily activities. Cognitive rehabilitation's major purpose is to help patients restore lost cognitive abilities or develop compensatory ways to manage cognitive deficiencies. Memory exercises focus training, problem-solving tasks, and communication skills training may all be included.

Cognitive therapy can be provided in settings, including rehabilitation centers, outpatient clinics or, at the patient's own residence. A team of healthcare professionals from disciplines such as therapists, speech therapists, neuropsychologists and rehabilitation specialists often collaborate to deliver these treatments. Research has shown that cognitive rehabilitation significantly improves function, independence and overall quality of life in individuals with impairments. However the effectiveness of the intervention depends on factors such as the type and severity of the impairment the patients motivation and active involvement in the rehabilitation process and the expertise and experience of the rehabilitation team. In environments known as platforms or virtual worlds specifically designed for rehabilitation purposes patients can engage in tailored activities. For instance someone recovering from a brain injury may participate in memory games and exercises to aid their memory recovery. The immersive nature of these environments enhances engagement and motivation while providing a safe space for skill development. Additionally metaverse platforms have benefits for connection and support, among individuals undergoing cognitive rehabilitation. Patients can join group therapy sessions. Interact with others participating in similar programs.

However it's important to highlight that incorporating the metaverse into rehabilitation should be seen as an approach rather, than a substitute, for established therapies and treatments. It has the potential to help and supplement traditional cognitive rehabilitation treatments in unique ways, but the overall treatment plan should be carefully customized to the individual's needs and conducted under the supervision of healthcare professionals. Furthermore, the metaverse must be designed with patient privacy and safety in mind, and healthcare personnel must be trained to use it successfully and ethically. Overall, the metaverse has the potential to improve the efficacy and accessibility of cognitive rehabilitation, and additional research in this area could lead to exciting new patient treatment approaches.

6. CONCLUSION

The metaverse participation feature enables patients to engage and stay motivated during their rehabilitation sessions. Offering rewards and tracking progress for instance adds enjoyment to the process. It also boosts adherence to treatment plans. Additionally within the metaverse patients can connect with friends and healthcare professionals fostering a community where information can be shared. Moreover healthcare providers can gather data on patients progress and performance through metaverse based rehabilitation. This data can then be utilized to adjust treatment plans monitor outcomes and identify patterns for enhancement. Although the metaverse holds potential it is important to integrate it into existing healthcare systems to enhance practices. Ultimately by providing enjoyable experiences the metaverse has the capability to revolutionize healthcare for individuals in need of rehabilitation. Some of its benefits include improved accessibility, an environment for practice sessions, heightened motivation levels, social interaction opportunities, as well, as insights derived from data analysis. Incorporating the metaverse into rehabilitation practices has the potential to enhance both effectiveness and efficiency in achieving healthcare outcomes.

REFERENCES

Aung, Y. M., & Al-Jumaily, A. (2017). *Augmented reality-based RehaBio system for shoulder rehabilitation.* In *2017 International Conference on Electrical and Electronic Engineering (ICEEE),* Istanbul. doi: 10.1109/ICEEE2.2017.8338852

Beristain-Colorado, M. P., Ambros-Antemate, J. F., Vargas-Treviño, M., Gutierrez-Gutierrez, J., Moreno-Rodriguez, A., Hernandez-Cruz, P. A., Gallegos-Velasco, I. B., & Torres-Rosas, R. (2020). Standardizing the Development of Serious Games for Physical Rehabilitation: Conceptual Framework Proposal. *IEEE Access : Practical Innovations, Open Solutions, 8,* 26119–26130. doi:10.1109/ACCESS.2020.2971707

Calabrò, R. S., Cerasa, A., Ciancarelli, I., Pignolo, L., Tonin, P., Iosa, M., & Morone, G. (2022). The Arrival of the Metaverse in Neurorehabilitation: Fact, Fake or Vision? *Biomedicines*, *10*(10), 2602. doi:10.3390/biomedicines10102602 PMID:36289862

Cho, K.-H., Park, J.-B., & Kang, A. (2023). Metaverse for Exercise Rehabilitation: Possibilities and Limitations. *International Journal of Environmental Research and Public Health*, *20*(8), 5483. doi:10.3390/ijerph20085483 PMID:37107765

Cooper, R. A., Ohnabe, H., & Hobson, D. A. (2006). *An Introduction to Rehabilitation Engineering*. CRC Press. doi:10.1201/9781420012491

Coulter, J. S. (1947). History and development of physical medicine. *Archives of Physical Medicine and Rehabilitation*, *28*(9), 600–602. PMID:20262280

Desai, K., Bahirat, K., Ramalingam, S., Prabhakaran, B., Annaswamy, T., & Makris, U. E. (2019). Augmented reality-based exergames for rehabilitation. *Journal of Medical Systems*, *43*(10), 316. doi:10.100710916-019-1489-2 PMID:31506773

Dionísio Corrêa, A. G., Ficheman, I. K., do Nascimento, M., & de Deus Lopes, R. (2012). *Contributions of an Augmented Reality Musical System for the Stimulation of Motor Skills in Music Therapy Sessions*. Learning Disabilities. 10.5772/30142

Elor, A., & Kurniawan, S. (2019). The Ultimate Display for Physical Rehabilitation: A Bridging Review on Immersive Virtual Reality. *Journal of interactive technology and pedagogy*, (15). doi:10.21985/jitp.v0i15.1285

Feng, H., Li, C., Liu, J., Wang, L., Ma, J., Li, G., Gan, L., Shang, X., & Wu, Z. (2019). Virtual reality rehabilitation versus conventional physical therapy for improving balance and gait in Parkinson's disease patients: A randomized controlled trial. *Medical Science Monitor*, *25*, 4186–4192. doi:10.12659/MSM.916455 PMID:31165721

Gaur, L., Afaq, A., Arora, G. K., & Khan, N. (2023). Artificial intelligence for carbon emissions using system of systems theory. *Ecological Informatics*, *102165*, 102165. doi:10.1016/j.ecoinf.2023.102165

Gaur, L., Rana, J., & Jhanjhi, N. Z. (2023). *Digital Twin and Healthcare: Trends, Techniques, and Challenges*. IGI Global. doi:10.4018/978-1-6684-5925-6

Gaur, L., Solanki, A., Wamba, S. F., & Jhanjhi, N. Z. (Eds.). (2021). *Advanced AI Techniques and Applications in Bioinformatics*. CRC Press. doi:10.1201/9781003126164

Hall, J. F. (2007). The History of Rehabilitation Medicine: A Brief Overview. *The Journal of the American Osteopathic Association*, *107*(9), 385–390.

Ibanez Valdes, L. F., Joseph, S. S., & Sibat, H. F. (2023). Rituximab in Refractory Myasthenia Gravis: A Systematic Review. *Clinical Schizophrenia & Related Psychoses*, *17*(1), 1–8.

Jee, Y.-S. (2023). Application of metaverse technology to exercise rehabilitation: Present and future. *Journal of Exercise Rehabilitation*, *19*(2), 93–94. doi:10.12965/jer.2346050.025 PMID:37163182

Kaswan, K. S., Gaur, L., Dhatterwal, J. S., & Kumar, R. (2021). AI-based natural language processing for the generation of meaningful information electronic health record (EHR) data. In L. Gaur, A. Solanki, S. F. Wamba, & N. Z. Jhanjhi (Eds.), *Advanced AI Techniques and Applications in Bioinformatics* (pp. 46–86). CRC Press. doi:10.1201/9781003126164-3

Laver, K. E. (2017). Virtual reality for stroke rehabilitation. *Cochrane Database of Systematic Reviews*, *11*(2). doi:10.1002/14651858.CD008349.pub4 PMID:29156493

Liu, L., Yin, H., & Chen, Z. (2020). *Using Self-Determination Theory to Explore Enjoyment of Educational Interactive Narrative Games: A Case Study of Academical.* Research Gate.

Mahbub, M. K., Biswas, M., Gaur, L., Alenezi, F., & Santosh, K. C. (2022). Deep features to detect pulmonary abnormalities in chest X-rays due to infectious diseases: Covid-19, pneumonia, and tuberculosis. *Information Sciences (New York)*, *592*, 389–401. doi:10.1016/j.ins.2022.01.062 PMID:36532848

Moon, I., An, Y., Min, S., & Park, C. (2023). Therapeutic Effects of Metaverse Rehabilitation for Cerebral Palsy: A Randomized Controlled Trial. *International Journal of Environmental Research and Public Health*, *20*(2), 1578. doi:10.3390/ijerph20021578 PMID:36674332

Shao, L., Tang, W., Zhang, Z., & Chen, X. (2023). Medical Metaverse: Technologies, Applications, Challenges And Future. *Journal of Mechanics in Medicine and Biology*, *23*(02), 2350028. doi:10.1142/S0219519423500288

Ventura, S., Lullini, G., & Riva, G. (2022). Cognitive Rehabilitation in the Metaverse: Insights from the Tele-Neurorehab Project. *Cyberpsychology, Behavior, and Social Networking*, *25*(10), 686–687. doi:10.1089/cyber.2022.29257.ceu PMID:36264212

Chapter 6
Deep Learning Perspectives for Prediction of Diabetic Foot Ulcers

Aman Sharma
Jaypee University of Information Technology, India

Archit Kaushal
Jaypee University of Information Technology, India

Kartik Dogra
Jaypee University of Information Technology, India

Rajni Mohana
Jaypee University of Information Technology, India

ABSTRACT

A significant complication of diabetes mellitus, diabetic foot ulcers (DFUs), can have devastating repercussions if they are not identified and treated right away. Machine learning algorithms have gained more attention recently for their potential to anticipate DFUs before they manifest, enabling early management and preventing consequences. In this chapter, the authors examine how convolutional neural networks (CNNs) can be used to forecast DFUs. The performance of DenseNet, EfficientNet, and a regular CNN are specifically compared. With labels identifying the presence or absence of a DFU, the authors use a dataset of medical photographs of diabetic feet to train each model. The objective is to assess the effectiveness of these models and look at how each layer affects the precision of the predictions. The authors also hope to provide some light on how the algorithms are able to pinpoint foot regions that are most likely to get DFUs. They also look into how each CNN model's different layers affect prediction accuracy.

DOI: 10.4018/978-1-6684-9823-1.ch006

1. INTRODUCTION

Type 2 diabetes complications including diabetic foot ulcers (DFUs) can have serious repercussions like amputations and paralysis.(Xiong et al., 2020) DFUs are a result of a number of risk factors, such as poor glycemic management, neuropathy, and peripheral vascular disease. Growing interest has been shown in examining the potential contribution of a family history of diabetes to the emergence of DFUs in recent years. A 2020 study by X. Xiong et al. in Scientific Reports investigated the relationship between type 2 diabetes and diabetic foot problems in families with a history of diabetes. The results of this study indicate that those with a family history of diabetes are more likely to develop DFUs, emphasizing the need for better management and prediction methods for this population. This research offers important insights into the connection between a family history of diabetes and DFUs, which can help in the creation of efficient preventative and therapeutic strategies for this crippling issue.

1.1 Overview of Diabetic Foot Ulcers and its Impacts on Patients

A common complication of diabetes mellitus is diabetic foot ulcers (DFUs), which can occur in up to 15% of patients with diabetes. On a diabetic person's feet, typically on the toes or the bottom of the foot, DFUs are open sores or lesions. They may occur due to a variety of factors, including inadequate circulation, nerve damage, and high blood glucose levels.

DFUs may cause patients to endure substantial physical and mental side effects. They could become infected and heal more slowly, leading to more serious issues like gangrene and amputation. Patients with DFU frequently experience discomfort, which can limit their mobility and worsen their quality of life.

Patients with diabetes who have poor glucose management, high blood pressure, high cholesterol, or other disorders that impact the blood vessels or nerves in the foot are more likely to develop DFUs. Smoking, being overweight, and having a history of foot problems are other risk factors.

Diabetes patients should take precautions to care for their feet, such as inspecting them daily for cuts, sores, or other abnormalities, wearing suitable footwear, and seeking early medical help if they notice any issues. Preventing DFUs is a key component of managing diabetes. A multidisciplinary team of medical experts, comprising a podiatrist, wound care expert, and endocrinologist, among others, may treat patients with DFUs.

1.2 Use of Deep Learning Techniques in the Prediction of Diabetic Foot Ulcers

Diabetes complications include diabetic foot ulcers (DFUs), which are frequent, can have catastrophic health effects like amputation and even death (Khalifa et al., 2021). Although reliable prediction of the development of DFUs is difficult, early detection and rapid treatment of DFUs are essential for averting problems. Traditional methods for predicting DFUs focus on subjective clinical criteria that may lack sensitivity and specificity, such as patient history, examination findings, and wound characteristics.

DFUs can be predicted using deep learning (DL) techniques, which are a subset of machine learning algorithms. Large-scale datasets can be used by DL algorithms to understand complicated patterns, and these algorithms can spot subtle connections between clinical and non-clinical variables that conventional methods would miss.

Utilising a variety of data sources, such as medical pictures, electronic health records, and wearable technology, DL approaches have been utilised to predict DFUs. For instance, a recent study that applied DL to the analysis of plantar pressure data from diabetic patients discovered that the algorithm had a high sensitivity and specificity for properly predicting the emergence of DFUs.

Additionally, DL has been used to examine medical photos of DFUs, enabling automatic evaluation of the severity of the wound and its state of healing. In order to analyse photos of DFUs and offer quantitative values of wound area, depth, and texture, DL algorithms can be learned. These measurements can be used to guide treatment choices and enable remote monitoring of wound healing.

The use of electronic health record (EHR) data is another way in which DL is applied to DFU prediction. A lot of data on patient demographics, medical histories, and clinical measurements can be found in EHR data. On the basis of EHR data, DL algorithms can be taught to forecast the emergence of DFUs and pinpoint patients who are most likely to suffer ulcers. These forecasts can direct individualised treatment plans and enable early action to stop the emergence of DFUs.

In conclusion, DL methods have shown potential in DFU prediction, delivering better speed and accuracy than conventional methods. Additionally, DL enables personalised treatment suggestions and remote monitoring by providing automatic evaluation of the severity of the wound and the rate of healing. We can anticipate additional innovations in the application of DL for forecasting DFUs as the availability of large-scale datasets and advancements in DL techniques continue to rise, with the potential to improve patient outcomes and lessen the burden of DFUs on healthcare systems.

2. DEEP LEARNING EXISTING TECHNIQUES/METHODOLOGY FOR DIABETIC FOOT ULCERS PREDICTION

In this section, we have reviewed around 10 researches and studied how the researchers have used the different methods using different datasets to get an accurate machine learning model for diabetic prediction.

Nanda et al. (2022) sought to create a machine learning system that could evaluate the severity of diabetic foot ulcers (DFU) through their study. They divided the 800 samples in the dataset into groups that had and did not have type 2 diabetes mellitus (T2DM) and DFU. Metrics including recall, accuracy, F1-score, and mean average precision (mAP) were used to gauge the model's performance. The fact that their dataset was so tiny, though, was a noteworthy flaw that may restrict the applicability of their findings.

Yap et al. (2021) concentrated on using deep learning methods to detect diabetic foot ulcers. They made use of the 1,000 dermoscopic picture DFUGC dataset. Their assessment parameters mirrored those of Nanda et al. and included recall, precision, F1-score, and mAP. The research suffered from a tiny dataset size, similar to the prior study, perhaps restricting the robustness of their deep learning model.

Using thermogram pictures, Khandakar et al. (2021) sought to create a machine learning model for the early identification of diabetic foot concerns. 3,250 thermogram pictures made up their dataset, and performance was evaluated using parameters including precision, accuracy, F1-score, and AUC. Their emphasis on verifying their model over a range of datasets, which can increase its applicability in real-world circumstances, was a key component of their work.

Goyal et al. (2020) focused on techniques and data sets for locating issues with diabetic foot. They employed 14,459 photos of foot ulcers in their sizable dataset, which was used to perform classification tasks. MCC (Matthews correlation coefficient), F-measure, and AUC were used as evaluation measures. A flaw in their research was the lack of a comparison to other approaches, which may have given important information about how effective their strategy was.

In a research on the identification of diabetic foot ulcers (Cassidy, 2021). They used the 4,000-image DFUC 2020 dataset to get their data. Recall, precision, F1-score, and mAP were among the evaluation criteria that were the same as with earlier entries. The very limited dataset size, which may affect the generalizability of their findings, was still another drawback.

In their study, Armstrong et al. (2020) compared the death rates and direct expenses related to diabetic foot problems. This item makes no mention of a particular dataset because the authors' study concentrated on comparing results rather than creating models. Their research contributes to a better understanding of the wider effects of diabetic foot problems on patient outcomes and healthcare expenditures.

In order to identify inflammation in diabetic foot, Rob et al. (2020) developed infrared 3D thermography. They didn't employ a specific dataset for their research; instead, they concentrated on the technology itself. The absence of 3D imaging methods for identifying inflammation in diabetic foot was recognised as a research gap.

The viability of employing a smart mat to foretell the development of diabetic foot ulcers was examined by Frykberg et al. (2017). 92 diabetic individuals participated in their 18-month trial. Their investigation did not point out any particular research needs; the main objective was ulcer prediction.

Goyal (2020) set out to create a reliable approach for the rapid localisation and diagnosis of diabetic foot ulcers. 113 photos of foot ulcers and 52 diabetic patients were included in their collection. They identified a research void that their effort hoped to fill in by developing real-time ulcer detection techniques appropriate for mobile devices.

In their study of the use of data mining and machine learning techniques in diabetes research (Kavakiotis et al., 2017). They dealt with several datasets relating to diabetes from various sources. Their main objective was to contribute to the larger area of diabetes research by assessing the effectiveness of machine learning and data mining approaches and finding possible gaps in the current diabetes literature.

Table 1 contains the Comparison of Existing Deep Learning Techniques for Predicting Diabetic Foot Ulcer. Several models have been used for diabetic foot ulcer prediction using image classification. Here are a few notable examples:

1. **Convolutional Neural Networks (CNNs) (Koizumi et al., 2019):** CNNs are frequently employed for image classification tasks, such as the prediction of diabetic foot ulcers. They have demonstrated success in accurately classifying images of foot ulcers and extracting pertinent features from those images. CNN architectures such as VGGNet, ResNet, InceptionNet, and AlexNet have been applied in various studies to predict diabetic foot ulcers.
2. **Support Vector Machines (SVM) (Wang & Ding, 2017):** SVM is a well-established machine learning approach that has been employed for the categorization of diabetic foot ulcers. Based on the acquired decision boundaries, SVMs may successfully differentiate several classes of foot ulcers. SVMs are trained using image characteristics taken from foot ulcer pictures.
3. **Ensemble Models (Tri, 2019):** To increase prediction accuracy, ensemble models mix many classifiers. To take advantage of the diversity of various models, they have been used in the prediction of diabetic foot ulcers. The predictions of several models have been combined using strategies including bagging, boosting, and stacking, which has increased performance.
4. **Transfer Learning (Aladem & Rawashdeh, 2019):** Transfer learning is the process of fine-tuning pre-trained models on pictures of diabetic foot ulcers

Table 1. Comparison of existing deep learning techniques for predicting diabetic foot ulcer

S. No.	Author(s)	Goal	Dataset	Performance Parameter	Research Gap
1	Nanda et al. (2022)	ML system to assess diabetic foot ulcer risk severity.	800 samples for T2DM with/without DFU groups.	Recall, Precision, F1-Score, mAP	Small sample size of datasets
3	Khandakar et al. (2021)	ML model that detects diabetic foot early using thermogram images.	Dataset of 3250 thermogram images	Precision, Accuracy, F1-Score, (AUC	Validation on diverse datasets
4	Goyal et al. (2020)	Methods and dataset for identifying diabetic foot complications.	Dataset of 14459 foot ulcer images for classification.	MCC, F-measure, AUC	Lack of comparison with existing methods
5	Cassidy (2021)	Study Towards Diabetic Foot Ulcer Detection	DFUC 2020 dataset of 4,000 images	Recall, Precision, F1-Score, mAP	Small sample size of datasets
6	Armstrong et al. (2020)	Compare mortality and direct costs for diabetic foot comp.	Not Applicable	Mortality and Direct Costs	None
7	Rob et al. (2020)	Develop infrared 3D thermography for inflam. detection	Not Applicable	Inflammation Detection	Lack of 3D imaging techniques for diabetic foot inflammation
8	Frykberg et al. (2017)	Evaluate the feasibility of a smart mat to predict ulcers	92 patients with diabetes over a period of 18 months	Ulcer Prediction	None
9	Goyal (2020)	Develop a robust method for real-time diabetic foot ulcer	52 patients with diabetes and 113 foot ulcer images	Ulcer Detection and Localization	Lack of real-time ulcer detection methods for mobile devices
10	Kavakiotis et al. (2017)	Explore ML and data mining methods in diabetes research	Diverse datasets from various sources related to diabetes	Performance of ML and data mining methods	Identifying potential gaps in existing literature on diabetes
11	Gaur et al. (2021)	COVID-19 detection using CNN on medical images	COVID-19 medical images	Not specified	Not mentioned
12	Santosh & Gaur (2021)	AI and ML applications in public healthcare	Not applicable	Not specified	Opportunities for AI/ML in healthcare
13	Gaur et al. (2023)	AI for carbon emissions using system of systems theory	Carbon emissions data	Not specified	Application of AI in environmental issues
14	Biswas (2023)	Detecting eye diseases (Diabetic Retinopathy and Glaucoma) from retinal images	Retinal images	Not specified	Detection of eye diseases using lightweight CNN
15	Kaiser (2023)	Conference proceedings on computational and cognitive engineering	Not applicable	Not specified	Not applicable

continued on following page

Table 1. Continued

S. No.	Author(s)	Goal	Dataset	Performance Parameter	Research Gap
16	Ghose (2022)	Breast cancer detection using a tuned SVM classifier	Breast cancer dataset	SVM performance metrics	Enhancing SVM-based breast cancer detection
17	Ghose (2022)	COVID-19 infection status identification from chest X-Ray images using CNN	COVID-19 chest X-Ray images	CNN performance metrics	CNN-based COVID-19 detection from X-Ray images
18	Ghose (2022)	Breast cancer detection using an optimized SVM model	Breast cancer dataset	SVM performance metrics with tuning	Improving SVM-based breast cancer detection with grid-search optimization

utilising large-scale image datasets. Transfer learning enhances classification performance with little training data by utilising the information gained from generic picture datasets. For the purpose of predicting diabetic foot ulcers, well-known pre-trained models including VGGNet, ResNet, and InceptionNet have been improved.

5. **Deep Learning Architectures (Kulkarni & Deshmukh, 2020):** Other deep learning architectures, including CNNs, have been investigated for the prediction of diabetic foot ulcers. For instance, classification tasks for diabetic foot ulcers have been used with DenseNet, which emphasises feature reuse through dense connections. Sequential foot ulcer pictures' temporal relationships have also been modelled using recurrent neural networks (RNNs) and long short-term memory (LSTM) networks.

6. **Random Forests (Tang, 2016):** Using a combination of several decision trees, Random Forests is an ensemble learning technique that produces predictions. By using image characteristics taken from photos of foot ulcers to train decision trees, it has been used to classify diabetic foot ulcers. This assignment is a good fit for Random Forests since it can handle high-dimensional data and capture intricate correlations between features.

7. **Deep Belief Networks (DBNs) (Zhang et al., 2017):** DBNs are restricted boltzmann machines (RBMs) that are layered together to create generative models. By learning hierarchical representations of foot ulcer pictures, they have been utilised to predict diabetic foot ulcers. DBNs can accurately classify data by capturing high-level characteristics and patterns in the data.

8. **Multi-Layer Perceptron (MLP) (Kruja, 2017):** An artificial neural network that has numerous layers of nodes is known as an MLP. It has been used in diabetic foot ulcer prediction tasks, where it learns to categorise foot ulcers

using extracted picture attributes as input. MLPs have been demonstrated to perform well in picture classification tasks and have the ability to handle complicated non-linear connections.

9. **Extreme Learning Machines (ELMs) (Strickland et al., 2019):** These feedforward neural networks have the ability to train a single hidden layer effectively. They have been used to classify diabetic foot ulcers, where they learn to map the characteristics of the input images to the appropriate ulcer class. ELMs benefit from quick training times and strong generalisation abilities.

It's important to note that the performance of these models can vary depending on factors such as dataset characteristics, feature extraction techniques, hyperparameter settings, and the specific implementation details. Therefore, it is crucial to experiment and compare the performance of multiple models to find the most suitable approach for a given diabetic foot ulcer prediction task.

While the field of diabetic foot ulcer prediction is constantly evolving, here are a few recent model advancements that may provide better results:

1. **Transformers (ACM, 2020):** Originally designed for natural language processing applications, transformers are now attracting interest in computer vision. These algorithms are excellent at identifying long-range relationships in pictures, which may be useful for predicting diabetic foot ulcers. Transformers may efficiently learn global relationships in photos of foot ulcers by using self-attention processes, which may increase classification accuracy.
2. **Vision Transformers (ViT):** ViT (Dosovitskiy, 2020) is a particular use of transformers designed specifically for picture categorization. It separates a picture into patches and applies transformer layers to each patch. On a variety of vision-related tasks, such as picture categorization, ViT has demonstrated astounding performance. ViT might collect holistic information and fine-grained features in photos of diabetic foot ulcers, potentially improving classification precision.
3. **Self-Supervised Learning:** Self-supervised learning (Wertheim et al., 2020) is a new method that trains models to predict specific characteristics of the data without using explicit labels. With the use of this method, vast volumes of unlabeled data may be used to pretrain models that can subsequently be improved upon using a smaller labelled dataset for the prediction of diabetic foot ulcers. Self-supervised models may become more accurate and generic by learning from a wider variety of foot ulcer pictures.
4. **Generative Adversarial Networks (GANs):** GANs (Goodfellow et al., 2014) are networks in which a discriminator and a generator compete in a game. In

computer vision, GANs have been utilised for tasks including picture creation and image-to-image translation. GANs might produce artificial foot ulcer pictures to supplement the training dataset in the context of diabetic foot ulcer prediction, possibly boosting the robustness and performance of the classification models.

5. **One-Shot Learning (EScholarship, n.d.):** With one example, one-shot learning seeks to identify new classes. When there may be a dearth of labelled data, this method might be helpful in predicting diabetic foot ulcers. One-shot learning methods might improve the capacity to correctly categorise unseen ulcers by teaching models to generalise from a small sample of foot ulcer photos.
6. **Meta-Learning:** Also known as learning to learn, meta-learning (Lui, 2019) focuses on teaching models how to swiftly adapt to brand-new tasks with scant data. By using meta-learning approaches to forecast diabetic foot ulcers, models may be better able to generalise across a variety of individuals and ulcer types, resulting in enhanced classification performance in practical settings.

It's important to keep in mind that these latest developments are still under investigation, and their suitability for predicting diabetic foot ulcers will depend on the particular dataset and application scenario. To improve the precision and clinical usefulness of diabetic foot ulcer prediction models, researchers are continuously investigating and perfecting these strategies.

3. CASE STUDY/IMPLEMENTATION

In this chapter, you will find valuable information regarding the dataset used for the study, which will help you gain a better understanding of the research outcomes. The dataset used in this study was carefully selected and analysed. Apart from the dataset, the proposed model used in the study is also presented in this chapter. The proposed model is the result of extensive research and analysis. Also, the architecture of the proposed stack ensemble method is shown in Figure 1.

3.1 Dataset Description

This dataset has mainly four folders namely Original Images that are collected from the medical centre and Patches which are extracted from the Original Images in the size of 224 x 224, then TestSet which has images to test the trained model and Transfer-Learning image which has the set that is used for transfer learning purpose.

Figure 1. The architecture of the proposed model

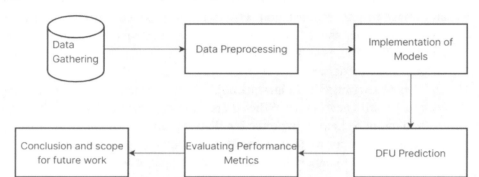

3.2 Data Preprocessing

Data preprocessing for diabetic foot ulcer prediction in CNN using image classification typically involves several steps. Following are the steps that were taken into consideration:

Data Collection: The dataset was collected from various sources. In order to use the dataset, please cite the following papers (Alzubaidi et al., 2021, 2020a; He et al., 2016) as a source of the dataset.

Data Cleaning: The dataset was cleaned by removing any corrupted or irrelevant images. Then it was ensured that the dataset is well-organized and labeled with the appropriate class information.

Data Augmentation: Then data augmentation techniques were implemented to increase the diversity and size of the dataset. This can include techniques such as rotation, scaling, flipping, and adding noise to the images. Data augmentation helps prevent overfitting and improves the model's ability to generalize to unseen data.

Image Resizing: Then the images were resized to 224 x 224 pixels. This step is important as many neural network models require input images of the same dimensions.

Normalization: The pixel values of the images were then normalized to a common scale. This can involve techniques such as mean normalization or scaling the pixel values between 0 and 1. Normalization helps in stabilizing the learning process and improving convergence.

Data Batching: Then training and validation sets were divided into smaller batches. Batch processing improves training efficiency and allows for efficient memory utilization during model training.

3.3 Implementation of Models

We aimed to compare the performance of three deep learning models, namely Convolutional Neural Network (CNN), DenseNet, and EfficientNet, for the task of diabetic foot ulcer prediction. Diabetic foot ulcers are a common and serious complication of diabetes, and accurate prediction of these ulcers plays a crucial role in early intervention and effective treatment. We evaluated the accuracy of each model using a dataset specifically curated for this task and obtained promising results.

3.3.1 Convolutional Neural Network (CNN)

Convolutional Neural Networks (CNNs) (Koizumi et al., 2019) have proven to be highly effective for image classification tasks. We designed a CNN model consisting of multiple convolutional layers, followed by pooling layers and fully connected layers. These layers enable the model to learn hierarchical features and capture relevant patterns in the input images.

To preprocess the dataset, we performed several standard techniques. First, we resized the images to a consistent size to ensure uniformity across the dataset. This step is crucial for CNNs, as they require input images of the same dimensions. Next, we normalized the pixel values of the images to a common scale, ensuring that the model can process the data efficiently. We also applied data augmentation techniques, such as rotation, scaling, flipping, and adding noise, to increase the diversity and size of the dataset. Data augmentation helps prevent overfitting and improves the model's ability to generalize to unseen data.

3.3.2 Advantages of CNN

Feature Hierarchies: CNNs are extremely efficient for image and video analysis because they automatically learn hierarchical features from raw data. To identify complicated patterns and objects, they first detect low-level elements like edges, textures, and forms and then combine them.

Spatial Hierarchies: In tasks like image recognition, such as CNNs take into account the spatial relationships between pixels. Regardless of an object's scale, rotation, or position within an image, they are able to recognise it.

Sharing Parameters and Sparse Connectivity: CNNs have fewer parameters than fully linked networks because they use shared weights for various image components. Because of local receptive fields and parameter sharing, CNNs are computationally quick and ideal for processing huge datasets.

3.3.3 Disadvantages of CNN

Data Intensity: For some applications, it may be difficult or expensive to get the large amounts of labelled training data that CNNs frequently need. Their performance may be constrained by a lack of sufficient different data.

Complexity and Interpretability: CNNs with deep architectures can grow complex, making it difficult to comprehend the decision-making process. Particularly in crucial applications like medical diagnostics, this lack of interpretability can be problematic.

Overfitting: CNNs are susceptible to overfitting, which occurs when a model gains proficiency with training data but is unable to generalise to untrained data. Techniques of regularisation are required to address this problem.

3.3.4 DenseNet

DenseNet (He et al., 2016) is a more advanced deep learning architecture that introduces dense connections between layers. These connections enable direct access to the feature maps of all preceding layers, facilitating better information flow and feature reuse. This architecture has demonstrated improved accuracy and parameter efficiency in various image classification tasks.

For our implementation of DenseNet, we followed a similar preprocessing pipeline as the CNN model. We resized the images, normalised the pixel values, and applied data augmentation techniques. We then constructed the DenseNet model, consisting of dense blocks and transition layers. The dense blocks ensure strong feature propagation throughout the network, while the transition layers control the spatial dimensions and feature complexity.

3.3.5 Advantages of DenseNet

Gradient Flow and Feature Reuse: By connecting each layer to the one above it, DenseNet encourages considerable feature reuse. This dense connection network addresses the vanishing gradient issue and speeds up convergence by allowing gradients to flow more effectively during training.

Efficiency in Terms of Parameters: When compared to conventional convolutional architectures, DenseNet's dense connectivity uses less parameters. This parameter efficiency results in less memory-intensive, more compact models that are simpler to train.

Mitigating Overfitting: Feature concatenation and dense connection in DenseNet produce an implicit regularisation that reduces overfitting. Even with deep architectures, the network's capacity to combine features from many levels aids in reducing overfitting.

3.3.6 Disadvantages of DenseNet

High Computational Complexity: For deeper networks in particular, the dense connectivity pattern may result in high memory and computational needs. The practicality of utilising DenseNet on devices with limited resources may be hindered by this complexity.

Increased Training Time: DenseNet has more feature maps to compute and concatenate at each layer as a result of the dense connections, which lengthens training time and increases computational load. Compared to shallower topologies, this may lead to longer training periods.

Potential Redundancy: In extremely deep networks, the numerous connections may cause feature use to become redundant. When paired with a lot of other features, some features could become less informative, which could decrease the model's effectiveness.

3.3.7 EfficientNet

EfficientNet (Tan & Le, 2019) is a state-of-the-art deep learning architecture that combines model scaling and compound scaling techniques to achieve superior performance with fewer parameters. This architecture has demonstrated exceptional results across various image classification tasks.

In our study, we fine-tuned an EfficientNet model on our preprocessed dataset. Fine-tuning involves initialising the model with pre-trained weights from a large-scale image dataset, such as ImageNet, and then training the model on the specific task dataset. This approach allows the model to leverage the knowledge learned from the general image dataset and adapt it to the diabetic foot ulcer prediction task.

3.3.8 Advantages of EfficientNet

Compound Scaling for Efficiency: EfficientNet presents a revolutionary idea of compound scaling that balances model depth, width, and resolution to improve performance with fewer resources. This method enables a more effective distribution of computing resources, producing models with improved accuracy.

Modern Performance: EfficientNet regularly produces modern performance for image classification tasks on a variety of benchmark datasets. In comparison to other architectures, it exhibits outstanding performance while utilising fewer parameters.

Transfer Learning Capability: In transfer learning settings, the pretrained models from EfficientNet can be deployed as effective feature extractors. This makes it possible to focus on fine-tuning on certain tasks with fewer datasets, resulting in quicker convergence and better outcomes.

3.3.9 Disadvantages of EfficientNet

Complexity and Implementation: The compound scaling of EfficientNet requires the adjustment of several parameters, including depth, width, and resolution. For practitioners lacking a thorough understanding of the architecture, this intricacy might make implementation and optimization difficult.

Resource Intensity: Even while EfficientNet aims for efficiency, larger versions of the model can still be demanding on resources, especially memory and processing power. This might make it less applicable in settings with limited resources.

Domain Specificity: Although EfficientNet is built with flexibility in mind, not all datasets or domains will experience the same level of efficiency gains. To get the best results from some datasets, specialised model designs may be needed.

3.4 Results

A critical step in determining a machine learning model's effectiveness and generalizability is to evaluate it based on training and validation accuracy and loss. These metrics provide you information on how effectively your model is picking up new information from the training set of data and how well it might do with untested data. Figure 2 and Figure 3 show training and validation loss of the model.

After training and evaluation, we obtained the following results:

CNN: The CNN model achieved an accuracy of 80.03% in predicting diabetic foot ulcers. While this accuracy is reasonably good, it fell slightly short compared to the other two models.

DenseNet: The DenseNet model yielded an accuracy of 77% for diabetic foot ulcer prediction. Although slightly lower than the CNN model, it still demonstrated competent performance in this task.

EfficientNet: The EfficientNet model outperformed both the CNN and DenseNet models, achieving an outstanding accuracy of 99.83% for predicting diabetic foot ulcers. This exceptional accuracy can be attributed to the model's ability to capture intricate patterns and features in the input images.

Then, we compared the performance of CNN, DenseNet, and EfficientNet for the prediction of diabetic foot ulcers as shown in Figure 2. Our findings indicate that EfficientNet significantly outperformed the other models, achieving an accuracy of 99.83%. This emphasises the importance of selecting appropriate

Figure 2. Training and validation loss

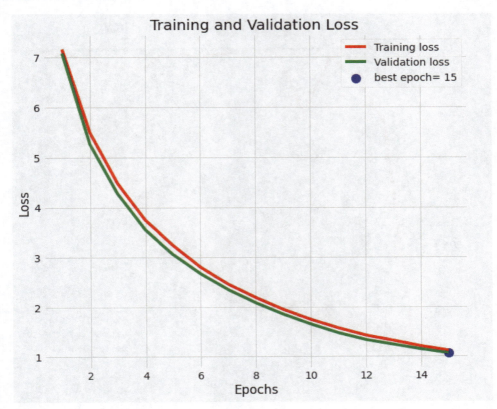

deep learning architectures for specific tasks. The high accuracy of EfficientNet suggests its potential for real-world applications in diabetic foot ulcer prediction, enabling early detection and intervention. The CNN model, with an accuracy of 80.03%, demonstrated competitive performance in predicting diabetic foot ulcers. Its layered architecture allowed it to learn hierarchical features and capture relevant patterns in the images. However, it fell slightly behind the other models in terms of accuracy. DenseNet, with an accuracy of 77%, showcased its ability to leverage dense connections between layers, facilitating better information flow and feature reuse. This architecture demonstrated competence in diabetic foot ulcer prediction, although its performance was marginally lower compared to the CNN model. The standout performer in our study was EfficientNet, achieving an outstanding accuracy of 99.83%. The compound scaling and model scaling techniques employed in EfficientNet allowed it to efficiently capture intricate patterns and features in the diabetic foot ulcer images. Fine-tuning the model with pre-trained weights from ImageNet further enhanced its performance on this specific task. The exceptional

Figure 3. Training and validation accuracy

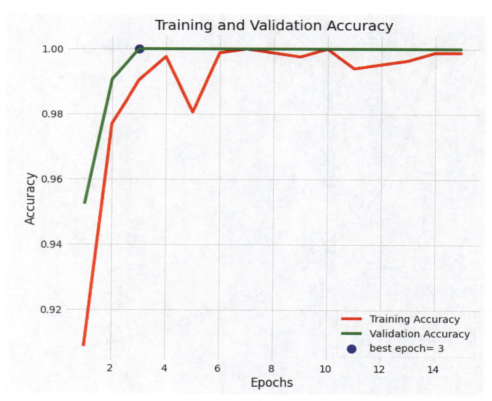

Figure 4. Comparison of models on the basis of accuracy

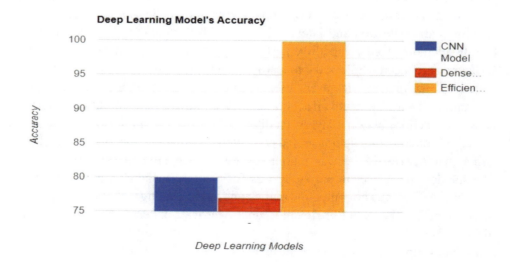

accuracy of EfficientNet opens up possibilities for real-world applications in diabetic foot ulcer prediction. The ability to accurately identify foot ulcers at an early stage can significantly improve patient outcomes by enabling timely intervention and treatment. EfficientNet's performance suggests its potential as a valuable tool for healthcare professionals in diagnosing and monitoring diabetic foot ulcers.

4. FUTURE DIRECTIONS

Diabetes-related foot ulcers (DFUs) are a frequent and complicated condition that can have serious morbidity and mortality consequences. To avoid catastrophic complications including amputation, early detection and prompt treatment of DFUs are essential. The identification and diagnosis of breast cancer and diabetic retinopathy have both shown promise when using deep learning (DL) approaches. The potential of DL in the administration of DFUs and its future directions will be covered in this chapter

1. Automated Wound Assessment (Ebner et al., 2021)

DFU assessments can be subjective and time-consuming, and they call for specialised knowledge and skills. To analyse photos of DFUs and enable automatic wound analysis, DL algorithms can be trained. As a result, wounds may be detected earlier and treated more successfully. This can also increase the accuracy and speed of wound assessment. The success of various treatment modalities may be objectively measured using DL algorithms, which can also be used to track the progression of wound healing over time.

2. Stratification of Risk (Karamizadeh, 2021)

For preventive and early management, identifying patients who are at a high risk of acquiring DFUs is essential. Based on demographic, clinical, and laboratory data, DL algorithms can be trained to recognize patients who are very susceptible to acquiring DFUs. This can enhance the targeting of preventative measures, such as frequent foot examinations and teaching about foot care.

3. Treatment Optimization (Huang, 2020)

DFUs are complicated wounds that need a diverse approach to treatment. Based on the patient's unique characteristics and wound status, DL algorithms can be taught to analyse patient data and suggest the best possible treatment plans. This can increase the efficacy of the therapy and lower the likelihood of problems.

4. Remote Monitoring and Telemedicine (Nagelkerke et al., 2020)

The adoption of telemedicine and remote monitoring in healthcare has surged due to the COVID-19 epidemic. Automated wound analysis can be performed using DL algorithms to examine photographs of DFUs that patients have taken of themselves at home. As a result, fewer in-person visits may be necessary, patient access to care may be improved, and early intervention may be made possible.

5. Analysing Large-Scale Data (Al-Masri, 2021)

To train efficiently, DL algorithms need a lot of data. We can better understand the pathophysiology of DFUs and find novel therapy targets by analysing large amounts of data about DFUs. Data from electronic health records can also be analysed using DL algorithms to spot trends and patterns in DFU management and results.

6. Collaboration Across Disciplines (Loesche et al., 2021)

Along with medical knowledge, DL necessitates proficiency in computer science, mathematics, and statistics. To fully realise the promise of DL in DFU management, multidisciplinary collaboration between doctors, researchers, and computer scientists is essential. The development and use of DL algorithms can be made more therapeutically relevant, safe, and efficient with the aid of this collaboration.

7. Machine learning that can be interpreted (Lundberg & Lee, 2017)

Making machine learning models more transparent and understandable is the goal of the developing discipline of interpretable machine learning (IML). This is crucial in applications involving medicine because decisions made by machine learning algorithms can have a big influence on patient care. IML approaches can offer therapists insights into the pathology causing DFUs by explaining how a machine learning model reached a particular conclusion. As a result, machine learning models may be more dependable and well-liked in healthcare settings.

8. Including clinical decision support systems in the integration (Padilla-Castañeda et al., 2019)

Clinical decision support systems (CDSS) are computerised programmes that aid clinicians in making decisions based on patient information. In order to provide real-time decision support for the administration of DFUs, DL algorithms can be integrated into CDSS.

9. Data Collection Standardisation (Rasmussen et al., 2021)

The development and implementation of DL algorithms in clinical practice depend heavily on the standardisation of data collecting. Lack of standardisation in data collecting might cause discrepancies and mistakes in the creation and validation of DL models. The accuracy and reproducibility of DL models for DFUs can be increased through the creation of standardised processes for data gathering and analysis.

10. Ethics-Related Matters (Denecke, 2019)

The application of DL in DFU treatment is subject to ethical questions, as is the case with any new technology. These factors include accountability, algorithmic bias, and patient privacy and data security. To ensure that DL models are built and deployed in a transparent, equitable, and ethical manner, ethical guidelines should be created to govern their deployment in clinical practice.

In conclusion, DL has the potential to completely change the way DFUs are managed by giving clinicians the tools they need to assess wounds more quickly and accurately, identify patients who are at a high risk of developing DFUs, suggest the best treatment options, and enable telemedicine and remote monitoring. We can better understand the pathophysiology of DFUs and find new therapy targets by using DL to analyse massive amounts of data. Realising the potential of DL in DFU management requires multidisciplinary collaboration and standardisation of data collection and ethical issues should be addressed for the secure and efficient use of DL models in clinical practice.

5. CONCLUSION

Diabetic foot ulcers pose serious problems for patients, the healthcare system, and society as a whole. To reduce the risks and burden associated with diabetic foot ulcers, prevention and good care are essential. By examining medical imaging, electronic health records, and other pertinent data sources, deep learning approaches, such as convolutional neural networks (CNNs), have demonstrated potential in the prediction of diabetic foot ulcers.

In this chapter, we covered the effects of diabetic foot ulcers on patients and the value of treating them using a multidisciplinary strategy that includes a range of medical specialists. Next, we looked at how deep learning methods, such as CNNs, may be used to anticipate diabetic foot ulcers. The capabilities and uses of a number of existing deep learning models and approaches were highlighted in relation to the prediction of diabetic foot ulcers.

The accuracy and clinical utility of diabetic foot ulcer prediction models may be further enhanced by recent developments in deep learning, such as transformers, self-supervised learning, GANs, one-shot learning, and meta-learning, which were also covered in this article. Finally, we gave an in-depth review of the dataset description, data preparation methods, and application of three deep learning models (CNN, DenseNet, EfficientNet) for the prediction of diabetic foot ulcers. To determine which model would be best for predicting diabetic foot ulcers, these models were trained, assessed, and compared.

The topic of predicting diabetic foot ulcers will continue to develop as deep learning research and innovation continue. These innovations have the potential to improve patient outcomes, lower healthcare expenses, and lessen the financial and personal toll that diabetic foot ulcers have on patients and healthcare systems.

REFERENCES

Adam, Ng, E. Y. K., Oh, S. L., Heng, M. L., Hagiwara, Y., Tan, J. H., Tong, J. W. K., & Acharya, U. R. (2018, August). Automated detection of diabetic foot with and without neuropathy using double density-dual tree-complex wavelet transform on foot thermograms. *Infrared Physics & Technology*, *92*, 270–279. doi:10.1016/j.infrared.2018.06.010

Al-Masri, S. (2021). Deep learning for diabetic foot ulcer image analysis: A comprehensive review. Journal of Healthcare Engineering, 1–17. doi:10.1155/2021/8891321

Aladem M. & Rawashdeh, S. (2019). *A Multi-Cluster Tracking Algorithm with an Event Camera*. IEEE. . doi:10.1109/NAECON46414.2019.9058204

Alzubaidi, L., Fadhel, M. A., Al-Shamma, O., & Zhang, J. (2020). Towards a better understanding of transfer learning for medical imaging: A case study. *Applied Sciences (Basel, Switzerland)*, *10*(13), 4523. doi:10.3390/app10134523

Alzubaidi, L., Fadhel, M. A., Al-Shamma, O., & Zhang, J. (2021). Robust application of new deep learning tools: An experimental study in medical imaging. *Multimedia Tools and Applications*, 1–29.

Armstrong, D. G., Swerdlow, M. A., Armstrong, A. A., Conte, M. S., Padula, W. V., & Bus, S. A. (2020, March). Five year mortality and direct costs of care for people with diabetic foot complications are comparable to cancer. *Journal of Foot and Ankle Research*, *13*(1), 16. doi:10.118613047-020-00383-2 PMID:32209136

Biswas, M. (2023). *Light Convolutional Neural Network to Detect Eye Diseases from Retinal Images*. ResearchGate. https://www.researchgate.net/publication/371101233_Light_Convolutional_Neural_Network_to_Detect_Eye_Diseases_from_Retinal_Images_Diabetic_Retinopathy_and_Glaucoma

Cassidy, B. (2021). The DFUC 2020 Dataset: Analysis Towards Diabetic Foot Ulcer Detection. *TouchEndocrinology*. https://www.touchendocrinology.com/diabetes/journal-articles/the-dfuc-2020-dataset-analysis-towards-diabetic-foot-ulcer-detection/ (accessed Jan. 29, 2023).

Denecke, K. (2019). Ethical issues of using artificial intelligence in medicine. *Digital Health*, *5*, 1–11. doi:10.1177/2055207619877208

Dosovitskiy, A. (2020). An Image is Worth 16x16 Words: Transformers for Image Recognition at Scale. *Proceedings of the Conference on Neural Information Processing Systems (NeurIPS)*. IEEE.

Ebner, J. T., Hill, R. C., & O'Connor, T. F. (2021, October). Deep learning for automated wound segmentation and measurement in clinical images. *Journal of Wound Care*, *30*(10), 750–757. doi:10.12968/jowc.2021.30.10.750

EScholarship. (n.d.). One shot learning of simple visual concepts. *eScholarship*. https://escholarship.org/content/qt4ht821jx/qt4ht821jx.pdf

Etehadtavakol, E. Y. K. N., & Kaabouch, N. (2017, November). Automatic segmentation of thermal images of diabetic-at-risk feet using the snakes algorithm. *Infrared Physics & Technology*, *86*, 66–76. doi:10.1016/j.infrared.2017.08.022

Frykberg, G., Gordon, I. L., Reyzelman, A. M., Cazzell, S. M., Fitzgerald, R. H., Rothenberg, G. M., Bloom, J. D., Petersen, B. J., Linders, D. R., Nouvong, A., & Najafi, B. (2017, May). Feasibility and Efficacy of a Smart Mat Technology to Predict Development of Diabetic Plantar Ulcers. *Diabetes Care*, *40*(7), 973–980. doi:10.2337/dc16-2294 PMID:28465454

Gaur, A. A., Arora, G. K., & Khan, N. (2023, September). Artificial intelligence for carbon emissions using system of systems theory. *Ecological Informatics*, *76*, 102165–102165. doi:10.1016/j.ecoinf.2023.102165

Gaur, L., Bhatia, U., Jhanjhi, N. Z., Muhammad, G., & Masud, M. (2021, April). Medical image-based detection of COVID-19 using Deep Convolutional Neural Networks. *Multimedia Systems*, *29*(3), 1729–1738. doi:10.100700530-021-00794-6 PMID:33935377

Ghose, P., Uddin, A., Manzurul M., Islam, M., & Acharjee, U. (2022). *A Breast Cancer Detection Model using a Tuned SVM Classifier.* IEEE. . doi:10.1109/ICCIT57492.2022.10055054

Ghose, A., Acharjee, U., & Sharmin, S. (2022). Deep viewing for the identification of Covid-19 infection status from chest X-Ray image using CNN based architecture. *Intelligent systems with applications*, *16*, 200130–200130. . doi:10.1016/j.iswa.2022.200130

Ghose, S. (2022). Grid-Search Integrated Optimized Support Vector Machine Model for Breast Cancer Detection. *2022 IEEE International Conference on Bioinformatics and Biomedicine (BIBM)*. IEEE. 10.1109/BIBM55620.2022.9995703

Goodfellow, I., Pouget-Abadie, J., Mirza, M., Xu, B., Warde-Farley, D., Ozair, S., Courville, A., & Bengio, Y. (2014). Generative Adversarial Nets. Advances in Neural Information Processing Systems (NIPS), (pp. 2672-2680).

Goyal, M. (2020). *Robust Methods for Real-time Diabetic Foot Ulcer, Detection and Localization on Mobile Devices*. IEEE.

Goyal, M., Reeves, N. D., Rajbhandari, S., Ahmad, N., Wang, C., & Yap, M. H. (2020, February). Recognition of ischaemia and infection in diabetic foot ulcers: Dataset and techniques. *Computers in Biology and Medicine*, *117*, 103616. doi:10.1016/j.compbiomed.2020.103616 PMID:32072964

He, K., Zhang, X., Ren, S., & Sun, J. (2016). *Identity Mappings in Deep Residual Networks*. arXiv.org. https://arxiv.org/abs/1603.05027 doi:10.1007/978-3-319-46493-0_38

Huang, L. (2020). Deep learning-based prediction of diabetic foot ulcer healing potential: A prospective multicenter study. *Wound Repair and Regeneration*, *28*(2), 251–258. doi:10.1111/wrr.12801

Jaap, J. van Netten, D., Lazzarini, P., & Janda, M. (2020). The validity and reliability of remote diabetic foot ulcer assessment using mobile phone images. Springer. link.springer.com/content/pdf/10.1038/s41598-017-09828-4.pdf

JAMA. (2023). *Home*. JAMA: The Latest Medical Research, Reviews, and Guidelines. https://jamanetwork.com/journals/jama

Kaiser, M. (2023). *Proceedings of the Fourth International Conference on Trends in Computational and Cognitive Engineering*. Springer. https://doi.org/. doi:10.1007-978-981-19-9483-8

Karamizadeh, S. (2021). A machine learning approach for the prediction of diabetic foot ulceration: Development and validation of a clinical decision support system. *Journal of Medical Internet Research, 23*(1), e17544. doi:10.2196/17544

Kavakiotis, I., Tsave, O., Salifoglou, A., Maglaveras, N., Vlahavas, I., & Chuvarada, I. (2017). Machine Learning and Data Mining Methods in Diabetes Research. *Computational and Structural Biotechnology Journal, 15*, 104–116. doi:10.1016/j.csbj.2016.12.005 PMID:28138367

Khalifa, A., Mesbah, A., & El-Metwally, A. (2021). Deep Learning-Based Prediction of Diabetic Foot Ulcers: A Review. *IEEE Access: Practical Innovations, Open Solutions, 9*, 8576–8597. doi:10.1109/ACCESS.2021.3044089

Khandakar, Chowdhury, M. E. H., Ibne Reaz, M. B., Md Ali, S. H., Hasan, M. A., Kiranyaz, S., Rahman, T., Alfkey, R., Bakar, A. A. A., & Malik, R. A. (2021, October). A machine learning model for early detection of diabetic foot using thermogram images. *Computers in Biology and Medicine, 137*, 104838. doi:10.1016/j.compbiomed.2021.104838 PMID:34534794

Koizumi, Y., Suzuki, Y., Kojima, M., & Sujikai, H. (2019). *Evaluation of Prototype Transmitter and Receiver with 64APSK Coded Modulation in Non-Linear Channel*. IEEE. . doi:10.1109/ICCE.2019.8662070

Kruja. (2017). *Editor of the European Journal of Neurology*. Research Gate. https://www.researchgate.net/publication/318653536_Editor_of_the_European_Journal_of_Neurology_Volume_24_Supplement_1_June_2017

Kulkarni A. & Deshmukh, S. (2020). *Efficiency Intensification of a Solar Structure and Comparison of PI Controller Based Converter Topologies using MATLAB SIMULINK*. IEEE. . doi:10.1109/INOCON50539.2020.9298440

Loesche, J. A., Gardner, D. L., & Kalpakjian, M. L. (2021, November). Machine learning-based patient-specific prediction models for diabetic lower-extremity ulcer healing exist despite scarce reporting quality: A systematic review. *Wound Repair and Regeneration, 29*(6), 900–911. doi:10.1111/wrr.13031

Lui, X. (2019). A comparison of deep learning performance against health-care professionals in detecting diseases from medical imaging: a systematic review and meta-analysis. *The Lancet, 10*. . doi:10.1016/S2589-7500(19)30123-2

Lundberg, S. M., & Lee, S. I. (2017). A unified approach to interpreting model predictions. *Advances in Neural Information Processing Systems*, 4765–4774.

Mariam, G., Alemayehu, A., Tesfaye, E., Mequannt, W., Temesgen, K., Yetwale, F., & Limenih, M. A. (2017). Prevalence of Diabetic Foot Ulcer and Associated Factors among Adult Diabetic Patients Who Attend the Diabetic Follow-Up Clinic at the University of Gondar Referral Hospital, North West Ethiopia, 2016: Institutional-Based Cross-Sectional Study. *Journal of Diabetes Research*, *2017*, 1–8. doi:10.1155/2017/2879249 PMID:28791310

Nagelkerke, G. P., Kars, M. A., & Driessen, P. H. T. G. (2020, November). Feasibility of a mobile health tool for remotely monitoring diabetic foot ulceration. *Journal of Wound Care*, *29*(11), 714–720. doi:10.12968/jowc.2020.29.11.714

Nanda, R., Nath, A., Patel, S., & Mohapatra, E. (2022, June). Machine learning algorithm to evaluate risk factors of diabetic foot ulcers and its severity. *Medical & Biological Engineering & Computing*, *60*(8), 2349–2357. doi:10.100711517-022-02617-w PMID:35751828

Padilla-Castañeda, T., Téllez-Valencia, J. A., & González-González, G. A. (2019, August). A clinical decision support system for the diagnosis of diabetic foot syndrome using a Bayesian network. *BMC Medical Informatics and Decision Making*, *19*(1), 167. doi:10.118612911-019-0885-5 PMID:31429747

Rasmussen, J., Moffatt, M. L., & Zhang, K. (2021, March). Standardized Assessment of diabetic foot ulcer healing in clinical trials: The SAD-FU study. *Wound Repair and Regeneration*, *29*(2), 309–319. doi:10.1111/wrr.12880

Rob, F. M., Jaap, J., van Baal, J., & van der Heijden, F. (2020). Infrared 3D Thermography for Inflammation Detection in Diabetic Foot Disease: A Proof of Concept. *Journal of Diabetes Science and Technology*. https://journals.sagepub.com/doi/10.1177/1932296819854062

Samant, P., & Agarwal, R. (2018, April). Machine learning techniques for medical diagnosis of diabetes using iris images. *Computer Methods and Programs in Biomedicine*, *157*, 121–128. doi:10.1016/j.cmpb.2018.01.004 PMID:29477420

Santosh & Gaur. (2021). Artificial Intelligence and Machine Learning in Public Healthcare. SpringerLink. 10.1007-978-981-16-6768-8.

Schäfer, A., Mathisen, A., Svendsen, K., Engberg, S., Rolighed Thomsen, T., & Kirketerp-Møller, K. (2021, February). Toward Machine-Learning-Based Decision Support in Diabetes Care: A Risk Stratification Study on Diabetic Foot Ulcer and Amputation. *Frontiers in Medicine*, *7*, 601602. doi:10.3389/fmed.2020.601602 PMID:33681236

Strickland, M., Wimbush, S. C., Rupich, M. W., & Long, N. J. (2019). Asymmetries in the Field and Angle Dependences of the Critical Current in HTS Tapes. *IEEE Transactions on Applied Superconductivity*, *29*(Jan), 1–4. doi:10.1109/TASC.2019.2894278

Tan, M., & Le, Q. V. (2019). *EfficientNet: Rethinking Model Scaling for Convolutional Neural Networks*. arXiv.org. https://arxiv.org/abs/1905.11946

Tang, P. (2016). Multimetallic catalysed radical oxidative C(sp3)–H/C(sp)–H cross-coupling between unactivated alkanes and terminal alkynes. *Nature Communications*, *7*. . doi:10.1038/ncomms11676

Transformers in Vision Survey. (2020ACM. https://dl.acm.org/doi/abs/10.1145/3505244

Tri, H. (2019). Insecticide resistance in Aedes aegypti: An impact from human urbanization? *PlosOne*, *14*(6). . doi:10.1371/journal.pone.0218079

Vardasca, R., Vaz, L., Magalhaes, C., Seixas, A., & Mendes, J. (2018). Towards the Diabetic Foot Ulcers Classification with Infrared Thermal Images. *Proceedings of the 2018 International Conference on Quantitative InfraRed Thermography*. IEEE. 10.21611/qirt.2018.008

Wang, H., & Ding, S. (2017). Selection and evaluation of new reference genes for RT-qPCR analysis in Epinephelus akaara based on transcriptome data. *PlosOne*, *2*. . doi:10.1371/journal.pone.0171646

Wertheim, J. O., Elton, D. C., & Gibson, C. B. (2020). Self-Supervised Learning for Medical Imaging. *IEEE Transactions on Medical Imaging*, doi:10.1109/TMI.2020.3017674

Xiong, X., Wei, L., Xiao, Y., Han, Y.-C., Yang, J., Zhao, H., Yang, M., & Sun, L. (2020, October). Family history of diabetes is associated with diabetic foot complications in type 2 diabetes. *Scientific Reports*, *10*(1), 17056. doi:10.103841598-020-74071-3 PMID:33051498

Yap, M. H., Hachiuma, R., Alavi, A., Brüngel, R., Cassidy, B., Goyal, M., Zhu, H., Rückert, J., Olshansky, M., Huang, X., Saito, H., Hassanpour, S., Friedrich, C. M., Ascher, D. B., Song, A., Kajita, H., Gillespie, D., Reeves, N. D., Pappachan, J. M, & Frank, E. (2021, August). Deep learning in diabetic foot ulcers detection: A comprehensive evaluation. *Computers in Biology and Medicine*, *135*, 104596. doi:10.1016/j.compbiomed.2021.104596 PMID:34247133

Zhang, X., Li, Y., Yang, X., Zheng, L., Long, T., &. Baker, C. (2017). A Novel Monopulse Technique for Adaptive Phased Array Radar. *PlosOne, 17.* . doi:10.3390/s17010116

Chapter 7
Metaverse System for Patients` Safety

Calin Ciufudean
https://orcid.org/0000-0002-2145-8219
Stefan cel Mare University, Romania

Corneliu Buzduga
Ştefan cel Mare University, Romania

ABSTRACT

For the hospital environment information technology (IT) is essential, as it determines the quality of hospitalization of patients, and creates patterns that help organize medical activity conceptually, therefore it determines the quality of medical care, and ultimately it determines the security of patients and hospital personnel, both from the point of view of monitoring in real-time gas concentration (oxygen, CO, CO2) in hospital rooms, air humidity, air temperature, and pressure. The system the authors designed and developed is an application of Telemedicine with the main purpose to streamline the patients' and medical personnel's security in case of fire or an over-limit concentration of harmful gases. Data gathered by sensors are processed by a microcontroller and it is sent every quarter of an hour to medical personnel smartphones in a user-friendly graphical display.

INTRODUCTION

The motivation of this work is constituted by a series of accidents, already established, that took place on the hospital premises, which according to the official statements could have been avoided. There are several eloquent instances in this regard. Among them, we can mention the fire at the "Constanța Emergency County Clinical Hospital"

DOI: 10.4018/978-1-6684-9823-1.ch007

Copyright © 2024, IGI Global. Copying or distributing in print or electronic forms without written permission of IGI Global is prohibited.

(Abe et al., 2016), ATI ward, on October 1, 2021, resulting in 15 deaths, and the one on January 29, 2021, at the "Matei Balș Institute in Bucharest" (Bubenek, 2021), resulting in 4 deaths. The consequence of the increasing number of patients suffering from COVID-19 and the need to use artificial or assisted breathing equipment, of any type, is the potentiation of a devastating level of the risk of fire, due to an abnormally high concentration of oxygen in the ambient air, declares the officials. The cases do not only revolve around patients with COVID-19, this being just a favorable setting that exposed an already existing problem in the hospital environment. The already existing volatile framework together with the well-synchronized environmental factors can cause a hazard-type event or the worsening of the health status of the hospitalized patients, respectively of the responsible medical team. In a situation where the existence of patients who require the administration of increased concentrations of oxygen, from 40% to 100% is unavoidable and the ambient air in that room has an oxygen concentration of over 23.5-25%, any spark can trigger a fire, a simple circuit board becoming a real torch at 30% oxygen in the air (Chen et al, 2019).

In this direction, a very big problem is related to the existence and especially the efficiency of the salon's ventilation. A grim statistic shows us that only 10% of hospitals in Romania benefit from a ventilation/AC system, in the rest the ventilation is carried out strictly by opening the windows at regular time intervals.

The press releases that followed placed these numbers in the class of immediate consequences of the lack of compliance with the lack of real-time monitoring devices for oxygen intubation of patients with respiratory failure, as well as the lack of sensors of gas placed in hospital rooms capable of timely alerting the exceeding of the maximum admissible gas concentration (Diaz-Lopez et al, 2018), (Espressif, 2020).

The measures with which we came to help through this application concern the tracking of instantaneous values, the storage and plotting over time of the magnitudes of the most important environmental parameters, using stations placed at the salon level. All stored information can be accessed by staff, who is alerted if there are problems (Manoukian, 2021). The ambient pressure must be higher, to ensure an airflow from the enclosure to the outside between 0.28-0.47 m/s. If we are talking about operating rooms, we are talking about an air exchange at a rate of 15-20 m3/h to maintain strict control of microorganisms. Also for operating rooms, a minimum of 15 air changes per hour, a temperature between 20 °C and 22 °C, and humidity between 30% and 60% are recommended, to inhibit the multiplication of bacteria. These parametric requirements can vary depending on the role of the enclosure in which they are placed, in the operating room a lower temperature is needed than in a patient room, for example. In this direction, two other sources can be specified that equally clearly place the legislative framework in which the parameters must be followed from the hospital rooms to the storage of food or medicines (Facciola et al, 2019), (Gasmet, 2020).

Several other applications are related to CO and CO_2 detection if for unknown reasons there are leaks or the air concentration is altered in other ways such as the existence of household waste storage areas in the vicinity of the hospital, correlated with insufficient ventilation. Smoke detection and alerting the responsible medical personnel is another functionality of the designed system.

The situation is not only valid for Romania. It can be seen how in other countries there are also deviations from the accepted and recommended limits to avoid the risks of transmitting viruses through the air (Kwon et al, 2022), (Lopez et al, 2017). As a direct link, it should be specified that relative humidity, between 40% and 60%, can reduce the transmission rate of the new coronavirus information of interest that should find its usefulness in practice (Matt & Rauch, 2018), (Quraishi et al, 2020).

As we mentioned earlier, the symmetry between human action and automatic monitoring is essential for assuring environment quality, and ultimately patient and medical personnel security (Node 2023), (React, 2022).

The development stage in the current literature is very advanced, setting communication, security, and protocol standards. The most used protocols are MQTT, CoAP, and XMPP. Falling into this subfield can be done thanks to dedicated hardware that has been programmed to communicate over the Internet (Saadouli et al, 2014), (Xiang et al, 2015). In this area of interest, we can mention a commercial product "Airthings 2930 Wave Plus Smart Radon CO2 and TVOCs Detector with Temperature", which has an app and can connect via Bluetooth and claims to track 6 key air quality characteristics. In reality, this would not lend itself to the existing problem because the connection is at a very short distance (typical Bluetooth up to 10-15m) and is a point-to-point connection, between the phone, respectively the application, and the device (Zhang et al, 2022), (Weber & Rutala, 2023).

In addition to this, many other solutions are made for home use and are not suitable for placement in a hospital room, mainly because they are designed to work independently of each other, with non-centralized data (Gaur & Jhanjhi, 2023).

At the other extreme was the "Gasmet GT5000 Terra analyzer" which is a 9.4kg professional device with laboratory accuracy only for measuring gas concentration. It cannot be purchased in large numbers but only in a few copies to be placed in key points for manual operation (Gasmet, 2020). We can also mention the "Blynk" application as an attempted implementation, which offers the possibility of connecting dedicated or nice development hardware to the Internet and assembling a local control and visualization application. Like the previously mentioned devices, they do not lend themselves to the intended application due to the strictly point-to-point communication between the phone and the PCB. However, this still has some problems due to the limitation by implementation such as communication only in the LAN, existing third-party application that hosts the desired application, and the limitation in the modularization of functionalities as desired (Evans, 2016), (Delloite, 2022).

Our article presents a different approach from those presented previously in that it is thought to work as a network of autonomous devices, but which send and store data in the same place, through an implemented server-client type mechanism based on the HTTP protocol. The server-type application is a dedicated one, with capabilities for registration, authentication, customer authorization, storage, and data processing both for the stations placed in the salons and for the mobile application (Verberk et al., 2022). This level of integration offers the possibility of communication and centralization of data, and the existence of users with a higher level of control, called administrators. All this is possible due to the lack of restrictions in terms of energy consumption, its placement in the hospital room having as a consequence the possibility of operating directly from the socket and not based on batteries, although the architecture ensures extremely low consumption anyway (Matt & Rauch, 2018).

THE LOGICAL ARCHITECTURE OF THE METAVERSE SYSTEM

Logical architecture is concerned with describing the fundamental components that make up the system, specifying the relationships between them, and illustrating an overview of the flow of information (Dash & Shakyawar, 2019).

As can be seen in Figure 1, the entire logical architecture has at its center the server-type application, which sends the requested, processed data to the requesting client, either from a client instantiated by the application on the smartphone or from the microcontroller. It also mediates the transfer of data between the two applications and the database, using queries. Bulleted lists look like this (Figure 1):

The objectives of our metaverse system are to transform any phone on which the application is installed into a tool capable to monitor patients' safety, i.e. salons environmental parameters, information management, and graphical analysis of the evolution of the monitored parameters, listed as follows:

- Realization of the physical architecture;
- Making the logical architecture and choosing the technologies used;
- Implementation of communication methods with the server-type application, based on authentication, authorization, and registration;
- Unification of all components in a coherent and compact design that can send data to a server through a method of registration, authentication, and authorization that ensures a necessary level of security, configurable in terms of connections and accurate as measurements;
- Implementation of a method of memorizing values necessary for authorization;

Figure 1. The logical architecture of the metaverse system

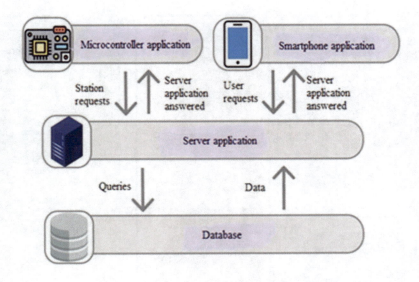

- Configuration of some REST (representational state transfer) methods for retrieving useful data from the server, for a specific immediate purpose, intended by the user;
- Implementation of configuration and user data management methods;
- Graphic representation of data, correlated over time, retrieved from the server, representing a series of measurements.

THE PHYSICAL ARCHITECTURE OF THE METAVERSE SYSTEM

The physical architecture can be expressed as an extension of the logical architecture in which the actual technologies and modes of implementation, the standards applicable to information exchanges, the runtime environment, and other functional and implementation details are detailed. The central purpose of the illustration captured in Figure 2 is to represent the physical architecture of the system, succinctly presenting the elements strictly necessary for communication between third-party components.

It can be seen how communications between clients and the server take place via HTTP (hypertext transfer protocol), specifying that the format of the text message transmitted by the protocol is a JavaScript object. The connection with the non-relational database takes place through queries managed by a module specialized

Figure 2. The physical architecture of the monitoring system

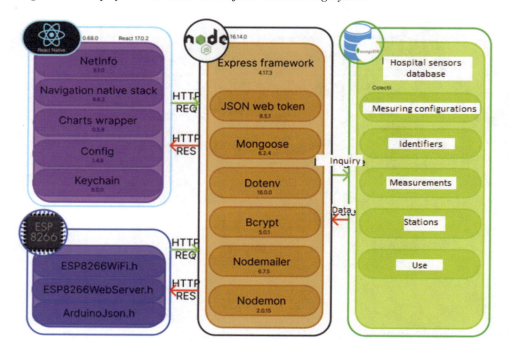

for this use. Figure 2 captures some important details, recalling the most important software libraries used, for the ESP8266 protocol client only the libraries needed to communicate with the server are shown, along with the versions used in the system. In the case of the database, the names of the database used and those of the collections that compose it are specified. We have chosen the graphical representation in order not to resort to an exhaustive enumeration of all software libraries, but to a selection of them, so that in future chapters we will address what is considered to be of interest. From a functional point of view, the architecture is centralized. The two distinct types of clients will send requests using the HTTP application layer protocol. Those requests will be taken asynchronously and processed by the server-side application, with an event-driven architecture, implemented in a JavaScript-based runtime environment, run outside the web browser. It is called Node.js and is based on the V8 JavaScript engine.

An important aspect worth remembering is the structure of the system following the MVC architectural template. In this particular situation, the models and controllers will be in the backend application (data access layer) and the views will be on the device supporting the frontend application (presentation layer) or client type.

THE HARDWARE SUPPORT OF THE METAVERSE SYSTEM

The hardware support of our monitoring station is shown in Figure 3, which depicts the principle diagram of the monitoring station installation, and in Figure 4 we show the electrical diagram of the installation of the monitoring station.

The development kit is used as a central hardware station control system for monitoring. This is an open-source Lua-based firmware development kit. This kit

Figure 3. Electric diagram of the metaverse station

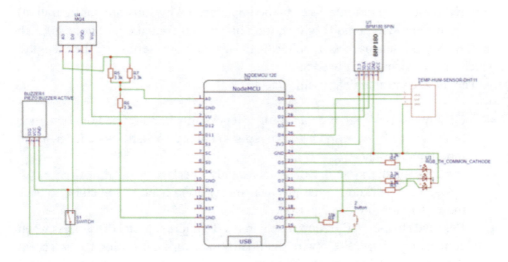

Figure 4. The command board of the metaverse system

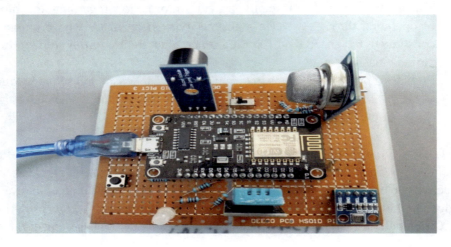

uses as a control element an ESP8266 microcontroller that integrates a Tensilica L106 processor, on 32 bits and in RISC (Reduced Instruction Set Computer) architecture, with a maximum frequency of 160MHz and which has a real-time operating system, ESP8266 RTOS SDK, based on FreeRTOS. The microcontroller, due to its integrated capabilities to work with the IEEE 802.11 standard and low power consumption, is most often preferred for IOT applications.

The kit features 17 General Purpose Inputs and Outputs (GPIOs), an Analog Digital Converter (ADC), UART, SPI, and I2C interface. In addition to those highlighted, functional features such as SDIO (Secure Digital Input/Output Interface is an interface that combines input/output capabilities with data storage), I2S, IR (infrared remote control interface can be implemented by software configuration) and the sniffer mode (a mode of operation in which the microcontroller can catch all IEEE 802.11 data packets, monitoring the network or determining their length), which the microcontroller used has.

The microcontroller deals with:

- Continuous retrieval of data and their reporting will be carried out on a time basis (with a fixed period between reports) or based on a drastic change in the monitored parameters;
- Integrity of the system will be constantly checked, also on a time basis, through a "watchdog" type mechanism, resetting itself if something blocks the system for too long a period;
- Responds to the user's requests sent to his IP (Internet protocol) address when connecting to the WIFI (wireless fidelity) network, according to the access data provided by him on the initial page, configuring the non-volatile runtime data of the microcontroller application itself;
- Transmits the data to a server in the time base and according to its configuration;
- The application will constantly provide information regarding the mode of operation through a "state manager" type mechanism, whose output is constituted by an RGB LED (red-green-blue light-emitting diode) in a periodic flashing state;
- Provides a physical mechanism to calibrate the gas sensor and sound warning of the dangerous gas concentration, as well as a way to stop it when necessary (for example during the calibration period).

The other components used are the buzzer, the gas sensor module, the temperature and humidity sensor module, and the atmospheric pressure module. The buzzer is an active one, fixed frequency, 2500Hz ($\pm$300Hz), with the control input in reverse logic. The humidity and temperature sensor is a DHT11 with 16-bit resolution, $\pm1°C$ (temperature) and $\pm1\%$ (humidity) accuracy and ideal measurement ranges between 0°C-50°C and 20%-90%. The atmospheric pressure and temperature sensor is a BMP180, which has a connection through the I2C interface with 7-bit addressing. It can measure pressures between 300hPa (225.0174 mmHg) and 1100hPa (825.0677 mmHg) and temperatures between -40°C and 85°C with an accuracy of ±2°C. The MQ7 gas sensor is a high-sensitivity sensor for CO and CO2 detection, but also good for measuring other gas variants, through software configuration. It can measure concentrations between 300ppm (parts per million) and 10000ppm, in the temperature range between -10°C and 50°C. In addition to the analog output, it also has a digital one, with an adjustable threshold using a potentiometer mounted on the board.

We mention that an important role in the system was played by the Ticker library, with the help of which we created fixed timing processes (tasks), implementing, among other things, a watchdog mechanism, and the EEPROM library, which even though the non-volatile memory made available to the programmer is flash, it helped to emulate and abstract the data storage mechanism.

THE SOFTWARE SUPPORT OF THE METAVERSE SYSTEM

The software support for making the mobile application is React Native software. This is a collection of open-source user interface software libraries created by Meta Platform. It can be used to develop applications for various platforms and operating systems, with the focus, in this case, on Android and iOS mobile platforms. The application between the two operating systems requires a few changes, depending on a few peculiarities, and has the advantage that the same application can be written simultaneously for both operating systems. React Native is run in a background process, called or periodically, that, directly on the end device, interprets JavaScript code written by the developer. It then communicates serialized data with the native platform through an asynchronous bridge. It runs in the background without requiring user interaction for this process (known as a batch job) (ESP, 2022).

The software support of database is NoSQL software, which includes collections and not tables and documents, not records, and does not itself impose restrictions on the number of columns or their values or on the content of documents, but the backend imposes through models what must be stored and how thus inserting in discussion and the notion of coercion. This type of database is very versatile, and object-oriented, which allows classic searches known from SQL databases but also new ones such as searches with regular expressions (regex). It is also very suitable for implementing the concept of load balancing, being able to replicate, if the current load stage requires it and it is correctly configured, thus there are several instances of the same database, which can be considered primary or secondary.

We considered the security of the system a very important matter, given its desired area of applicability and the originally proposed field. As a result, we have implemented several mechanisms for data protection, authentication and authorization, and modification of configuration parameters.

The first measure taken is at the microcontroller level. The wireless access point managed by the microcontroller has a visual interface for configuring the connection data with the server and some other important data. It is secured with a password which itself is part of the configurable parameters. All that data is written in the non-volatile memory of the microcontroller and is not indexed by fixed addresses, but varies with the length of the stored information, only their order is important. This in itself is also a method of keeping data safe from people who should not have access to it. Storing data this way excludes keeping passwords statically in code, but also offers the possibility of changing them if needed. Another parameter stored this way is also a station ID. It must be generated by a user with administrator rights and provided to the person configuring the station. If a valid ID is not entered when configuring it, when it connects to the server and tries to register it will receive an error and fail, thus requiring an administrator's consent to register a station.

Registration is performed only if no station is found with the name or, a parameter whose duplicate is not allowed in the entire database. The methods explained above are only valid for the monitoring station client. In addition, there are two security methods, valid for all users. One of them is the encrypted storage of the password in the database. This procedure is carried out at the same time as the registration and at each authentication the compatibility of the password sent with the encrypted password corresponding to the user who wants to authenticate will be tested. Once the registration and/or authentication procedure of the user is successful, two tokens will be provided to him to avoid the continuous sending of the password and the user, a method by which the message could be intercepted and decoded, thus having the password clear. Those tokens contain information about the user, concatenated with a secret key that is encrypted. One of them has an expiration period, also containing data about when it was created and the other does not. When the first one expires, the second one will be sent and in response, in addition to the other data requested by the user, he will also receive a new token to replace the expired one. The password encryption and token exchange method are implemented for both the client represented by the microcontroller and the clients in the mobile application, whether they are normal users or administrators.

MICROCONTROLLER APPLICATION

In this chapter, we will discuss some particularities related to the implementation of the system, such as the logic of the procedures, user interfaces, methods, and functions. Other aspects like the physical and logical architecture of both hardware and software along with use cases have been clarified previously.

The microcontroller application is an automated one, which once properly configured runs independently of the user interface.

An interrupt mechanism is implemented in this application to manage the gas sensor calibration button. Once pressed, the on/off button will change the value of a logic variable that will cause the next cycle to perform a calibration sequence of the MQ7 gas sensor. To remove noise from the button signal line the system ignores consecutive pulses that came in a time interval shorter than 200 milliseconds. At the same time, two timers were programmed and configured with the same period, 1000 milliseconds. One is intended to reset the microcontroller if for 1 minute (counts up to 60 per 1000 millisecond cycle) it has not completed a full program cycle, concluding that it has stalled. The second timer implements a mechanism for framing the behavior of the microcontroller in an operating mode and displaying with the help of the RGB LED to the user a color code to notify if there is a problem and what it is. The interrupt will have the role of taking the data from a utility function to turn on or off the LED as a whole and when it turns on, only the necessary color from the spectrum will be commanded. The utility function will use binary variables in which it will be stored whether or not there are errors in the application. They are updated everywhere in the program where needed and on call have the actual values as a result of polling.

At the time of evaluation, a decision will be made depending on the logical values of the variables received as parameters, resulting in the status color. The colors are guided by their standard and signify certain errors or modes of operation.

For correct operation, the most serious errors have been prioritized so that the least priority is the initialization state; after its completion, it will be replaced by the normal operation state (see Table 1).

Table 1. Meaning of colour standard for microcontroller status

Priority level	Color	Meaning
1	Magenta	Problems with sensors or accessing non-volatile memory
2	Red	Problems managing the local server
3	Yellow	Wi-Fi connection problem
4	Blue	Problem connecting to the server
5	Green	Normal operating mode
6	White	Running the initialization sequence

Regarding saving and retrieving data from the non-volatile memory, we mention that this process is of extreme importance in terms of the system's behavior, the entire data reporting procedure is based on the data stored and modified in this way. The configuration can be modified using a user interface that is available when connecting to the monitoring station via Wi-Fi. It constantly works in STA+AP (station and access point) mode which enable it to process the access/navigation routes of a connected user. This procedure is logically independent of the main program but depends on it in terms of timing, the web page being delivered when the client interaction function (local server management) is called from within the main cycle. The stored and displayed information can be changed and saved only when the changes are validated. After they are validated, an information page will appear with the new changes; the microcontroller will reset and resume the procedure. Resetting was required to perform the initialization routines correctly, with possible configurations including access point name, password, and other information that only initialization depends on. When entering the page with parameters to configure, the fields will be populated with the last saved values to preserve some of the parameters and minimize human error. Authentication is done by username and password and authorization is done by cookies.

All pages were built to be accessible both on a laptop and a mobile phone, being a responsive design, including for screen minimization and screen rotation.

The settings page contains a series of data that can be confused with each other as follows:

- The first set of data, the SSID and Password, refers to the data of the Wi-Fi network that the microcontroller can connect to access the Internet. To ensure that the SSID field is filled in correctly, the current network will be scanned and only an available network will be allowed to be selected, after which the password must be filled in correctly (ESP, 2022). After the reset it will be noted if correct data was provided by connecting or not connecting to the server;
- The second set of data refers to the access point data, AP SSID and AP Password, actually denoting the new network name and password, created and managed by the microcontroller to fix the configurations. Very important is that the program is designed in such a way that the local server management component does not strictly depend on an internet connection, being able to do without it. The clue that proves the connection is whether or not the map with the declared location of the station is loaded;
- The following set of data; User and Password identify the login data for authentication in the local server configuration page;

- The address is a field that will be filled with the location of the station assembly and has an interactive map attached for viewing. This is sent, upon registration, to the server which will append it as current station information;
- The data set made up of the Address and Port of the server are configurable data that allow hosting the web server of the entire system anywhere, following only the modification of these parameters for a faster reporting of the measured data;
- The last set of data consists of the ID, User, and Password of the station and is data for registration and authentication of the station on the central server. They must be modified when creating a new station, the name requiring being unique and the identifier, in addition to being unique, also has to have been previously generated by an administrator and then provided for use by the station. In other conditions, the station will never record and have no associated measurements. The microcontroller communication mechanism with the server has been implemented with the help of a function that uses the REST API (Application Programming Interface) to set the server, port, route, method, authorization code, and information in JSON format to send the request. The global and fixed variables that have been inserted into these code sequences only pertain to the tokens received as an authentication response after a registration, authentication, or regeneration operation of an expired JWT. The two tokens generated in the backend and stored only in program memory in the C++ application are:
- JWT (JSON Web Token) is the token that expires and needs to be refreshed no longer usable after;
- REF (Refresh Token) is the non-expiring token and is sent only when the first token needs to be refreshed, in response to its expiration.

To be able to work with the non-synchronicity specific to web applications in the C++ application, and not complicate the implementation with call-backs by reference to a function, we implemented a second function for receiving the response, which waits a fixed time before checking if it received an answer and what it is. The communication architecture is modular and intended to work with the current server instance to avoid redundant re-initializations of some objects, which is why most of the functions work either with parameters received by reference or with pointers to the respective values and dynamic allocation.

THE MOBILE APPLICATION

The mobile app, built in React Native, is a user interface that separates users by their roles. They have different capabilities and are given selection options, even visually providing different information not just functionally limiting. To be able to communicate with the server, we implemented similar to the microcontroller application, a modular method of sending requests to the server. This, too, was designed so that, regardless of the nature of the request, if the object received as a response it receives one of the two tokens for authorization, it saves them locally, encrypted, using the keychain library. A particularity that generated some problems was the possibility to save in the keychain only in string format. The implemented solution was that whenever writing the object is converted into a string and when reading the string is converted back to a JSON object. This way the object value key can be used without having trouble isolating any values, and save nested objects as needed.

The response received following the request, from the server, was processed on each page separately, as needed, resending if it was the case that the token was expired with the help of the refresh one. The screen that raised the most problems was the one showing the measurements for a particular station. The problems arose from handling a very large amount of data and graphing it in a time-dependent system. The graphics component documentation specified that one could organize the information in a coordinate system where the abscissa is the time axis, with just a few tweaks. We managed to implement a time-scalable variant, which, however, took the date and time provided by the database forming a vector to represent precisely the time axis, which we provided to the component. We depicted this information in Figures 5, a, b, and c, where measurements were made between the 5th of June and

Figure 5. The screen for displaying a station's measurements from the mobile app

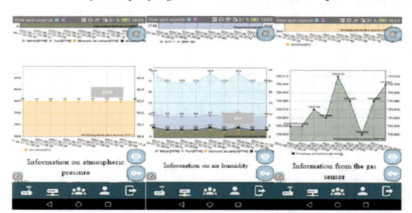

the 25th of June 2022 in our laboratory of Discrete Event Systems. We notice that in Figure 5, c the gas sensor is the above-mentioned one, i.e. MQ7 sensor capable to measure the concentration of CO_2 and CO, and the measured values which are shown in the figure are deliberately provoked by us for testing the system response.

SERVER APPLICATION

The server side of the application is responsible for handling all requests from clients. This management includes route and data processing, authorization, access code generation, database access and querying, and more. From this perspective, we can refer to the backend as a service provider. The MVC standard that is the basis for dividing the current system into controllers, models, and routes has already been exposed previously. When any of the clients register, it is initially checked if its name is unique and in the case of the station, if it has a unique identifier, both between generated and unused and between used ones. If all these conditions are validated, the password will be encrypted, the user will be stored in the database and the two tokens will be generated. They will contain, encrypted, the user's name and a unique, randomly generated key stored in the 64-character environment variables. These two values will be sent to the client in response to registration (Koleck et al., 2019).

If we were talking about an authentication, upon receiving the data, the received password will be evaluated against the stored one and it will be determined if there is a match (it is not equal because it is not stored in the clear). If everything is fine, the procedure with the tokens is identical to that of registration.

In the case of authorization, the situation is a little more complicated. One of the authorization tokens will be inserted in the request sent by the client. The backend will have to decompose the Header and take the value it is interested in, evaluate it, and see if they match. It will also determine if it is an expired code but the refresh code is good, it will inject a new JWT token into the sent request, which the next step in the server application will send as a response, in addition to the other data, to the client. It is very important to specify that the authorization is a step that is taken before any other procedure, on any route, which is why it does not send the response, but only allows or not for the operation to go forward, as the client would like. Controllers also manage database access through models. They request a series of data that they process so that they are as suitable as possible to the client's request and in a format that is as predictable as possible. Most of the instructions in controllers are based on this type of mechanism.

An instruction that is slightly out of the pattern is the one that deals with inserting a station's measurements into the database. After the insert is done, the backend performs a series of queries. First of all, it retrieves the configuration data, after which it checks if any of the data reported by the station, for measurement, deviates from the allowed range. If this happens, all the email addresses of the users (ignoring duplicates) associated with the station that recorded those measurements will be retrieved. After this step, an email will be drafted in which the problem encountered is passed and sent to the obtained list. For the operation of sending e-mails from the application, some settings were required, the activation of two-step authentication and the generation of a password for applications from the used e-mail account.

CONCLUSION

The paper "Metaverse system for patients` safety" falls into a niche of the Internet of Things applications dedicated to devices intended for the medical field, being focused on monitoring air quality both from the point of view of gas concentration and humidity, temperature, and pressure.

The system we propose is based on a mobile phone application and its operating requirements:

- Start-up, after the welcome page, the user can either log in or register;
- After inserting the data and validating it, the user will be shown only the information of interest to his role;
- Navigation between pages will be intuitive and informative, but above all personalized, according to the data associated with the user over time;
- Observation of data about time and calibration methods will be carried out both in numerical and graphic format, to facilitate the process of evaluating the information;
- The user will be notified as soon as a station of interest to him reports a series of data among which a deviation from the allowed values can be identified;
- The management mechanism will be provided that is only available to certain users and at their request.

Compared to other similar systems the presented system is more versatile and therefore is more flexible considering the communication protocols and statistic environmental data processing, also the system is ultra-portable and by far is chipper and that makes it affordable for a large category of medical care units. The system is far from perfect, so a series of future improvements will be performed:

The addition, from a software point of view, of several sets of configurations and the possibility of choosing between them, because, as we have observed in practice and from the specialized literature, some parameters differ between the uses of the rooms, from those of storage during surgery or maternity.

Providing more relevant statistical data from the application related to the evolution of parameters over time, recommendations based on the weather outside, explaining certain variations by correlating them, and trying to anticipate in-order planning activities.

For the server and database of application micro-services and load-balancers were introduced. Splitting into micro services would ideally lend itself to implementing more advanced data processing to get more advanced statistics so that upon receiving a set of data, obtained as a result of a measurement, it will be checked if it deviates from the accepted intervals and, if necessary, all interested users will be alerted by the station that provided them.

We underline that future development of our work will consider implementing a machine learning application capable to anticipate events; respectively capable to deliver prognoses concerning the air quality evolution in the hospital saloons based on the previously gathered data (Bi et al., 2019). This development of the metaverse system is meant to implement symmetry between human action and automatic monitoring as an essential issue for assuring environment quality, and ultimately patient and medical personnel security.

REFERENCES

Abe, T. K., Beamon, B. M., Storch, R. L., & Agus, J. (2016). Operations research applications in hospital operations: Part II. *IIE Transactions on Healthcare Systems Engineering*, *6*(2), 96–109. doi:10.1080/19488300.2016.1162880

Adams, J., Mauldin, T., Yates, K., Zumwalt, C., Ashe, T., Cervantes, D., & Tao, M.-H. (2022). Factors related to the accurate application of NHSN surveillance definitions for CAUTI and CLABSI in Texas hospitals: A cross-sectional survey. *American Journal of Infection Control*, *50*(1), 111–113. doi:10.1016/j.ajic.2021.07.007 PMID:34303723

Alotaibi, Y. K., & Federico, F. (2017). The impact of health information technology on patient safety. *Saudi Medical Journal*, *38*(12), 1173–1180. doi:10.15537mj.2017.12.20631 PMID:29209664

Bi, Q., Goodman, K. E., Kaminsky, J., & Lessler, J. (2019). What is machine learning? A primer for the epidemiologist. *American Journal of Epidemiology*, *188*, 2222–2239. doi:10.1093/aje/kwz189 PMID:31509183

Bubenek, S. I. (2021). *Incendiu la Institutul Matei Bals, Societatea Romana de Anestezie si Terapie Intensiva, [Fire at the Matei Bals Institute, Romanian Society of Anesthesia and Intensive Care]*. SRATI. https://www.srati.ro/noutati/comunicat-de-presa-incendiu-institutul-matei-bals

Chen, W., Guo, H., & Tsui, K.-L. (2019). A new medical staff allocation via simulation optimization for an emergency department in Hong Kong. *International Journal of Production Research*, *58*, 1–20.

Dash, S., Shakyawar, S. K., Sharma, M., & Kaushik, S. (2019). Big data in healthcare: Management, analysis and future prospects. *Journal of Big Data*, *6*(54), 54. doi:10.118640537-019-0217-0

Delloite (2022). *The hospital of the future; How digital technologies can change hospitals globally*. Deloitte. https://www2.deloitte.com/content/dam/Deloitte/global/Documents/Life-Sciences-Health-Care/us-lshc-hospital-of-the-future.pdf

Diaz-Lopez, D. M., Lopez-Valencia, N. A., Gonzalez-Neira, E. M., Barrera, D., Suarez, D. R., Caro-Gutierrez, M. P., & Sefair, C. (2018). A simulation-optimization approach for the surgery scheduling problem: A case study considering stochastic surgical times. *International Journal of Industrial Engineering Computations*, *9*(4), 409–422. doi:10.5267/j.ijiec.2018.1.002

Evans, R. S. (2016). Electronic health records: Then, now, and in the future. *Yearbook of Medical Informatics*, *25*(S 01, Suppl 1), S48–S61. doi:10.15265/IYS-2016-s006 PMID:27199197

Facciola, A. (2019). The role of the hospital environment in the health-care associated infections: A general review of the literature. *European Review for Medical and Pharmacological Sciences*, *23*, 1266–1278. PMID:30779096

Gasmet. (2022). *Emission Monitoring Book*. GT500 Terra, gasmet.com.

Gaur, L., & Jhanjhi, N. Z. (2023). *Metaverse Applications for Intelligent Healthcare*. IGI Global.

Koleck, T. A., Dreisbach, C., Bourne, P. E., & Bakken, S. (2019). Natural language processing of symptoms documented in free-text narratives of electronic health records: A systematic review. *Journal of the American Medical Informatics Association*, *26*(4), 364–379. doi:10.1093/jamia/ocy173 PMID:30726935

Kwon, H., An, S., Lee, H.-Y., Cha, W. C., Kim, S., Cho, M., & Kong, H.-J. (2022). Review of Smart Hospital Services in Real Healthcare Environments. *Healthcare Informatics Research*, *28*(1), 3–15. doi:10.4258/hir.2022.28.1.3 PMID:35172086

Lopez, J.-L. C. (2017). An IoT Approach for Wireless Sensor Networks Applied to e-Health Environmental Monitoring. *The 2017 IEEE International Conference on Internet of Things (iThings-2017)*. IEEE.

Manoukian, S., Stewart, S., Graves, N., Mason, H., Robertson, C., Kennedy, S., Pan, J., Kavanagh, K., Haahr, L., Adil, M., Dancer, S. J., Cook, B., & Reilly, J. (2021). Bed-days and costs associated with the inpatient burden of healthcare-associated infection in the UK. *The Journal of Hospital Infection*, *114*, 43–50. doi:10.1016/j.jhin.2020.12.027 PMID:34301395

Matt, D.T., Arcidiacono, G., Rauch, E. (2018). Applying Lean to Healthcare Delivery Processes - a Case-based Research. *International Journal on Advanced Science, Engineering and Information Technology*, *8*(123).

Quraishi, S. A., Berra, L., & Nozari, A. (2020). Indoor temperature and relative humidity in hospitals: Workplace considerations during the novel coronavirus pandemic. [EPub.]. *Occupational and Environmental Medicine*, *77*(7), 508–512. doi:10.1136/oemed-2020-106653 PMID:32424023

Saadouli, H., Masmoudi, M., Jerbi, B., & Dammak, A. (2014). An optimization and simulation approach for Operating room scheduling under stochastic durations. *Proceedings - International Conference on Control, Decision and Information Technologies*. IEEE. 10.1109/CoDIT.2014.6996903

Verberk, J. D. M., Aghdassi, S. J. S., Abbas, M., Nauclér, P., Gubbels, S., Maldonado, N., Palacios-Baena, Z. R., Johansson, A. F., Gastmeier, P., Behnke, M., van Rooden, S. M., & van Mourik, M. S. M. (2022). Automated surveillance systems for healthcare-associated infections: Results from a European survey and experiences from real-life utilization. *The Journal of Hospital Infection*, *122*, 35–43. doi:10.1016/j.jhin.2021.12.021 PMID:35031393

Weber, D. J., & Rutala, W. A. (2023). Understanding and Preventing Transmission of Health-Care Associated Pathogens Due to the Contaminate Hospital Environment. *Infection Control and Hospital Epidemiology*, *34*(5), 449–452. doi:10.1086/670223 PMID:23571359

Xiang, W., Yin, J., & Lim, G. (2015). An ant colony optimization approach for solving an operating room surgery scheduling problem. *Computers & Industrial Engineering*, *85*, 335–345. doi:10.1016/j.cie.2015.04.010

Xiao, Y., & Yoogalingam, R. (2021). Reserved capacity policies for operating room scheduling. *Operations Management Research*, *14*(1-2), 107–122. doi:10.100712063-020-00172-x

Zhang, Z., Xie, X., & Geng, N. (2021). Promise surgery start times and implementation strategies. *IEEE International Conference on Automation Science and Engineering*. IEEE.

Chapter 8
Ethical Considerations in the Use of the Metaverse for Healthcare

Loveleen Gaur
https://orcid.org/0000-0002-0885-1550
Taylor's University, Malaysia

Devanshi Gaur
Florida International University, USA

Anam Afaq
Amity University, Noida, India

ABSTRACT

The promotion of augmenting and enhancing healthcare in the ethical metaverse setting should be guided by the fundamental bioethical principles of beneficence, nonmaleficence, autonomy, and justice, focusing on minimising risks and adverse outcomes. Implementing a patient-centred strategy and establishing responsible regulatory measures are essential for harnessing the advantages of metaverse technology in the healthcare sector while effectively tackling the associated problems. The chapter explores the ethical considerations surrounding using metaverse technology within the healthcare sector.

1. INTRODUCTION

In the contemporary era of swift and constant transformations, technology emerges as an all-encompassing entity that propels alterations in nearly every aspect of human existence (Gaur et al., 2023; Sharma et al., 2022). The rapid progression of technology consistently reveals novel solutions and prospects, affecting almost all industries with its capacity for transformation (Afaq and Gaur, 2021; Chaudhary, Gaur and Chakrabarti, 2022). Among the various industries, healthcare stands out as a primary benefactor of technology improvements (Bhandari et al., 2022; Biswas et al., 2022). The integration of advanced technologies, including artificial intelligence, data analytics, and telemedicine, has significantly transformed the provision of healthcare services, diagnostic procedures, and patient treatment (Ahmed, Biswas, et al., 2022; Protic et al., 2022). The advancement in healthcare technology not only improves the standard of medical services but also holds the potential to extend the accessibility and customisation of healthcare to an unprecedented level (Bandyopadhyay et al., 2023; Sahu et al., 2023). The metaverse, a networked virtual reality environment, plays a significant role in redefining the future of healthcare within the dynamic framework of healthcare technology. This transformative influence is unprecedented in its impact (Afaq et al., 2023a; Chaudhary, Gaur, Jhanjhi, et al., 2022).

The metaverse, a networked virtual reality environment, is bringing about significant transformations in numerous sectors, including healthcare (Gaur, Afaq, Solanki, et al., 2021; Jain et al., 2021). The metaverse presents a novel domain for implementing intelligent healthcare applications, utilising immersive technologies and artificial intelligence to augment patient experiences, increase medical training, and facilitate customised care. The metaverse holds immense potential for transformative advancements in healthcare, encompassing a wide range of applications such as telemedicine, virtual consultations, medical simulations, and mental health support. Integrating virtual reality, artificial intelligence, and other sophisticated technologies in the healthcare sector offers a promising domain known as the metaverse. This emerging frontier holds the potential to revolutionise the delivery and experience of healthcare services. Particularly the outbreak of COVID-19 has expedited the incorporation of technology inside the healthcare sector to an unprecedented extent (Afaq et al., 2023b; Tyagi et al., 2022). Telemedicine and remote monitoring technologies have emerged as crucial instruments in the management of patient care and the mitigation of physical interaction (Bandyopadhyay et al., 2023; Gaur, Afaq, Singh, et al., 2021). The digital transformation facilitated not just enhanced responsiveness to the pandemic but also underscored the imperative for pioneering healthcare solutions (Gaur, Singh, et al., 2021; Ghose et al., 2023).

With the integration of technology into the healthcare sector, the metaverse has emerged as a prominent player, assuming a heightened level of importance (Gaur and Afaq, 2020). The metaverse has significant opportunities for enhancing patient care, medical training, and research. However, it raises a novel array of ethical concerns requiring meticulous scrutiny and contemplation. The potential impact of the metaverse on healthcare is significant, since it has the capacity to bring about a transformative shift (Afaq et al., 2021; Gaur, Solanki, et al., 2021). This can be achieved through the facilitation of immersive telehealth encounters, fostering connections between patients and healthcare professionals within virtual environments, and establishing a robust platform for medical education and simulations (Anshu and Gaur, 2018; Rana et al., 2022). In light of the COVID-19 pandemic, the metaverse emerges as a potentially advantageous domain for the healthcare sector, presenting novel avenues to tackle health-related obstacles within an interconnected and digital realm (Ghose et al., 2022; Mathur and Gaur, 2021).

The metaverse of healthcare presents various ethical considerations that pertain to the conscientious utilisation of technology, safeguarding patient privacy and data security, promoting fair access to virtual healthcare services, and upholding the welfare and self-determination of patients inside virtual environments (Afaq et al., 2022; Bhandari et al., 2022). As the integration of the metaverse into healthcare practises progresses, healthcare practitioners, technology developers, policymakers, and ethicists must engage in collaborative efforts to effectively address the ethical difficulties that arise and ensure the preservation of patient safety, privacy, and dignity at the utmost level (Ahmed, Shaharier, et al., 2022; Biswas et al., 2023).

This introduction emphasises the significance of incorporating ethical principles inside the healthcare metaverse. It establishes a foundation for delving into the distinct ethical concerns that emerge in this swiftly progressing field (Fernandez and Hui, 2022). The comprehensive examination of these ethical considerations will play a crucial role in fully harnessing the transformative capabilities of the metaverse in the healthcare field, all the while ensuring the preservation of patients' trust and the confidence of healthcare stakeholders (Kaddoura and Al Husseiny, 2023).

The metaverse in healthcare introduces distinct ethical considerations that necessitate meticulous attention to guarantee the safety of patients, protection of privacy, and equitable availability of healthcare services.

2. KEY ETHICAL CONSIDERATIONS IN THE METAVERSE OF HEALTHCARE

2.1. Informed Consent

For patients to engage in virtual trials, telemedicine consultations, or utilise metaverse applications, they must offer informed consent. It is imperative for healthcare providers to effectively communicate the fundamental aspects of the metaverse encounter, as well as the associated hazards and advantages, to patients before their involvement (Anshari et al., 2022). The principle of informed consent holds significant ethical importance within the healthcare metaverse, as it guarantees that patients possess the essential knowledge required to autonomously and knowledgeably determine their involvement in virtual healthcare services, research endeavours, or any other undertakings that incorporate virtual reality, augmented reality, or similar advanced technologies (Kshetri, 2022). Within the framework of the metaverse, the concept of informed consent involves providing explicit and thorough information to individuals regarding the inherent characteristics of their virtual encounters, potential advantages, and potential hazards. It is imperative to ensure that patients are adequately informed regarding the nature of the data gathered during their virtual interactions, the intended purposes for which it will be utilised, and any potential third parties with whom this data may be disclosed (Benjamins et al., 2023). The healthcare metaverse comprises various essential elements pertaining to informed consent.

- **Full Disclosure:** Giving patients extensive details about the goals, aims, and consequences associated with their involvement in metaverse experiences is imperative. The information outlines the technological methods utilised, potential adverse effects or discomfort, and expected outcomes (Chengoden et al., 2023).
- **Voluntary Participation:** Voluntary involvement in medical research or treatment necessitates that patients possess the autonomy to make independent decisions, free from undue influence, coercion, or pressure exerted by healthcare practitioners or researchers (Song and Qin, 2022).
- **Capacity to Understand:** Ensuring that patients possess the cognitive ability to comprehend the information presented to them and subsequently make well-informed decisions is of utmost importance. Patients with cognitive or intellectual impairments may require specific attention (Yang, Zhou, et al., 2022).
- **Withdrawal of Consent:** Patients can revoke their agreement at any moment without encountering adverse repercussions. Individuals should be provided with knowledge regarding their entitlement and the appropriate methods to exercise it.
- **Opportunity for Questions:** Patients must be able to inquire and obtain an explanation before granting their consent. Healthcare providers or researchers must be readily accessible to attend to any inquiries or uncertainties.
- **Documentation:** The documentation of informed consent is necessary to ensure its validity and adherence to ethical standards. This can be achieved through written or technological means. It is recommended that patients be provided with a duplicate of the consent form to maintain their privacy (Zhang et al., 2023).
- **Ongoing Communication:** In specific instances, it may be imperative to maintain continuous communication with patients throughout their virtual encounters, mainly when some updates or modifications could potentially impact their engagement.

The metaverse can uphold ethical ideals of autonomy, respect for individuals, and transparency by implementing a process where patients must express informed consent before participating in virtual healthcare activities. Establishing ethical principles surrounding informed consent fosters a sense of confidence between healthcare practitioners and patients, hence facilitating the appropriate and advantageous use of the metaverse within healthcare environments.

2.2. Data Privacy and Security

The metaverse collects and analyses extensive patient data, encompassing various aspects of health-related information. Implementing rigorous data privacy and security safeguards is necessary to safeguard patients' sensitive information from unauthorised access and breaches. The preservation of patients' sensitive health information and the ethical use of technology are of utmost importance in safeguarding data privacy and security inside the healthcare metaverse (Musamih et al., 2023). Protecting patient data from unauthorised access, breaches, or misuse becomes imperative as the metaverse incorporates virtual reality, augmented reality, and other advanced technologies inside healthcare environments. The metaverse of healthcare presents several crucial factors to be taken into account when addressing data privacy and security:

- **Data Encryption:** It is imperative to employ encryption techniques to safeguard patient data conveyed through the metaverse. This measure aims to thwart unauthorised interception.
- **Access Controls:** The metaverse should enforce limitations on the accessibility of patient data, permitting only licenced healthcare experts and workers access. Creating robust access controls and authentication mechanisms is imperative to guarantee that only persons with proper authorisation may access sensitive information (Bansal et al., 2022).
- **Anonymisation and De-Identification:** It is advisable to anonymise or de-identify patient data whenever feasible to safeguard patient privacy. This practice mitigates the potential of personal data being correlated with particular individuals (Skalidis et al., 2022).
- **Consent Management:** It is imperative to ensure that patients provide informed consent before utilising their data within the metaverse. Healthcare professionals must uphold patients' preferences regarding the sharing of data, participation in research, and choice of treatment options.
- **Secure Storage:** It is imperative to ensure that patient data in the metaverse is securely maintained in data storage facilities with robust security measures, including suitable encryption protocols and stringent access controls.

Establishing and maintaining regular data backups and implementing comprehensive disaster recovery strategies is imperative to guarantee data availability and integrity (Mozumder et al., 2022).
- **Data Minimisation:** Gathering and preserving the minimal essential data for particular metaverse undertakings is necessary. To mitigate the potential for data breaches, it is advisable to remove superfluous data.
- **Regular Audits and Assessments:** It is imperative to conduct security audits and assessments to detect vulnerabilities and effectively mitigate security concerns within the metaverse (Yang, Siau, et al., 2022).
- **User Training:** Healthcare professionals and workers utilising the metaverse must undergo comprehensive training to acquire knowledge and skills about data privacy and security best practices. This training is essential to mitigate the risk of inadvertent data breaches effectively.
- **Data Breach Response Plan:** Healthcare businesses must possess a delineated data breach response plan to efficiently and expeditiously address any security events that may arise. This entails the obligation to inform individuals who have been impacted and pertinent authorities in accordance with data protection legislation (Sparkes, 2021).
- **Compliance with Regulations:** Healthcare providers utilising the metaverse must adhere to pertinent data protection and privacy legislation. Such regulations include the Health Insurance Portability and Accountability Act (HIPAA) in the United States and the General Data Protection Regulation (GDPR) in the European Union.
- **Secure Communication Channels:** It is imperative to ensure the security of communication channels employed inside the metaverse, encompassing virtual consultations and telemedicine sessions, to safeguard patient data during transmission (Wang et al., 2022).

Establishing data privacy and security measures within the healthcare metaverse is vital to foster patient trust and safeguard their confidential health data. Healthcare businesses may effectively utilise the metaverse's capabilities to enhance patient care and experiences while maintaining the utmost privacy and security by implementing comprehensive data protection procedures.

2.3. Equitable Access

It is imperative to prioritise implementing measures to guarantee fair and equal access to metaverse applications and virtual healthcare services. The consideration of inclusivity is crucial to effectively accommodate those who have impairments, encounter language problems, or face limited access to technology. Equitable access within the healthcare metaverse pertains to the just and comprehensive dissemination of virtual healthcare services and resources to all individuals, irrespective of their demographic characteristics, geographical position, socioeconomic standing, or technological aptitude. The objective is to guarantee equitable access for all individuals to avail themselves of the capabilities and breakthroughs in healthcare the metaverse provides. The following are a few fundamental elements of equitable access inside the healthcare metaverse:

- **Digital Inclusion:** It is imperative to undertake endeavours aimed at narrowing the digital gap and ensuring the availability of metaverse applications and virtual healthcare services to persons who encounter technological obstacles, including older adults, individuals with impairments, and those residing in rural or low-income regions (Suh et al., 2023)
- **Accessibility:** The prioritisation of accessibility should be a key consideration in designing virtual healthcare platforms and applications inside the metaverse to accommodate those who experience visual, aural, or cognitive disabilities. Implementing this method is paramount to facilitate all individuals' optimal use of technology (Tan et al., 2022).
- **Language Diversity:** To accommodate linguistically diverse populations and mitigate potential comprehension or engagement obstacles, healthcare content inside the metaverse must be accessible in multiple languages.
- **Affordability:** Ensuring acceptable and accessible costs for virtual healthcare services in the metaverse is crucial to mitigate financial barriers that may impede persons' access to vital healthcare resources.
- **Education and Training:** It is imperative to prioritise initiatives to provide individuals with comprehensive education and training on optimally utilising metaverse apps. This will enable them to harness the potential of virtual healthcare experiences and make well-informed decisions about their health (Mbunge et al., 2022).
- **Cultural Sensitivity:** Cultural sensitivity is a crucial aspect to consider while developing healthcare material and facilitating experiences in the metaverse. It is imperative to approach these endeavours with respect for varied cultural practises and beliefs to foster inclusivity and prevent the perpetuation of biases.
- **Remote and Underserved Areas:** The utilisation of virtual healthcare services inside the metaverse can serve as a pivotal mechanism for extending healthcare access to those residing in geographically isolated or underserved regions, hence granting them the opportunity to avail healthcare resources that would otherwise be inaccessible.
- **Health Disparities:** Health disparities can be effectively addressed through the utilisation of the metaverse since it allows for the targeting of vulnerable

populations and the provision of customised healthcare experiences that cater to their unique requirements (Athar et al., 2023).
- **Equitable Research Opportunities:** In the context of virtual clinical trials and research studies done within the metaverse, it is imperative to make deliberate endeavours towards incorporating diverse and representative participant communities. This is crucial to safeguard the generalizability of research findings.
- **Outreach and Awareness:** It is recommended that healthcare professionals and organisations actively participate in outreach and awareness endeavours to educate individuals about the accessibility and advantages of virtual healthcare services within the metaverse.

Healthcare practitioners can foster fairness, social justice, and equal opportunity principles by strongly emphasising equitable access within the healthcare metaverse. This approach enables all individuals to participate equally and benefit from virtual healthcare experiences. The aforementioned method aligns with a patient-centred care model that expands the scope of healthcare services and enables individuals to manage their health and overall well-being actively (Wei, 2023).

2.4. Authenticity and Accountability

In the metaverse, healthcare providers must uphold the integrity of their identity and assume responsibility for their activities. The verification of credentials for healthcare practitioners and institutions is of paramount importance. Authenticity and accountability play a crucial role in ensuring the responsible and reliable utilisation of technology within the healthcare metaverse, hence facilitating the delivery of virtual healthcare services. The above principles prioritise preserving integrity in interactions, data, and identities within the metaverse while adhering to professional norms and ethical rules.

Authenticity:

- **Identity Verification:** Identity verification is a crucial process in the metaverse, wherein healthcare practitioners and experts are required to authenticate their identity and validate their credentials. This step is essential for establishing confidence and credibility within the virtual environment. Patients need to possess a sense of assurance in their interactions with healthcare providers who are both legal and qualified.
- **Authentic Experiences:** Authenticity inside the metaverse involves providing true and realistic healthcare experiences. It is imperative that

virtual interactions, medical simulations, and educational content faithfully mirror authentic healthcare circumstances and practises.
- **Transparent Communication:** Healthcare providers utilising the metaverse ought to communicate openly and honestly with patients regarding the inherent characteristics of virtual experiences, the potential constraints, and the advantages they offer (Agac et al., 2023).

Accountability:

- **Responsibility for Actions:** Healthcare professionals and organisations utilising the metaverse are obligated to assume responsibility for their activities and decisions within virtual healthcare environments. This entails guaranteeing the precision and dependability of information disseminated to patients.
- **Data Governance:** Data governance is a crucial aspect of accountability within the metaverse, as it pertains to the responsible and ethical use of patient data to ensure its security. Healthcare organisations must have explicit data governance policies and implement corresponding practices to safeguard patient privacy and mitigate the risk of data exploitation (Hollensen et al., 2023).
- **Informed Consent:** Obtaining informed permission from patients is essential to ensuring accountability. Healthcare practitioners must uphold patients' autonomy and preferences, ensuring they understand the ramifications of their engagement in virtual healthcare services.
- **Quality Assurance:** Healthcare companies ought to use quality assurance techniques to evaluate the efficacy and safety of virtual healthcare encounters within the metaverse.
- **Ethical Considerations:** Ethical considerations are crucial in virtual healthcare practices, emphasising accountability. Adhering to moral rules and principles is essential in ensuring the responsible and ethical delivery of virtual healthcare services. Healthcare providers must place patient well-being as a top priority and make decisions that are in the best interests of their patients (Camilleri, 2023).

Data Transparency:

- **Openness about Data Use:** Healthcare providers must maintain transparency and communicate clearly to patients regarding the intended utilisation of their data inside the metaverse. Patients must comprehensively comprehend how their information enhances their healthcare or research endeavours.
- **Optimal Data Sharing:** The responsible and compliant data sharing in the metaverse should adhere to patients' consent and necessary data protection

legislation. Patients must possess knowledge and provide informed consent about disseminating their data for explicit objectives.

Establishing authenticity and accountability within the metaverse of healthcare plays a crucial role in fostering patient trust, elevating the overall quality of virtual healthcare encounters, and promoting the ethical utilisation of technology in healthcare environments. By adhering to these principles, healthcare professionals and organisations may guarantee the successful incorporation of the metaverse into healthcare while simultaneously protecting patient welfare and privacy (Agarwal and Alathur, 2023).

2.5. Virtual Reality Safety

Preserving patients' emotional and psychological well-being during virtual encounters is imperative. It is essential for virtual reality (VR) experiences to refrain from eliciting painful feelings or intensifying pre-existing mental health issues. Safety in virtual reality within the healthcare metaverse pertains to the actions and deliberations undertaken to safeguard individuals' physical and psychological welfare in virtual reality (VR) encounters within healthcare environments. Virtual reality (VR) is a potent instrument capable of generating immersive and authentic simulations. However, its utilisation without due care and responsibility may have detrimental consequences. The following are essential components of safety considerations in virtual reality inside the healthcare metaverse (Dwivedi et al., 2023).

Physical Safety:

- **Avoiding Obstacles:** To ensure patient safety, individuals utilising virtual reality (VR) devices must be situated inside a secure physical setting devoid of any potential obstructions or dangers that may inadvertently arise during their immersion in the virtual realm.
- **Properly Secured Equipment:** It is imperative to ensure that VR equipment, including headsets and controllers, is appropriately fastened to minimise the risk of slippage or accidental dislodgement during virtual experiences.
- **Clear Instructions:** Providing patients with explicit advice regarding utilising virtual reality (VR) equipment is imperative to mitigate the risk of strain or pain (Hwang and Chien, 2022).

Motion Sickness and Discomfort:

- **Gradual Exposure:** In certain instances, users may encounter symptoms of motion sickness or discomfort while engaging with virtual reality (VR)

technology. Healthcare practitioners ought to prioritise the progressive exposure of patients to virtual reality (VR) experiences to mitigate the potential adverse consequences of such disclosure (Song and Qin, 2022).
- **Comfortable Settings:** It is recommended that patients be actively encouraged to take periodic breaks when engaging in prolonged virtual reality (VR) sessions. Furthermore, it is essential to ensure that patients have convenient access to comfortable seating arrangements or designated rest places.

Psychological Well-being:

- Healthcare professionals should exercise caution when utilising virtual reality (VR) for exposure therapy or other psychological interventions. Ensuring patients are not subjected to distressing content without explicit agreement and preparedness is imperative.
- Healthcare providers should exercise diligent oversight of patients' emotional responses during virtual reality (VR) encounters and be prepared to offer appropriate assistance if required (Yaqoob et al., 2023).

Consent, Autonomy and Data Privacy:

- The acquisition of informed consent is crucial for patients before participating in virtual reality (VR) experiences. This process entails providing patients with a comprehensive explanation of such incidents' potential impacts and hazards.
- The right to withdraw should be granted to patients, allowing them the autonomy to discontinue their participation in virtual reality (VR) experiences at any given moment, particularly if they experience feelings of discomfort or overwhelming sensations (Yang, Siau, et al., 2022).
- **Protecting Patient Data:** Healthcare businesses must adopt robust data privacy and security protocols to safeguard patient data acquired during virtual reality (VR) encounters.

2.6. Bias in AI Algorithms

The development of AI-driven healthcare applications within the metaverse necessitates a cautious approach to mitigate biased algorithms, which could perpetuate health disparities and yield unequal treatment recommendations. Bias in artificial intelligence (AI) algorithms within the healthcare metaverse pertains to systematic and unjust inaccuracies or prejudices embedded within the algorithms employed for decision-making or providing suggestions. Artificial intelligence (AI) algorithms are specifically engineered to analyse extensive volumes of data and derive logical inferences. However, it is essential to acknowledge that these algorithms may unintentionally include biases inherent in the data or be subject to the biases of their developers. The cautious development of AI-driven healthcare applications inside the metaverse is necessary to address the potential presence of biased algorithms (Thomason, 2022). These algorithms can unintentionally perpetuate health inequities and result in unequal treatment recommendations. The bias in artificial intelligence (AI) algorithms within the healthcare metaverse refers to systematic and unjust inaccuracies or prejudices inherent in the algorithms used for decision-making or offering advice. Artificial intelligence (AI) algorithms are purposefully designed to evaluate large quantities of data and draw logical conclusions. Nevertheless, it is crucial to recognise that these algorithms have the potential to inadvertently incorporate intrinsic biases present in the data or be influenced by the prejudices of their creators (Venugopal et al., 2023).

2.7. Patient Autonomy

Although AI-driven personalised healthcare offers numerous advantages, patients must retain autonomy when making decisions regarding their treatment plans and preferences for data sharing. The concept of patient autonomy within healthcare in the metaverse pertains to the idea that individuals are entitled to exercise their judgement and choices about their medical care and treatment inside virtual healthcare environments. The significance of upholding patients' rights to autonomy and the ability to make healthcare decisions based on their values, beliefs, and individual preferences is underscored. The metaverse of healthcare encompasses several crucial elements of patient autonomy:

- **Informed Consent:** The principle of informed consent necessitates that patients receive comprehensive information regarding the nature of virtual healthcare services, including the potential advantages, disadvantages, and alternative options. Implementing informed consent protocols guarantees that patients are equipped with comprehensive information, enabling them to make informed choices regarding their engagement in virtual healthcare encounters (Iwanaga et al., 2023).
- **Choice and Decision-Making:** It is imperative to afford patients the autonomy to make informed choices regarding their participation in virtual healthcare services. Individuals own the prerogative to determine the degree of their involvement and can revoke their consent at any moment.
- **Personalised Healthcare:** The metaverse can facilitate Personalised healthcare experiences, leveraging patient data and preferences. Promoting patient autonomy is encouraged by providing personalised treatment

alternatives and acknowledging patients' decisions about their healthcare (Dwivedi et al., 2023).
- **Preferences for Data Sharing:** Individuals own the entitlement to exercise control over the utilisation of their data within the metaverse. Users should be able to explicitly indicate their preferences about sharing their data and expect it to be managed according to their stated preferences.
- **Treatment alternatives:** Patients must be provided with comprehensive information regarding treatment alternatives, enabling them to actively participate in decision-making and select the strategy that best aligns with their goals and values (Moro, 2023).
- **Transparent Communication:** It is imperative for healthcare practitioners operating inside the metaverse to engage in open and transparent communication with patients. This entails ensuring patients comprehensively comprehend their health issues, treatment plans, and virtual healthcare encounters (Surveswaran and Deshpande, 2023).
- **Preservation of Privacy:** The safeguarding of patient privacy within the metaverse is intricately linked to the principle of patient autonomy. Individuals are entitled to maintain the confidentiality of their health information, and their data must be managed in compliance with data protection legislation.
- **Collaborative Decision-Making:** Using the metaverse can enable collaborative decision-making processes between healthcare practitioners and patients, allowing patients to actively engage in care planning and effectively communicate their treatment choices.

2.8. Medical Accuracy and Validity

To prevent the dissemination of disinformation and the provision of misleading advice, the content and medical information given within the metaverse must adhere to the principles of accuracy, evidence-based practice, and validation by trustworthy sources. The concepts of medical correctness and validity within the metaverse of healthcare pertain to the dependability and trustworthiness of medical information, diagnoses, and treatments presented in virtual healthcare encounters. The significance of guaranteeing that the material and medical advice provided within the metaverse adhere to evidence-based practises, remain current, and align with established medical standards is underscored. The metaverse of healthcare encompasses several crucial medical accuracy and validity elements (De Felice et al., 2023).

- **Evidence-Based Information:** Medical information disseminated within the metaverse must be grounded on evidence-based practises, substantiated by rigorous scientific research and subjected to peer review. The document must

accurately represent the present understanding of medical information and be subject to periodic revisions in light of emerging findings.
- **Credible Sources:** Healthcare practitioners and organisations functioning within the metaverse should rely on reliable and trustworthy sources when seeking medical information. The sources mentioned above encompass medical publications, clinical recommendations, and content authored by experts.
- **Medical Expertise:** Including proficient healthcare practitioners within the metaverse is vital since they possess the qualifications to offer precise medical counsel, diagnoses, and treatment suggestions derived from their extensive expertise and training. The precision of medical simulation in mimicking authentic medical processes and situations is paramount in facilitating successful learning and practice during medical training scenarios. The accuracy and authenticity of data utilised to train algorithms in AI-driven healthcare applications are crucial to guarantee dependable forecasts and treatment suggestions. The validation of AI algorithms employed for clinical decision support in the metaverse is vital to ensure their precision and reliability in aiding healthcare professionals in diagnosis and treatment planning (Fan et al., 2023).
- **Regulatory Compliance:** Medical applications within the metaverse must adhere to pertinent healthcare legislation and standards to uphold patient safety and promote the ethical use of technology. The importance of transparency in algorithms is evident in AI-driven healthcare apps, as they should provide clear and comprehensive information regarding the process by which they reach their findings. This transparency enables healthcare professionals to understand the underlying rationale behind the AI-generated recommendations thoroughly.
- **Continuing Education:** It is imperative for healthcare providers inside the metaverse to actively participate in ongoing learning endeavours to remain abreast of medical breakthroughs and uphold their proficiency in delivering precise and reliable medical guidance (Inceoglu and Ciloglugil, 2022).

2.9. Patient Empowerment

The empowerment of patients through knowledge and control of their health data is crucial for enabling them to make informed decisions regarding their healthcare. In virtual healthcare settings, patient empowerment refers to facilitating patients to actively manage their health and make well-informed choices about their medical care. This approach underscores the significance of involving patients as collaborative partners in their healthcare journey, fostering autonomy, and equipping them with the necessary resources and information to participate in their health and well-being actively. Essential components of patient empowerment in the metaverse of healthcare encompass:

- **Access to Information:** Patients within the metaverse must be granted the opportunity to obtain credible and easily understandable health-related information. Virtual healthcare experiences should offer patients educational resources and information that facilitate their comprehension of health issues, treatment alternatives, and preventive measures.
- **Shared Decision-Making:** Using the metaverse can enhance decision-making processes between patients and healthcare professionals. Promoting open dialogue between patients and healthcare providers regarding their treatment preferences, goals, and concerns is imperative. This approach enables a cooperative decision-making procedure that is in accordance with the patient's values and preferences.
- **Personalised Healthcare:** Virtual healthcare experiences within the metaverse can be tailored to accommodate the precise needs of individual patients, encompassing their medical history, preferences, and essentialities. Implementing customisation tactics has influenced patient engagement and satisfaction in healthcare encounters favourably.
- **Self-Management Tools:** Patient empowerment can be facilitated by providing self-management tools and applications within the metaverse. The technologies mentioned above include medication trackers, symptom monitoring systems, and lifestyle management software, which empower individuals to participate in their healthcare actively.
- **Health Literacy:** Including health literacy is of utmost importance when developing virtual healthcare experiences, as it is essential to effectively communicate information in a manner that is understandable and readily available to patients with varying levels of health literacy.
- **Virtual Support Groups:** Virtual support groups can augment patient empowerment by fostering relationships among virtual world individuals facing comparable health challenges. These groups facilitate the exchange of personal experiences among participants and offer mutual support to one another (Tlili et al., 2022).
- **Real-Time Monitoring:** Real-time monitoring is a crucial feature of the metaverse, enabling continuous health data tracking. This capability gives patients essential insights into their present health condition and advancement. Providing access to this dataset facilitates individuals in monitoring their well-being and making informed decisions.
- **Mindfulness and Well-Being:** In the metaverse, individuals can partake in mindfulness practises and employ relaxation techniques, which have

demonstrated efficacy in improving mental well-being and mitigating stress. The immersive environment facilitates the empowerment of patients in managing their emotional well-being.
- **Virtual Coaching:** Virtual coaching has emerged as a promising approach in the metaverse, offering patients the opportunity to receive direction and support in pursuing health-related objectives. This form of coaching facilitates behaviour modification and fosters sustainable enhancements in long-term well-being (Zhang et al., 2022).
- **Feedback and Engagement:** It is recommended to motivate patients to actively participate in providing feedback regarding their virtual healthcare experiences within the metaverse. The user's feedback has the potential to enhance the quality of services and foster greater patient engagement.
- **Ethical Use of AI:** Using artificial intelligence (AI) algorithms in the realm of diagnosis and treatment planning necessitates a commitment to transparency, explainability, and a primary focus on augmenting the capabilities of healthcare professionals rather than supplanting their expertise. The ethical utilisation of artificial intelligence (AI) in the healthcare metaverse pertains to the prudent and conscientious implementation of AI technology inside virtual healthcare encounters. The process entails assuring ethical norms, protecting patient rights, and prioritising patient well-being in developing, deploying, and utilising AI algorithms and systems. The ethical use of artificial intelligence (AI) within the healthcare metaverse encompasses several crucial elements. Data Privacy and Security: AI algorithms must respect patient privacy by securely handling and protecting sensitive health data collected within the metaverse. Data should be anonymised or de-identified whenever possible to minimise the risk of re-identification (Rospigliosi, 2022).
- **Transparency and Explainability:** The principle of transparency and explainability in designing AI systems for healthcare emphasises the importance of enabling healthcare providers and patients to comprehend the decision-making process of algorithms. Explainable artificial intelligence (AI) plays a crucial role in fostering trust and enhancing the quality of decision-making processes.
- **Bias Mitigation:** Efforts should be undertaken to identify and mitigate biases present in AI algorithms to promote equal and just healthcare results. Implementing bias detection and mitigation measures is crucial at the development and testing stages.
- **Informed Consent:** The acquisition of informed consent is crucial for patients participating in virtual healthcare encounters incorporating artificial intelligence (AI). This consent should encompass the disclosure of AI

technologies employed, the utilisation of patient data, and the potential ramifications associated with AI-generated suggestions.
- **Human Oversight:** The inclusion of human oversight and expertise should be maintained as a vital component of decision-making in healthcare, notwithstanding the potential for AI to enhance many procedures within the field. Healthcare providers must maintain authority over AI-generated.
- **Continuing Education**: Healthcare workers must get continuous education and training on artificial intelligence (AI) technologies and their ethical implications. This is necessary to guarantee the responsible application of AI in virtual healthcare environments.
- **Equitable Access:** The objective of integrating artificial intelligence (AI) into the healthcare metaverse should ensure fair and equal availability of virtual healthcare encounters to patients from diverse backgrounds, regardless of their geographical location or socioeconomic standing.
- **Safety and Reliability:** Safety and dependability are crucial considerations when implementing AI algorithms for clinical decision support. These algorithms must undergo thorough testing and validation to ascertain their effectiveness in assisting healthcare practitioners with accurate diagnoses and treatment plans.
- **Regulatory Compliance:** It is imperative for virtual healthcare experiences incorporating artificial intelligence (AI) to strictly comply with pertinent healthcare legislation and norms to safeguard patient well-being and prevent the occurrence of unethical conduct.
- **Patient Autonomy:** Patient autonomy is crucial in AI, as it aims to enhance patients' ability to make informed decisions regarding their healthcare by equipping them with relevant information and insights. It is essential to ensure that patient preferences and choices are respected throughout this process.
- **Minimisation of Harm:** Efforts should be undertaken to mitigate any harm resulting from AI-driven recommendations, particularly in situations where decisions may have substantial implications for the health and well-being of patients (Manto and D'Oria, 2023).

Healthcare professionals can optimise the capabilities of artificial intelligence (AI) inside the healthcare metaverse by adhering to ethical rules and principles. This approach enables the improvement of patient care, the enhancement of medical training, and the advancement of research. Simultaneously, it ensures patient safety, privacy, and trust preservation. Incorporating ethical issues is crucial in developing and implementing AI technologies within virtual healthcare settings, as it facilitates the responsible and advantageous integration of these technologies into healthcare practices.

The inclusion of these ethical considerations is crucial in the development of a conscientious and reliable healthcare metaverse. Effective utilisation of the metaverse for the betterment of patients and the preservation of healthcare ethics necessitates a collaborative effort among healthcare providers, technology developers, policymakers, and patients.

3. CONCLUSION

Incorporating modern technology into healthcare settings necessitates careful attention to ethical considerations to ensure responsible and trustworthy integration within the metaverse of healthcare. With the continuous development of the metaverse, which encompasses virtual reality and augmented reality technologies, there is a growing need to emphasise the importance of safeguarding patient well-being, autonomy, and privacy, all while upholding ethical values.

Patient empowerment is enhanced when virtual healthcare experiences provide tailored, evidence-based information and encourage collaborative decision-making. Promoting equal access to the metaverse contributes to the cultivation of inclusion. At the same time, the ongoing surveillance and assessment processes aid in identifying and mitigating unintended repercussions and potential prejudices.

The ethical utilisation of artificial intelligence (AI) within the metaverse necessitates implementing transparent, explainable algorithms without bias. It is also imperative to prioritise protecting patient data privacy and incorporate human oversight in decision-making procedures. The principle of patient autonomy promotes the active involvement of individuals in their healthcare decision-making process and empowers them to make well-informed decisions. Healthcare practitioners can enhance patient trust and confidence in virtual healthcare encounters, promoting improved patient outcomes and enhanced healthcare delivery through ethical issues. Ethical principles within the healthcare metaverse serve the dual purpose of safeguarding patients' well-being and fostering progress in medical education, scientific inquiry, and therapeutic approaches.

In the future, healthcare stakeholders must demonstrate unwavering dedication to maintaining ethical standards, complying with regulatory obligations, and actively pursuing continuous education. These efforts are crucial to guarantee the ethical utilisation of technology within the healthcare metaverse. By implementing this approach, the metaverse has the potential to bring about a paradigm shift in the healthcare field. Offering patient-centric, inclusive, and empathetic virtual encounters can fundamentally alter how healthcare services are provided, thereby shaping the future of healthcare delivery.

REFERENCES

Afaq, A., & Gaur, L. (2021). The Rise of Robots to Help Combat Covid-19. *2021 International Conference on Technological Advancements and Innovations (ICTAI)*, (pp. 69–74). IEEE. 10.1109/ICTAI53825.2021.9673256

Afaq, A., Gaur, L., & Singh, G. (2022). A Latent Dirichlet allocation Technique for Opinion Mining of Online Reviews of Global Chain Hotels. *2022 3rd International Conference on Intelligent Engineering and Management (ICIEM)*, (pp. 201–206). IEEE. 10.1109/ICIEM54221.2022.9853114

Afaq, A., Gaur, L., & Singh, G. (2023a). Social CRM: Linking the dots of customer service and customer loyalty during COVID-19 in the hotel industry. *International Journal of Contemporary Hospitality Management, Emerald Publishing Limited*, *35*(3), 992–1009. doi:10.1108/IJCHM-04-2022-0428

Afaq, A., Gaur, L., & Singh, G. (2023b). A trip down memory lane to travellers' food experiences. *British Food Journal, Emerald Publishing Limited*, *125*(4), 1390–1403. doi:10.1108/BFJ-01-2022-0063

Afaq, A., Gaur, L., Singh, G., & Dhir, A. (2021). *COVID-19: transforming air passengers' behaviour and reshaping their expectations towards the airline industry. Tourism Recreation Research*. Routledge. doi:10.1080/02508281.2021.2008211

Agac, G., Sevim, F., Celik, O., Bostan, S., Erdem, R. and Yalcin, Y.I. (2023). Research hotspots, trends and opportunities on the metaverse in health education: a bibliometric analysis. *Library Hi Tech*. Emerald Publishing Limited. doi:. doi:10.1108/LHT-04-2023-0168

Agarwal, A. and Alathur, S. (2023). Metaverse revolution and the digital transformation: intersectional analysis of Industry 5.0. *Transforming Government: People, Process and Policy*. Emerald Publishing Limited. . doi:10.1108/TG-03-2023-0036

Ahmed, S., Biswas, M., Hasanuzzaman, M., Mahi, M. J. N., Islam, M. A., Chaki, S., & Gaur, L. (2022). A Secured Peer-to-Peer Messaging System Based on Blockchain. *2022 3rd International Conference on Intelligent Engineering and Management (ICIEM)*, (pp. 332–337). IEEE. 10.1109/ICIEM54221.2022.9853040

Ahmed, S., Shaharier, M. M., Roy, S., Lima, A. A., Biswas, M., Mahi, M. J. N., Chaki, S & (2022). An Intelligent and Multi-Functional Stick for Blind People Using IoT. *2022 3rd International Conference on Intelligent Engineering and Management (ICIEM)*, (pp. 326–331). IEEE. 10.1109/ICIEM54221.2022.9853012

Anshari, M., Syafrudin, M., Fitriyani, N. L., & Razzaq, A. (2022). Ethical Responsibility and Sustainability (ERS) Development in a Metaverse Business Model. *Sustainability MDPI*, *14*(23), 15805. doi:10.3390u142315805

Anshu, K., & Gaur, L. (2018). Managing Customers Online Recovery – An Insight for E-Retailers Using Conjoint Analysis. *2018 4th International Conference on Computational Intelligence & Communication Technology (CICT)*, (pp. 1–7). IEEE. 10.1109/CIACT.2018.8480207

Athar, A., Ali, S. M., Mozumder, M. A. I., Ali, S., & Kim, H.-C. (2023). Applications and Possible Challenges of Healthcare Metaverse. *2023 25th International Conference on Advanced Communication Technology (ICACT)*, (pp. 328–332). IEEE. 10.23919/ICACT56868.2023.10079314

Bandyopadhyay, A., Ghosh, S., Bose, M., Kessi, L., & Gaur, L. (2023). Supervised Neural Networks for Fruit Identification. In K. C. Santosh, A. Goyal, D. Aouada, A. Makkar, Y.-Y. Chiang, & S. K. Singh (Eds.), *Recent Trends in Image Processing and Pattern Recognition* (pp. 220–230). Springer Nature Switzerland. doi:10.1007/978-3-031-23599-3_16

Bansal, G., Rajgopal, K., Chamola, V., Xiong, Z., & Niyato, D. (2022). Healthcare in Metaverse: A Survey on Current Metaverse Applications in Healthcare. *IEEE Access : Practical Innovations, Open Solutions*, *10*, 119914–119946. doi:10.1109/ACCESS.2022.3219845

Benjamins, R., Rubio Viñuela, Y., & Alonso, C. (2023). Social and ethical challenges of the metaverse. *AI and Ethics*, *3*(3), 689–697. doi:10.100743681-023-00278-5

Bhandari, M., Parajuli, P., Chapagain, P., & Gaur, L. (2022). Evaluating Performance of Adam Optimization by Proposing Energy Index. In K. C. Santosh, R. Hegadi, & U. Pal (Eds.), *Recent Trends in Image Processing and Pattern Recognition* (pp. 156–168). Springer International Publishing. doi:10.1007/978-3-031-07005-1_15

Biswas, M., Chaki, S., Ahammed, F., Anis, A., Ferdous, J., Siddika, A. M., & Shila, D. A. (2022). Prototype Development of an Assistive Smart-Stick for the Visually Challenged Persons. *2022 2nd International Conference on Innovative Practices in Technology and Management (ICIPTM)*. IEEE. 10.1109/ICIPTM54933.2022.9754183

Biswas, M., Chaki, S., Mallik, S., Gaur, L., & Ray, K. (2023). Light Convolutional Neural Network to Detect Eye Diseases from Retinal Images: Diabetic Retinopathy and Glaucoma. in M.S. Kaiser, S. Waheed, A. Bandyopadhyay, M. Mahmud, & K. Ray (Eds.), *Proceedings of the Fourth International Conference on Trends in Computational and Cognitive Engineering*, Springer Nature Singapore, Singapore, pp. 73–83. 10.1007/978-981-19-9483-8_7

Camilleri, M.A. (2023). Metaverse applications in education: a systematic review and a cost-benefit analysis. *Interactive Technology and Smart Education*, Emerald Publishing Limited. doi:. doi:10.1108/ITSE-01-2023-0017

Chaudhary, M., Gaur, L., & Chakrabarti, A. (2022). Comparative Analysis of Entropy Weight Method and C5 Classifier for Predicting Employee Churn. *2022 3rd International Conference on Intelligent Engineering and Management (ICIEM)*, (pp. 232–236). IEEE. 10.1109/ICIEM54221.2022.9853181

Chaudhary, M., Gaur, L., Jhanjhi, N. Z., Masud, M., & Aljahdali, S. (2022). Envisaging Employee Churn Using MCDM and Machine Learning. Intelligent Automation & Soft Computing, 33(2). doi:10.32604/iasc.2022.023417

Chengoden, R., Victor, N., Huynh-The, T., Yenduri, G., Jhaveri, R. H., Alazab, M., Bhattacharya, S., Hegde, P., Maddikunta, P. K. R., & Gadekallu, T. R. (2023). Metaverse for Healthcare: A Survey on Potential Applications, Challenges and Future Directions. *IEEE Access : Practical Innovations, Open Solutions*, 11, 12765–12795. doi:10.1109/ACCESS.2023.3241628

De Felice, F., Rehman, M., Petrillo, A., & Baffo, I. (2023). A metaworld: Implications, opportunities and risks of the metaverse. *IET Collaborative Intelligent Manufacturing, The Institution of Engineering and Technology*, 5(3), e12079.

Dwivedi, Y.K., Hughes, L., Wang, Y., Alalwan, A.A., & Ahn, S.J., Balakrishnan, J., & Barta, S. (2023). Metaverse marketing: How the metaverse will shape the future of consumer research and practice. *Psychology & Marketing*. John Wiley & Sons.

Fan, X., Wang, H., & Wang, L. (2023). P-2.8: Metaverse: Origin, Current Applications and Prospects for Future Development. *SID Symposium Digest of Technical Papers*, John Wiley & Sons, Ltd. 10.1002dtp.16342

Fernandez, C. B., & Hui, P. (2022). Life, the Metaverse and Everything: An Overview of Privacy, Ethics, and Governance in Metaverse. *2022 IEEE 42nd International Conference on Distributed Computing Systems Workshops (ICDCSW)*, (pp. 272–277). IEEE. 10.1109/ICDCSW56584.2022.00058

Gaur, L., & Afaq, A. (2020). Metamorphosis of CRM: incorporation of social media to customer relationship management in the hospitality industry. In *Handbook of Research on Engineering Innovations and Technology Management in Organizations* (pp. 1–23). IGI Global. doi:10.4018/978-1-7998-2772-6.ch001

Gaur, L., Afaq, A., Arora, G. K., & Khan, N. (2023). Artificial intelligence for carbon emissions using system of systems theory. *Ecological Informatics*, 76, 102165. doi:10.1016/j.ecoinf.2023.102165

Gaur, L., Afaq, A., Singh, G., & Dwivedi, Y. K. (2021). Role of artificial intelligence and robotics to foster the touchless travel during a pandemic: A review and research agenda. *International Journal of Contemporary Hospitality Management, Emerald Publishing Limited*, *33*(11), 4079–4098. doi:10.1108/IJCHM-11-2020-1246

Gaur, L., Afaq, A., Solanki, A., Singh, G., Sharma, S., Jhanjhi, N. Z., My, H. T., & Le, D.-N. (2021). Capitalising on big data and revolutionary 5G technology: Extracting and visualising ratings and reviews of global chain hotels. *Computers & Electrical Engineering*, *95*, 107374. doi:10.1016/j.compeleceng.2021.107374

Gaur, L., Singh, G., & Agarwal, V. (2021). Leveraging Artificial Intelligence Tools to Combat the COVID-19 Crisis. In P. K. Singh, G. Veselov, V. Vyatkin, A. Pljonkin, J. M. Dodero, & Y. Kumar (Eds.), *Futuristic Trends in Network and Communication Technologies* (pp. 321–328). doi:10.1007/978-981-16-1480-4_28

Gaur, L., Solanki, A., Wamba, S. F., & Jhanjhi, N. Z. (2021). *Advanced AI Techniques and Applications in Bioinformatics*. CRC Press. doi:10.1201/9781003126164

Ghose, P., Biswas, M., & Gaur, L. (2023). BrainSegNeT: A Lightweight Brain Tumor Segmentation Model Based on U-Net and Progressive Neuron Expansion. In F. Liu, Y. Zhang, H. Kuai, E. P. Stephen, & H. Wang (Eds.), *Brain Informatics* (pp. 249–260). Springer Nature Switzerland. doi:10.1007/978-3-031-43075-6_22

Ghose, P., Sharmin, S., Gaur, L., & Zhao, Z. (2022). Grid-Search Integrated Optimized Support Vector Machine Model for Breast Cancer Detection. *2022 IEEE International Conference on Bioinformatics and Biomedicine (BIBM)*, (pp. 2846–2852). IEEE. 10.1109/BIBM55620.2022.9995703

Hollensen, S., Kotler, P., & Opresnik, M. O. (2023). Metaverse – the new marketing universe. *Journal of Business Strategy, Emerald Publishing Limited*, *44*(3), 119–125. doi:10.1108/JBS-01-2022-0014

Hwang, G.-J., & Chien, S.-Y. (2022). Definition, roles, and potential research issues of the metaverse in education: An artificial intelligence perspective. *Computers and Education: Artificial Intelligence*, *3*, 100082. doi:10.1016/j.caeai.2022.100082

Inceoglu, M. M., & Ciloglugil, B. (2022). Use of Metaverse in Education. In O. Gervasi, B. Murgante, S. Misra, A. M. A. C. Rocha, & C. Garau (Eds.), *Computational Science and Its Applications – ICCSA 2022 Workshops* (pp. 171–184). Springer International Publishing. doi:10.1007/978-3-031-10536-4_12

Iwanaga, J., Muo, E. C., Tabira, Y., Watanabe, K., Tubbs, S. J., D'Antoni, A. V., & Rajaram-Gilkes, M. (2023). Who really needs a Metaverse in anatomy education? A review with preliminary survey results. *Clinical Anatomy*. John Wiley & Sons. doi:10.1002/ca.23949 PMID:36087277

Jain, M., Singh, G., & Gaur, L. (2021). Green Internet of Things: Next-Generation Intelligence for Sustainable Development. In P. K. Kapur, G. Singh, & S. Panwar (Eds.), *Advances in Interdisciplinary Research in Engineering and Business Management* (pp. 359–367). doi:10.1007/978-981-16-0037-1_28

Kaddoura, S., & Al Husseiny, F. (2023). The rising trend of Metaverse in education: Challenges, opportunities, and ethical considerations. *PeerJ Computer Science*, 9, e1252. PMID:37346578

Kshetri, N. (2022). Policy, Ethical, Social, and Environmental Considerations of Web3 and the Metaverse. *IT Professional*, 24(3), 4–8. doi:10.1109/MITP.2022.3178509

Manto, A., & D'Oria, M. (2023). Some Ethical and Educational Perspectives on Using Artificial Intelligence in Personalized Medicine and Healthcare. In A. Cesario, M. D'Oria, C. Auffray, & G. Scambia (Eds.), *Personalised Medicine Meets Artificial Intelligence: Beyond "Hype", Towards the Metaverse* (pp. 261–269). Springer International Publishing. doi:10.1007/978-3-031-32614-1_18

Mathur, S., & Gaur, L. (2021). Predictability, Power and Procedures of Citation Analysis, in D. Goyal, A.K. Gupta, V. Piuri, M. Ganzha, & M. Paprzycki (Eds.), *Proceedings of the Second International Conference on Information Management and Machine Intelligence*. Springer Singapore, Singapore. 10.1007/978-981-15-9689-6_6

Mbunge, E., Muchemwa, B., & Batani, J. (2022). Are we there yet? Unbundling the potential adoption and integration of telemedicine to improve virtual healthcare services in African health systems. *Sensors International*, 3, 100152. doi:10.1016/j.sintl.2021.100152 PMID:34901894

Moro, C. (2023). Utilising the metaverse in anatomy and physiology. *Anatomical Sciences Education*. John Wiley & Sons. PMID:36545794

Mozumder, M. A. I., Sheeraz, M. M., Athar, A., Aich, S., & Kim, H.-C. (2022). Overview: Technology Roadmap of the Future Trend of Metaverse based on IoT, Blockchain, AI Technique, and Medical Domain Metaverse Activity. *2022 24th International Conference on Advanced Communication Technology (ICACT)*, (pp. 256–261). IEEE. 10.23919/ICACT53585.2022.9728808

Musamih, A., Yaqoob, I., Salah, K., Jayaraman, R., Al-Hammadi, Y., Omar, M., & Ellahham, S. (2023). Metaverse in Healthcare: Applications, Challenges, and Future Directions. *IEEE Consumer Electronics Magazine*, *12*(4), 33–46. doi:10.1109/MCE.2022.3223522

Protic, D., Gaur, L., Stankovic, M., & Rahman, M. A. (2022). Cybersecurity in smart cities: Detection of opposing decisions on anomalies in the computer network behavior. *Electronics. MDPI*, *11*(22), 3718. doi:10.3390/electronics11223718

Rana, J., Gaur, L., & Santosh, K. (2022). Classifying Customers' Journey from Online Reviews of Amazon Fresh via Sentiment Analysis and Topic Modelling. *2022 3rd International Conference on Computation, Automation and Knowledge Management (ICCAKM)*, (pp. 1–6). IEEE. 10.1109/ICCAKM54721.2022.9990124

Rospigliosi, P. (2022). Adopting the metaverse for learning environments means more use of deep learning artificial intelligence: this presents challenges and problems. *Interactive Learning Environments*. Routledge. doi:. doi:10.1080/10494820.2022.2132034

Sahu, G., Gaur, L., & Singh, G. (2023). Investigating the impact of personality tendencies and gratification aspects on OTT short video consumption: a case of YouTube shorts. *2023 3rd International Conference on Innovative Practices in Technology and Management (ICIPTM)*. IEEE. 10.1109/ICIPTM57143.2023.10118122

Sharma, S., Singh, G., Gaur, L., & Afaq, A. (2022). Exploring customer adoption of autonomous shopping systems. *Telematics and Informatics*, *73*, 101861. doi:10.1016/j.tele.2022.101861

Skalidis, I., Muller, O., & Fournier, S. (2022). CardioVerse: The cardiovascular medicine in the era of Metaverse. *Trends in Cardiovascular Medicine*. doi:10.1016/j.tcm.2022.05.004 PMID:35568263

Song, Y.-T., & Qin, J. (2022). Metaverse and Personal Healthcare. *Procedia Computer Science*, *210*, 189–197. doi:10.1016/j.procs.2022.10.136

Sparkes, M. (2021). What is a metaverse. *New Scientist*, *251*(3348), 18. doi:10.1016/S0262-4079(21)01450-0

Suh, I., McKinney, T., & Siu, K.-C. (2023). Current Perspective of Metaverse Application in Medical Education, Research and Patient Care. *Virtual Worlds*, *2*(2), 115–128. doi:10.3390/virtualworlds2020007

Surveswaran, S., & Deshpande, L. (2023). *A Glimpse into the Future*. AI in Clinical Medicine. doi:10.1002/9781119790686.ch47

Tan, T. F., Li, Y., Lim, J. S., Gunasekeran, D. V., Teo, Z. L., Ng, W. Y., & Ting, D. S. W. (2022). Metaverse and Virtual Health Care in Ophthalmology: Opportunities and Challenges. *Asia-Pacific Journal of Ophthalmology*, *11*(3), 237–246. doi:10.1097/APO.0000000000000537 PMID:35772084

Thomason, J. (2022). Metaverse, token economies, and non-communicable diseases. *Global Health Journal*, *6*(3), 164–167. doi:10.1016/j.glohj.2022.07.001

Tlili, A., Huang, R., Shehata, B., Liu, D., Zhao, J., Metwally, A. H. S., Wang, H., Denden, M., Bozkurt, A., Lee, L.-H., Beyoglu, D., Altinay, F., Sharma, R. C., Altinay, Z., Li, Z., Liu, J., Ahmad, F., Hu, Y., Salha, S., & Burgos, D. (2022). Is Metaverse in education a blessing or a curse: A combined content and bibliometric analysis. *Smart Learning Environments*, *9*(1), 24. doi:10.118640561-022-00205-x

Tyagi, A., Gaur, L., Singh, G., & Kumar, A. (2022). Air Quality Index (AQI) Using Time Series Modelling During COVID Pandemic. In G. Sanyal, C.M. Travieso-González, S. Awasthi, C.M.A. Pinto, & B.R. Purushothama (Eds.), *International Conference on Artificial Intelligence and Sustainable Engineering*. Springer Singapore, Singapore. 10.1007/978-981-16-8546-0_36

Venugopal, J.P., Subramanian, A.A.V. & Peatchimuthu, J. (2023). The realm of metaverse: A survey. *Computer Animation and Virtual Worlds*. John Wiley & Sons, Ltd. doi:. doi:0.1002/cav.2150

Wang, G., Badal, A., Jia, X., Maltz, J. S., Mueller, K., Myers, K. J., Niu, C., Vannier, M., Yan, P., Yu, Z., & Zeng, R. (2022). Development of metaverse for intelligent healthcare. *Nature Machine Intelligence*, *4*(11), 922–929. doi:10.103842256-022-00549-6 PMID:36935774

Wei, W. (2023). A buzzword, a phase or the next chapter for the Internet? The status and possibilities of the metaverse for tourism. *Journal of Hospitality and Tourism Insights*. doi:. doi:10.1108/JHTI-11-2022-0568

Yang, D., Zhou, J., Chen, R., Song, Y., Song, Z., Zhang, X., Wang, Q., Wang, K., Zhou, C., Sun, J., Zhang, L., Bai, L., Wang, Y., Wang, X., Lu, Y., Xin, H., Powell, C. A., Thüemmler, C., Chavannes, N. H., & Bai, C. (2022). Expert consensus on the metaverse in medicine. *Clinical EHealth*, *5*, 1–9. doi:10.1016/j.ceh.2022.02.001

Yang, Y., Siau, K., Xie, W. & Sun, Y. (2022). Smart health: Intelligent healthcare systems in the metaverse, artificial intelligence, and data science era. *Journal of Organizational and End User Computing (JOEUC)*. IGI Global.

Yaqoob, I., Salah, K., Jayaraman, R., & Omar, M. (2023). Metaverse applications in smart cities: Enabling technologies, opportunities, challenges, and future directions. *Internet of Things*, *23*, 100884. doi:10.1016/j.iot.2023.100884

Zhang, G., Dai, Y., Wu, J., Zhu, X., & Lu, Y. (2023). Swarm Learning-based Secure and Fair Model Sharing for Metaverse Healthcare. *Mobile Networks and Applications*. doi:10.100711036-023-02236-1

Zhang, X., Chen, Y., Hu, L., & Wang, Y. (2022). The metaverse in education: Definition, framework, features, potential applications, challenges, and future research topics. *Frontiers in Psychology*, *13*, 6063.

Chapter 9
Metaverse for Healthcare:
Possible Potential Applications (Virtual Reality Technologies), Opportunities, Challenges, and Future Directions

Hafiz Asif
Islamia University of Bahawalpur, Pakistan

Misbah Firdous
Islamia University of Bahawalpur, Pakistan

Rabia Zahid
Islamia University of Bahawalpur, Pakistan

Ahsan Zahid
Islamia University of Bahawalpur, Pakistan

Uzma Bashir
Islamia University of Bahawalpur, Pakistan

Muhammad Hasnain
https://orcid.org/0000-0003-1705-7751
Islamia University of Bahawalpur, Pakistan

Waseem Afzal
Islamia University of Bahawalpur, Pakistan

ABSTRACT

2021 is known as the first Year of the Metaverse, and around the world, internet giants are eager to devote themselves to it. Metaverse is the augmented virtual world formed by convergence of virtual and physical space. Users interact within this created world, meeting each other virtually, immersing themselves in performing virtual activities, which subsequently could lead to real experiences. Conventionally, the healthcare "industry" is conservative in deploying future ready technology. Demonstrating significant improvement in healthcare outcomes using the metaverse will be difficult to prove. This overview discusses the untapped potential of metaverse applications in healthcare, and also points out the advantages, disadvantages, limitations, and challenges in actual deployment of the metaverse in clinical practice in the real world. This alone will ultimately lead to the development of a business model, insurance reimbursement, and behavioral modification necessary for accepting and using a hitherto unused method in patient care.

DOI: 10.4018/978-1-6684-9823-1.ch009

1. METAVERSE

The application of metaverse in healthcare is just one example of how it is a new concept for the disruptive changes predicted in many areas of our lives. For many years, diagnosing patient problems, prescribing medical treatments, and performing surgical procedures on patients have all involved direct physical contact between patients and doctors. The introduction of telemedicine services has little altered this state (Yang et al., 2022). The recent rapid developments in technology offer limitless possibilities to improve healthcare. From virtual health to mental health and from reality management to virtual management, the metaverse has the potential to change healthcare (Kavanagh, 2021).

Although not two new initiatives, AI and data science in hospital management provide novel possibilities. The earliest artificial intelligence (AI) program, MYCIN, was utilized as early as the 1970s to assist in the treatment of blood infections (Davenport & Kalakota, 2019). The handling of a vast amount of data on patients with blood infections has been done using data science. Incorporating collected data, data science contributes in the analysis and investigation of patients' blood issues. The American Association for Artificial Intelligence (AAAI) was established in 1979 (Schrodt, 2019).

Intelligent Systems in Medicine, the first worldwide AI journal, was established in 1980. AI was used in clinical contexts between 1980 and 1990, from developing minimally-invasive procedures to exploring the idea of virtual presence during surgery (Yang et al., 2022). Automated Endoscopic System for Optimal Positioning (AESOP), a voice-activated endoscope, was introduced in 1994 with the aid of data science and machine learning techniques, enabling surgeons to view inside the bodies of the patients (Oniani et al., 2021).

The FDA recognized the implementation of algorithms to find tumors in medical photographs in 1998, despite the introduction of deep learning methods in data science. The American robotics company Computer Motion created the ZEUS Robotic Surgical System (ZRSS) in 2001 to aid in surgery. Three robotic arms on the ZRSS, including the upgraded AESOP, can be remotely operated by the surgeon (Yang et al., 2022). The Da Vinci Surgical System was created by the new business in 2003 after Computer Motion and Intuitive Surgical merged. This is not a robotic system. Scientists developed the platform to do robotically supported surgery that is minimally invasive (Morrell et al., 2021). A panel on clinical data mining, knowledge-based healthcare, and temporal data mining was organized at the Artificial Intelligence in Medicine Europe (AIME) symposium in Amsterdam, the Netherlands, in 2007 (Yang et al., 2022). Without a question, data science and AI are vital tools for the healthcare industry. Researchers in artificial intelligence in medicine (AIM) are working to create a wide range of AI-inspired approaches to address a variety of significant clinical and biological issues. Deep neural learning technology has significant potential in smart health and intelligent healthcare management, as shown by the fact that the deep neural networks introduced in 2012 have demonstrated good performance properties relative to those of more conventional AI (Yang et al., 2022).

Development in data science and AI for medical applications has significantly increased in recent years. Remote illness assessment, virtual health screening, telemedicine and many other creative and intelligent healthcare applications are emerging thanks to the use of artificial intelligence in the metaverse and data science applications in primary care (Liang & Liu, 2018). Examples of such applications include the three-dimensional immersive remote monitoring of seriously ill patients, blood glucose monitoring, clinical patient data analysis, heart rate observing, boosting capabilities for recording physical activity, and other new and previously inconceivable medical and health services (Chen & Zhang, 2022). For instance, the technology company Oculus, which Meta recently acquired, has been assisting in orthopedic surgery (Chen & Zhang, 2022).

Google Glass is assisting new mothers who are having trouble breastfeeding. AccuVein, a medical technology business, uses augmented reality to make life easier for both patients and nurses. These programs and equipment can also help medical practitioners and enhance their abilities (Chimakurthi, 2019). AR can increase the surgical efficiency of surgeons. AR healthcare apps can help save lives and treat patients effectively, whether they are performing a minimally invasive treatment or identifying a tumor in the liver (Bohr & Memarzadeh, 2020).

Applications of AI and data science are also emerging, being tested, and expanding quickly in hospital management. The STATISTA website revealed the worldwide healthcare (Humayun, 2020). AI market's growth rate from 2014 to 2021 and forecast that growth would be 55% in that year shown in figure 1. Furthermore, according to Sage Growth Partners, 75 percent of hospital executives believe that AI is a crucial tool for the medical hospital setting in light of the COVID-19 epidemic, and 90 percent of hospitals around the world have an AI plan in place (Tyagi & Saxena, 2022). Investment in AI for medical diagnostics is also anticipated to increase, from $505 million in 2020 to $387,87 billion in 2025. In order decrease doctors' workloads, government measures will continue to drive up demand for AI solutions in the medical industry (Yang et al., 2022).

Clinical document management is another area for AI and data science in hospital management.

Approximately 1.2 billion clinical documents are generated each year in the United States. Out of these, 20% of the data are structured, and structured data can be easily stored electronically and analyzed (Yang et al., 2022). Further, nearly 80% of the data are in the form of notes written by doctors, medical images, and clinical

Figure 1. AI market's growth rate from 2014 to 2021

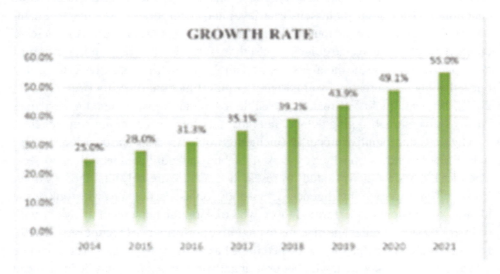

documents. Thus, data science can be applied to analyze and study a large number of clinical documents and data in the medical field to reduce the workload of the healthcare worker (Yan et al., 2019).

1.1 Medical Metaverse

Technologies related to the metaverse have created new opportunities for developments in medicine. Technology improvements are being embraced by medical education and healthcare practices to enhance patient care (Singh et al., 2020). Metaverse technologies are being used by a wide range of subspecialties, including cardiology, emergency medicine, gynaecology, gastrointestinal, ophthalmology, oncology, and radiology. Innovations in the metaverse, notably XR (virtual, augmented, and mixed reality) technology, are also advantageous to the fields of mental health (López-Ojeda & Hurley, 2023). One of the most often used developments in mental health interventions is virtual reality technology. Specific phobias, anxiety, posttraumatic stress disorder (PTSD), attention deficit hyperactivity disorder, depression, substance use disorders, and eating disorders have all been successfully treated with VR exposure treatment (VRET) and AR exposure therapy (Emmelkamp & Meyerbröker, 2021).

When a patient is receiving treatment, VRET uses comprehensive psychotherapeutic paradigms that offer multisensory virtual reality (VR) adventures to increase their level of experiential involvement. After military trauma, VRET therapies are successful in lowering PTSD symptoms in active-duty and combatants

(Emmelkamp & Meyerbröker, 2021). The immersive qualities of XR, which enable encounters at a digital multi-sensorial level and incorporate a seamless human-computer interaction, contribute to its therapeutic advantages in part. A researcher claimed that "the metaverse guides us past the assumption that body, mind and spirit are separate" because the metaverse uses technology (such as VR and AR) to correct one's dysfunctional reality by employing virtual (functional) reality (Cerasa et al., 2022). Innovations in VR make it possible to imitate transcendental experiences (such as diversion, bringing delight and pleasant affect in a relaxing atmosphere).

Higher-order cognitive processes (including problem solving and decision making) may differ depending on which aspects of the body an individual feels they possess. This idea is demonstrated in a study by researchers using extremely intelligent ("Albert Einstein") and average-intelligence virtual body robots. Participants who took on the identity of Einstein outperformed those who took on the persona of an avatar with ordinary IQ and a similar age in terms of cognitive performance (Yampolskiy, 2019). In studies of social behavior, the owned body has been shown to have a comparable effect. These tests looked at whether pro- or antisocial behaviors may be influenced by acting as specific avatars (i.e., players in video games) and the avatars' actions (194 subjects). Players who selected heroic-themed portraits were encouraged to act more sociably. According to the authors, after playing a villain or superhero in the virtual world, volunteers imitated those actions while engaging with other players in the actual world (Bediou et al., 2018). The researchers also emphasized that role-playing activities promoted behaviors compatible with the priming acts (i.e., the avatar's heroic or evil activities). The use of avatars in therapy may encourage patient participation. Avatars drive these processes, making the virtual environment a platform for simulation, observation, and modelling. Increased treatment seeking through anonymity, decreased communication barriers, facilitated expression and client identity exploration, and improved interventional settings due to therapists' ability to regulate and influence the therapeutic conditions within the simulation are all additional advantages of avatar-integrated therapies (Kwame & Petrucka, 2020).

1.2 Metaverse in Medical Domain

The development of future the skills of medical professional's expertise and knowledge bases is significantly impacted by the application of digital reality in the healthcare sector. Technology like the Microsoft HoloLens is an example of a surgical assistance tool that surgeons use to facilitate and expedite surgical procedures (Galati et al., 2020). In addition to pre-operative images from MRI, CT and 3D scans, AR headsets are used to view critical immediate patient information such as body temperature, heart rate, breathing rate and blood pressure (Cornejo et al., 2022). Nurses and doctors are currently using augmented reality to enhance vein detection. For many people, even those with dark skin or tiny blood veins, this eliminates the problem of identifying a vein (Ren et al., 2022). In the healthcare sector, visual-driven technology like X-rays and CT scans etc. shown in figure 2 is widespread. Simply put, they enable medical practitioners to see inside patients' bodies and assist in the detection, diagnosis, and treatment of patients. The technology of the metaverse was adopted by several medical institutes.

Figure 2. Metaverse in medical domain

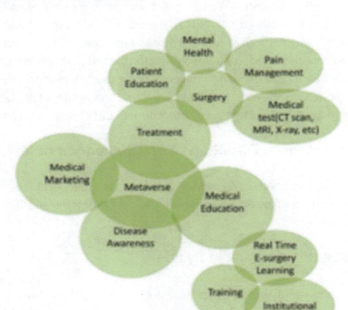

- A. Metaverse Activities role in Healthcare
    - Augmented reality surgery, telepresence, remote surgery
    - 3D human anatomy models for planning, diagnosis, and education
    - Healthcare facility architecture
    - Treatment planning, medical therapy
    - Pain management; virtual patients
    - Haptic assistance in rehabilitation
    - Visualization of large medical datasets
    - Preventive medicine and patient education
    - Surgery simulation
    - Virtual patients (Musamih et al., 2022)
- B. General Patient Treatment Proposed Process Using Metaverse Technology

Applications-based treatment to expedite training without creating wonder or risk, metaverse is used. It is applied in the field of medicine to treat a variety of disorders. Future metaverse technology will play a useful function in enhancing the effectiveness of the medical industry. The usage of the technology known as Metaverse can improve patient and learner satisfaction (Mozumder et al., 2022). The Metaverse is a crucial technology for the development process that makes use of specialized and cutting-edge software and hardware, and it offers an applicable answer in the medical industry. We can gather the patient's history and specify the precise goal of the necessary treatment. To generate 3D virtual data that generates a 3D virtual world, various hardware and software are required. The required medical data is created and identified using the best method feasible in the metaverse virtual reality and augmented reality. This process can be used to plan the treatment and ultimately aids in carrying out the actual treatment (Mozumder et al., 2022). Figure 3 depicts the general patient treatment procedure using Metaverse technology.

1.3 Future Research Directions and Challenges of Metaverse

The application of metaverse, AI, and data science in smart health and intelligent healthcare systems is discussed, along with the new problems and future research areas it encounters.

1.3.1 Challenge 1: Explicable Systems

Even if they provide diagnoses that are more accurate than those provided by human doctors, the majority of current AI, machine learning, and deep learning

Figure 3. General patient treatment procedure using metaverse technology

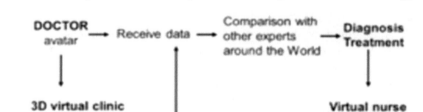

systems are unable to explain how they arrived at a certain conclusion. We cannot directly see any models or pieces of data because machine learning's internal processing—often referred to as the "black box"—does not include traditional machine learning algorithms like decision trees, simple statistical machine learning models like logistic regression, and many others (Chengoden et al., 2022). Patients have a limited comprehension of and low faith in AI and data science systems as a result of the diagnoses that the systems provide not being able to be articulated by human doctors. In all forms of partnerships, trust is essential and acceptance is a requirement. According to the Health Insurance Portability and Accountability Act (HIPAA), it is difficult to use machine learning and deep learning to patients (Chang et al., 2022). Some contend that applications including as medication discovery and development, patient population management, and arranging appointments may be better suited for the use of AI technologies than diagnostic and treatment planning. However, given the promise of AI, machine learning and deep learning are required to develop an AI that can be explained and have its inner workings made open and transparent. Until the working methods are transparent, regulatory compliance may limit AI uses in smart health.

Research Direction. 1: It is challenging to explain and comprehend how AI and data science employing machine learning operate and what they perform since they are opaque. The expansion and adoption of AI depend heavily on research on explainable AI (Adadi & Berrada, 2018).

1.3.2 Challenge 2: Relationship Among Patients and Hospitals

The complicated interactions among patients and hospitals present another inherent difficulty in a medical hospital setting. Patients may still feel unsatisfied despite the fact that AI and data science technologies might decrease costs and waiting times for them. This could be because of a number of things, including health results, unmet expectations, and disconcerting communication. Patients who argue about their rights, cast doubt on the validity of the data, and lack faith in the doctors will eat up crucial time that could be better spent helping the patients.

Research Direction. 2: Intelligent avatars can assist in explaining some of the medical symptoms, causes, treatment alternatives, and therapy processes because the majority of individuals lack medical expertise on disease diagnosis and treatment. For instance, virtual worlds like metaverse may be employed to model hospital floor plans and replicate operating rooms and procedures. With metaverse, AI, and data science, telemedicine and subsequent care can also be considerably facilitated and improved. Another crucial research field is healthcare education programs that employ AI to customize and offer health education to patients (Ward, 2018).

1.3.3 Challenge 3: Trust

Patients may find AI systems and health robotics less trustworthy because they lack human emotions like empathy and compassion. Patients frequently put their trust in their doctors rather than the more precise AI systems because of this. Therefore, if AI is engaged, healthcare providers face the additional issue of gaining patients' trust. The growth of smart health also depends on enhancing the accuracy of diagnosis and treatments, decreasing incorrect and misdiagnosed diagnoses, and fostering trustworthy interactions between people and AI.

Research Direction. 3: How can we make AI systems that mimic or develop human emotions like empathy and compassion? In the short term, it may be challenging for AI to emulate genuine empathy and compassion, but it is possible. AI that possesses "emotional" intelligence is crucial in the healthcare industry. However, such imitation must not transcend the line into unethical and dishonest behavior (Musamih et al., 2022).

1.3.4 Challenge 4: Data Security and Privacy

A huge database is used for machine learning by many AI systems. A vast amount of data is also necessary for data science. Many sensitive and personal data may need to be gathered in order to build the database. In such cases, data security and privacy are crucial concerns. It is necessary to practice and regulate informed consent, privacy, and data protection. These databases are also vulnerable to attacks and hacking. There are numerous private and sensitive data at risk. The bad news is that these hacking and attacks will be more sophisticated and advanced. On the dark web, patient data and information are highly prized. Modern, cutting-edge security measures are needed for hospitals and other medical facilities' data security requirements.

Research Direction 4: Data privacy and security are always areas for improvement, particularly in the healthcare industry. In order to improve security and privacy and stop data breaches, AI and data science can be helpful. The advancement of smart health is dependent on research in these fields(Y. Wang et al., 2022).

1.3.5 Challenge 5: Ethical Issues

The ethical use of data in AI and data science must be taken into account in addition to the legal use of the data obtained. Additionally, ethical behaviour is expected of developed AI systems, and ethical standards must also be upheld by creators. New laws must be passed to govern AI data protection, liability determination, and monitoring in terms of legal matters. For the application of AI and data science in the healthcare setting, legislation like to HIPAA should be drafted. There is an urgent need for laws, rules, and regulations pertaining to the ethical usage of AI.

Research Direction. 5: It is impossible to neglect the ethical component of the metaverse, AI, and data science developments. In reality, a large portion of the AI community believes that the ethical application of AI is of the utmost importance. Another crucial area for research is using AI to teach AI professionals about ethical issues. Ethics in AI are desperately needed (Kaddoura & Al Husseiny, 2023).

Table 1. The application of metaverse, enabling technologies along with the challenges and future directions

Enabling Technology	Contributions	Challenges	Future Directions
Blockchain, XAI, Teleoperation, 6G	A framework for blockchain and XAI assisted telesurgery is proposed. 6G TI channel is also used.	Real metaverse set up is required for testing the framework	Different XAI models can be compared and the optimal technique can be chosen
XR, MR	Eye MG Holo: An immersive 4D pedagogical tool for learning about various ophthalmologic structures is proposed.	Cost effectiveness: Approximately 3500 USD for a HoloLens 2	Can be used for surgical simulation training
XR, VR, AR	A training in lung cancer surgery using metaverse is explained. The smart operating room was set up in Seoul National University Bundang Hospital, South Korea.	Advanced imaging and other high-end equipments are required for accomplishing the task	Can be extensively used for surgical training and other health related applications
AR, VR	Cardioverse is introduced for the diagnosis and prevention of cardiovascular diseases	Legal Regulations, security and privacy, user rights	Moral and credibility aspects need to be considered
ML	A hybrid Structural Equation Modelling- Machine Learning approach is proposed to predict the intention of specific users to employ metaverse in healthcare education. Application of metaverse in UAE is taken into consideration	Only personal innovativeness and user satisfaction is taken into account. Perceived Ease of Use and Perceived Usefulness only were considered	Focus to be given on other medical aspects as well
VR	Immersion, collaboration and interaction could be greatly improved with the intervention of the Metaverse in online pedagogy	Only small group size was considered for evaluation	To understand the detrimental effect of adoption of metaverse in medical education
AR, VR	To provide counselling services to post-operative patients	Set up needs to be changed for addressing a large group of patients	Can be adopted for ICU
Wearable devices, IoT	A technique for providing social skills training for children affected with Autism Spectrum Disorder is proposed	Obtaining consent from guardians	Children of all categories can be considered for the study
AI, VR, Robotics	Adoption of the Metaverse in spine care with respect to education, diagnosis, consultation, surgery and research	Affordable advanced care facilities	Other advanced technologies can be incorporated

1.4 Metaverse Medical Intervention

MeTAI will have a significant impact on how practitioners and people use medical data and tools to comprehend diseases, choose medicines, and carry out interventions. We can design sophisticated surgical procedures and other treatments, for instance, using such a virtual environment. The trial-and-error method can be used repeatedly to practice operations when done virtually. This works well with modern surgical technologies like da Vinci (https://www.davincisurgery.com), which let a surgeon operate from a nearby room or from a different continent using high-speed internet. In MeTAI, surgeons can perform various procedures (like plastic surgery) on avatars (Hamet & Tremblay, 2017). Another illustration is radiotherapy. By using patient-specific computer simulations to regularly modify treatment strategies, MeTAI would extend this practice to all medical treatments. Before and during a course of therapy, biological reactions to radiation delivery could be simulated in order to optimize the treatment response based on the patient's genetic information and data from prior patients' responses. Currently, computational constraints and biological model uncertainties render this approach unusable for standard treatment planning. By utilizing libraries of simulators and clinical knowledge that are made immediately useful by their incorporation in the metaverse, injury to organs at risk during radiation therapy could potentially be significantly decreased in the future. None of these potential advantages are free, and early adoption of MeTAI may cause busy practitioners stress or distraction (G. Wang et al., 2022).

There will be a demand for training and certifying practitioners as MeTAI gets established and implemented. It may feel peculiar at first for a surgeon or interventional radiologist to employ new equipment or robots. This is comparable to the risk offered by an aeroplane with new sorts of automation, which could cause an accident if the pilot is inexperienced. To help with the introduction of new systems, surgical robotic simulations and curriculum were created. Using VR and AR technologies, certain medical schools are launching cadaver-free anatomy instruction initiatives. Additionally, the metaverse's human-computer interactions have inspired computer scientists to create the Metaverse Knowledge Center (https://metaverse.acm.org/). Some businesses are developing in this field. For instance, OSSO VR (https://www.ossovr.com) is creating ways for individuals to explore new surgical techniques using VR. MeTAI is naturally compatible with team training and co-development through metaversed interactions that are comparable to those in the real world, as well as interactive and continuous learning and multi-institutional projects. Particularly intriguing is embodied AI, which teaches AI agents through interactions as well as data. In MeTAI, avatars can be promoted to embodied AI agents, which facilitates the reversible value alignment and allows avatars to express preferences for radiation dosage, healthcare costs, and the side-effect profiles of diverse medicinal selections. These avatar personalities also allow for the creation of interest groups, metaverse-based surveys, and policymaking (Miller, 2020).

1.4.1 How Could the Metaverse Transform Patient Therapy?

Virtual environments, such as the Metaverse, may also play a bigger part in patient therapy in the future for a variety of psychiatric problems. Exposure to fear, for example, has been used to cure certain phobias, and so virtual worlds might be used to gradually expose patients in a safe context. In tailored virtual experiences, such therapeutic strategies may also be applied to other disorders such as obsessive-compulsive disorder, anxiety, or depression. The Metaverse's potential collaborative capacity would also allow therapist- or patient-led support groups to easily discover one another and gather from all over the world in a more engaging environment than a text-based support group. There are various potentially useful uses for realistic virtual simulations, many of which are still in the early phases of development as technology advances to meet the challenge. Haptic sensors that simulate patient movement within a virtual environment, for example, could have applications in movement rehabilitation and alleviating Parkinson's symptoms, while distracting virtual reality experiences have shown some success in replacing pain medications when changing burn victims' wound dressings or in easing blood collection from children (Mozumder et al., 2022).

The immersive virtual healthcare business was allegedly valued at roughly $1.2 billion in 2021, with a projected value of over $12 billion by 2028. Within the last year, Meta has made massive investments in making the Metaverse a reality. However, the healthcare industry will have to wait some time before reaping the full benefits. One major barrier to Metaverse adoption is the requirement for virtual reality headsets and maybe additional haptic technologies, which means that the typical patient, particularly older generations, is unlikely to have the necessary equipment (Schoonjans, 2021).

2. HEALTHCARE

Healthcare remains one of the most important determinants of the global human population's general, physical, social, and mental well-being. Any healthcare system's primary goal is to direct its resources towards activities that promote, restore, maintain, and improve healthcare services. It also makes a significant contribution to the effective management of a country's economy and industrialization. As a result of being highly revealed to technological evolution, this sector has seen rapid growth and revolution in order to improve the experience of interaction between carers, patients, and related stakeholders (Søvold et al., 2021). Digital healthcare has revolutionized the healthcare industry, but still faces challenges such as long-term chronic ailments, accelerating costs, aging population, insufficient workforce, and limited resources. The recent pandemic, COVID-19, has added immense pressure to the global healthcare sector and related workforce, infrastructure, and supply chain management. This has accelerated rapid change across the healthcare ecosystem and has compelled stakeholders to adapt the technologies used in this sector (Dang et al., 2021).

The Metaverse is a healthcare system that provides immersive, interactive and recreational services tailored to individual patient needs. It is composed of advanced technology revolutions such as VR, AI, AR, digital twinning, telepresence and blockchain, which have a huge impact on healthcare. It creates the experience of a virtual world using the Internet, where human gestures and emotions are simulated (Jaung, 2022). The four federation of the Metaverse applications in healthcare are depicted in Figure 4.

Figure 4. Four federation of the metaverse applications in Healthcare

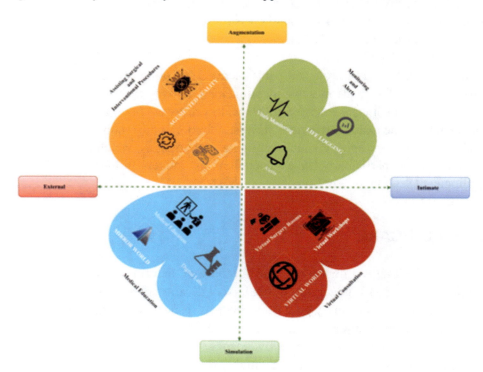

2.1 Potential Opportunities for E-Healthcare

Research on metaverse applications and potential opportunities for e-healthcare and e-education has revealed that the use of VR and AR in the healthcare industry and education sector is essential for enhancing patient services, remote medical education and training, and mental health treatment. This technology has revolutionized how we seek help from friends, family, co-workers, or healthcare professionals during a mental breakdown. Metaverse is a technology that allows mental health professionals to review the diagnosis and understand the anatomy of a brain MRI. It has been found that virtual reality can be used to treat PTS, reduce depression, and ease trauma pain. This technology could expand access and reduce costs, and a new era of care delivery can be unleashed in tackling the rising demand for mental health therapy (Chengoden et al., 2023). Virtual therapy improves overall access by providing a more realistic experience and eliminating the risks of visiting real-world physical sites. For example, Applied VR has FDA approval for successfully reducing chronic pain, which affects more than 100 million Americans. VR and the metaverse for healthcare is still in its infancy and has the potential to digitally empower the younger generation to take control of their health and educate themselves and their counterparts in a safe social virtual environment. Furthermore, the current situation suggests that metaverse VR has excellent virtualization and the opportunities to be integrated with healthcare, education, and training. Furthermore, it was revealed that after the pandemic, virtual meetings to be held remotely are expected to reach 75% by 2024 in terms of collaboration for training, education, and providing healthcare care services (Slater et al., 2020). During the COVID-19 epidemic, numerous well-established teleconference solutions were widely used to communicate in both personal and professional settings. Popular platforms, such as Zoom, Skype, and Google Meet, have been used in the education context and blackboard Collaboration. Due to these platforms' inadequacies in terms of presence, existing companies with expertise in VR, AR, and XR are accelerating development in this field. Furthermore, 60.9 percent of the 298 respondents who took part in the VR survey obtained their VR equipment during the epidemic, in addition to playing games and watching films, 46.0 percent of respondents who used VR for business and 37.2 percent of respondents who used it for education, respectively (Lee et al., 2022). Furthermore, metaverse's Horizon Workrooms is a leading collaboration tool that allows people to collaborate virtually regardless of their physical location. In terms of education and training, it was discovered that the metaverse would aid in the delivery of high-quality education and training from top experts around the world, as well as the benefit of allowing safe simulations of situations that would be dangerous in a practical setting (Dutta et al., 2022). In addition, according to 72% of the 3080 participants, switching to digital education made it harder for them to follow the curriculum. It was found that the reason VR is getting more attention is because of the metaverse, a three-dimensional virtual reality where users can fully immerse themselves in the environment in terms of visuals and motion. Virtual reality, for example, was found to be crucial for education and training and to provide the advantages of flexible training schedules regardless of location. However, it was found in many studies that implementing VR in education had a positive effect (Lee et al., 2022).

2.2 Future Directions of Healthcare

Furthermore, we think that in the future, the advancement of metaverse technologies may support the provision of educational and mental health services in hostile environments. Since there is no assurance that violent conflict won't break out again, it is essential to review and summarize the evidence from these studies in order to expand the use of metaverse in conflict settings, close the treatment gap, and expand mental health services there. As the researcher noted, it is necessary to develop strategies that can function in ambiguous circumstances. This attempt will serve as the foundation for upcoming metaverse research projects in light of the humanitarian crisis (Dwivedi et al., 2022). Along with the development of armed conflict in recent decades, the range of e-health health technologies to address geographic, epidemiologic, and clinical inequities in conflict has also increased. More research is required to develop an evidence base that will support the continued deployment of eHealth services in these circumstances. The passion for innovation will continue to burn in the future by making these immersive services available to people living in unstable and conflict-ridden environments. Additionally, a number of intricate and varied issues must be addressed, such as whether or not someone could develop an addiction. Will those who have mental illnesses be harmed by it? On the other hand, will it make mental health services accessible to people with disabilities, low incomes, or those residing in violent conflict? Is it conceivable that it will alter the approach taken to treating psychiatric disorders? In terms of the effects of digital addiction to the metaverse, it is currently challenging to define what it is, exactly what its implications are, and what conclusions can be drawn (Reardon et al., 2019).

2.3 Potential Application for Healthcare

When compared to the "handicraft workshop model," where the diagnosis and treatment vary from doctor to doctor and hospital to hospital, the Metaverse significantly aids in providing comprehensive healthcare. In a scenario involving comprehensive healthcare, choices would be made in accordance with the advice of the expert and the findings of the various Metaverse enabling technologies (Davenport & Kalakota, 2019). Numerous medical uses of the Metaverse exist, including research, physical examination, diagnosis, and insurance. Virtual physiotherapy, virtual biopsy, virtual counselling, and virtual alert response are just a few of the Metaverse's possible applications that could take off in the near future. A virtual biopsy is a non-invasive method of obtaining and analyzing an image to characterize tissues. Patients undergoing rehabilitation could be guided through exercises and movement by means of virtual physiotherapy (Silver et al., 2021).

- **Medical diagnosis**: Medical diagnosis is the process of figuring out a patient's condition from their symptoms. The use of the Metaverse in healthcare greatly aids in the accurate diagnosis of a patient's medical conditions with the aid of a variety of cutting-edge technologies like AR, VR, extended digital twins, blockchain, 5G, and so forth. The existing medical IoT can also be improved by the metaverse, which does so by overcoming its limitations in terms of human-computer interaction, connectivity, and integration with and between the real world and virtual world. Utilizing the MIoT through AR/VR glasses can aid in holographic construction, imitation, real-world interaction, and integration, simplifying the challenging issues encountered in the healthcare industry. Medical professionals from the real world and the virtual world can communicate and make wise decisions in the Metaverse environment, leading to accurate disease diagnosis (Bashir et al., 2023). Thus, delivering high-quality healthcare requires that the treatment plan adhere to the guidelines established by the relevant regulatory bodies. Blockchain technology integration in the Metaverse enables efficient health-based digital asset storage and exchange across multiple platforms, allowing medical professionals to diagnose various medical conditions more accurately and wisely. Here, we use a "nonmutagenic multidimensional Hash Geocoding" method to effectively index multidimensional data. Implementing the Metaverse in assessment will significantly aid in the improvement of the overall quality of all the other phases, as diagnosis is the essential and fundamental process in evaluating the level of therapy and prescription drugs to be provided (Wong et al., 2021).
- **Patient monitoring**: The healthcare industry will greatly benefit from the Metaverse thanks to the convergence of telepresence, digital twinning, and blockchain, particularly in terms of patient monitoring. Remote medical care is offered through telemedicine, also known as telepresence in medicine. In emergency situations, test dummies of patients can be used to determine how treatments will affect patients long before they actually receive them. In order to store and transfer medical data securely and to ensure that it is not compromised or put at risk, blockchain technologies are used because it is the most sensitive and significant type of data. If all three of these elements are made to function well together, patient monitoring can be provided in an efficient manner (Piacevoli, 2023). By combining these technologies into one, the Metaverse offers a solution. Through the provision of medical advice followed by a voice call or video call with the patient, COVID-19 has forced

medical professionals to consider providing high-quality healthcare even when it is provided remotely. However, with the scientific development of the Metaverse, the healthcare industry will greatly benefit from the ability to create virtual worlds wherever is crucial and provide treatments to the poor even when they are thousands of miles apart. When it comes to patient monitoring, the Metaverse environment is crucial and helpful because it can give the feeling of "being there." This facilitates communication not only between patients and healthcare professionals but also between patients and their families. By having quality interactions between patients, healthcare professionals, and family members, patient monitoring using the Metaverse can therefore significantly improve a patient's health condition and thereby create an optimal environment for the patient (Liu et al., 2020).

- **Medical education:** The Metaverse represents a significant major shift in medical education. The innovators of the Metaverse in the field of medical education are IoT, blockchain, AI, AR, and VR. A digital virtual world that encompasses the boundaries of the physical world is created by the Metaverse using AI and blockchain. These technologies enable medical students to concentrate during sessions, participate in discussions, interact in-depth, and engage in activities with greater enjoyment—all while working in a busy clinical setting. In the traditional method of instruction, the instructor would make the medical students visit a patient, then present and discuss the pertinent medical information with the group of students. With the rise of these digital integration and 3D technologies, clinical teaching has undergone a significant change. Now, a group of medical students are presented with a patient in virtual reality (Almarzouqi et al., 2022).

- **Surgeries:** A crucial piece of medical technology, particularly in surgery, is the metaverse. Currently, surgeons simulate actual surgical procedures using tools like VR headsets and haptic gloves, which improves readiness and reliability in the operating room. By providing surgeons with easy access to data, AR can make surgeries more convenient for them to perform. By projecting 3D virtual models onto the patient's body, augmented reality (AR) can give surgeons quick, simple, and hands-free access to patient information (Athar et al., 2023). In the Metaverse, professors and lecturers could demonstrate complex surgeries in three dimensions. The Metaverse could also be used to offer post-operative patients counselling services. The AR system consists of a head-mounted wearable device that records a person's facial features and makes maxillofacial bone surgery easier. By overlaying the patient details, the product design aids practitioners in creating a virtual plan. For the past 20 years, spine surgeons have had to adapt minimally invasive spine surgery (MISS), which has a high radiation exposure rate (Chengoden et al., 2023). The digital transformation in spine surgery is being accelerated by a lack of navigational cues and indirect visualization. Only 2D flat monitors are capable of displaying the 3D reconstructed images used in spine surgery. Digital transformation in spine surgery is supported by 3D hologram viewing technologies with advanced spatial imagination. In order to analyze posture, surface topography is used. It is becoming more popular due to its accurate diagnostics and low radiation exposure. Patients' data is collected using wearable sensors, which also make patient monitoring easier. Patients, doctors, and students will benefit from the use of these Metaverse enabling technologies in the field of healthcare systems. The factors accelerating the digital transformation in spine are a lack of navigational cues and indirect visualization (Vadalà et al., 2020).

- **Medical therapeutics & theranostics:** Medical therapeutics may be defined as the branch of medicine concerned with illness treatment. Digital therapies (DTx) are a type of digital medicine that provides evidence-based treatment interventions. According to the Digital Therapeutics Alliance, digital therapeutics are devices that "provide evidence-based therapeutic treatments to patients that are powered by high quality software programs to prevent, regulate, or treat a medical ailment or disease." This entails the employment of various digital technologies to maintain patients' physical and emotional well-being (Hong et al., 2021). However, medical theranostics is a combination of the terms therapeutics and diagnostics. With the support of the underlying technologies, the Metaverse's intervention in therapeutics and theranostics can lead to important advances in the area of medicine. Because digital therapeutics does not require the use of drugs to treat a patient, it is becoming increasingly important in the field of healthcare. One such technology is computer vision, which can process, analyze, visualize, and understand movies and pictures. The Metaverse is the prospect of medicine, capable of advancing telemedicine by combining technologies such as XR, AR, VR, AI, computer vision and blockchain. Using a conventional electronic health record (EHR), a digital twin of a patient can be created, from which a 3D simulation can be obtained. Thus, EHRs have a significant impact in the health sector (Ning et al., 2021).

2.4 Open Issues and Challenges

Current healthcare technology trends have adopted telehealth services in an effective and productive way, guaranteeing the best service to patients via the use of current telemedicine tools. The Metaverse is a new term that predicts disruptive changes in many spheres of life. However, the Metaverse's adoption in the healthcare domain will improve the current patient health monitoring service by changing the way patients interact with healthcare systems by adding interactive features in a virtual world using technologies such as VR for medical training, AR in surgical procedures, and so on (Ferorelli et al., 2020). Although the Metaverse appears to be a promising solution for the healthcare domain, it still faces some challenges, including;

- **Data privacy concerns:** The Metaverse strives to deliver an exceptional user experience for the patient in a virtual environment by integrating the physical and virtual worlds through the advancement of telecommunication and virtual technologies. The patient's physiological reactions and body motions will be managed and monitored by the Metaverse. Furthermore, the Metaverse can collect personal information such as brainwaves, biometric data, health information, and individual patient preferences while interacting with various services (Lee et al., 2021).
- **Information security concerns:** While providing health services, large healthcare enterprises will collect sensitive information in a variety of ways, with or without the patients' consent. The Metaverse will be able to deliver an exceptional virtual experience for doctors to treat patients with various health issues remotely using various electronic devices, creating a tremendous quantity of digital data, with the use of distinct communication and virtual technologies. Because the Metaverse is a hybrid of modern technologies, the patients' current health conditions are transmitted via the communication channel, and the doctor's responses are also transmitted via the same channel. However, electronically generated medical data contains sensitive information about patients, and protecting it from external breaches or attackers at various stages of the process is a difficult task. Malware invasions and data breaches are facilitated by AR/VR gadgets (Abouelmehdi et al., 2018).
- **Interoperability issues:** Healthcare interoperability denotes the ability of healthcare providers and other systems to electronically share patients' information without hindrance, i.e., one provider's electronic health record system should be able to transfer patient data to another provider's system using modern technologies and electronic equipment, standardizing and availability of sensitive information related to various patients. Interoperability becomes a difficult issue as the amount of health data and updated devices in the healthcare area grows. By combining diverse hardware and software components with wearable equipment in a virtual environment, the Metaverse will open the door to new problems in healthcare. Every Metaverse-based healthcare service should ensure the security and consistency of sensitive data by interacting with the various components, beginning with data sensing and ending with data processing. To minimize severe and unexpected

repercussions while transferring devices from traditional healthcare services to the virtual world, proper communication standards and data adoption techniques must be developed (Jabbar et al., 2020).

- **High cost of technology:** Healthcare technology is continually developing as a result of new medical advances, leading to digital transformations by combining robotic surgery and VR in various medical services. The combination of augmented reality and virtual reality is largely employed in medical training and surgical operations to execute difficult surgery with high precision. These software and hardware components will help medical devices and equipment work better. The rise of Metaverse-focused enterprises has accelerated the development of superior AR and VR-based technologies to improve the entire surgical environment in a worldwide market. To effectively transform the current healthcare system with the Metaverse, high-tech wearables such as glasses, gloves, sensors, and other hardware components that can properly assess the status of the patients are required. However, the cost of wearables is very high, and in order to gain new capabilities, we will also need to purchase new equipment as technology advances (Singh et al., 2021).

- **The personal touch is lost:** The current digital revolution of healthcare systems, including telemedicine and remote tracking of patient's technologies, creates a schism between patient and clinician. Physicians can recommend remote therapy after gathering the relevant patient history and current symptoms, or by reviewing digital health information without actually seeing the patients. However, by providing effective and efficient interactive options, the Metaverse will offer a fully interactive virtual digital world for both patients and healthcare professionals. Most patients perceive a loss of distinctive bonding of face-to-face rapport as a result of the new digital form of therapy. The digital style of treatment causes the individual to feel lonely and has an impact on the rate of recovery (Győrffy et al., 2020).

3. CONVENTIONAL RADIOGRAPHY

Beginning with traditional x-ray technology, is there anything new under the sun? In the future years, this oldest radiologic modality may undergo the most change. For more than a century, x-ray tubes employed a thermionic cathode to "boil off" electrons, which required a lot of power. Nonthermionic electron emission using "cold cathode" technology, on the other hand, looks to be practical for medical radiography. Cold cathode x-ray tubes provide the promise for quick digital operation, low power consumption, and prolonged durability while preserving good spatial resolution and a tiny focus spot size. A system like this might enhance access to medical imaging in impoverished countries. Consider the combination of cold cathode x-ray technology with digital tomosynthesis, which gives greater diagnostic assessment above traditional radiography alone. The resulting low-cost equipment might assist in reaching the majority of the world's population, who now lacks meaningful access to medical imaging (McCain et al., 2018).

- **Abdominal CT:** CT is the single most significant advancement in medicine during the last half-century. This imaging revolution will continue in the near future with the introduction of photon-counting CT. Higher spatial resolution, improved dose efficiency, reduced motion blur and artefacts, and improved multi-energy/spectral imaging are all expected improvements. Overall, dual-energy CT may be considered a letdown in the field of abdominal radiology. The advantages of dual-energy CT may be overshadowed by the additional expense and difficulty, at least for some providers. Given the added benefits of photon-counting CT, the overall balance may swing in favor of greater acceptance by radiologists and radiological clinics. However, efficiency and cost-effectiveness issues must be addressed (Wagenius, 2021). The creation of reliable virtual non-contrast CT images using dual-energy CT has proven difficult, with up to 20 HU over- and underestimation compared to actual non-contrast series. Initial attempts at virtual non-contrast images with photon-counting CT have also been mixed, but show promise that needs to be investigated further. Deep learning AI technologies should be used to delicate CT image enhancement techniques in order to maximize picture quality and radiation dosage levels. In terms of CT image interpretation, innovative three-dimensional volumetric presentations, such as cinematic rendering, offer stunning portrayals of abdominal pathologic characteristics. However, it is unclear whether we will ever move to true volumetric interpretation. Over a 20- to 30-year horizon, I have no idea how such a great test can optimize beyond the incremental gains outlined herein (Ulhaq et al., 2020).
- **Abdominal US:** The evolution of abdominal US technology may proceed along two diverging pathways. One cutting-edge method will serve high-end imaging professionals, such as devoted radiologists and sonographers. The other, simpler version will be for extended normal clinical usage, primarily serving non-radiology workers in the trenches. The particular abdominal imager will increasingly rely on analytic and quantitative evaluation. The initial work with quantitative US-based detection of diffuse liver disease is an excellent illustration of what is to come in the future. Although promising, these early attempts at statistical US-based evaluation need more research and improvement before they can replace more accurate CT and MRI approaches

(Starekova & Reeder, 2020). Nonetheless, US imaging has a global presence. As a result, it is the imaging modality most adapted to addressing global health challenges associated with hepatic steatosis and metabolic syndrome. Although MRI (and CT) are currently more accurate in assessing liver-specific progression to fibrosis and cirrhosis than US techniques, further advances in US techniques beyond elastography appear likely. The complicated signal returning to the ultrasonic transducer (the device that delivers and receives mechanical energy predicated on the piezoelectric effect) will be further evaluated and leveraged utilizing deep learning AI for abdominal US evaluation in general (Pirmoazen et al., 2020). American technology will continue to get more streamlined, intuitive, and helpful to non-radiologist providers. Image acquisition will be aided by AI-driven pattern recognition software, which will direct the user to anatomic landmarks and standardized pictures. Eventually, these streamlined photos might be automatically examined for pathologic anomalies, accommodating operators throughout the world with limited resources, experience, and access. If they become commonplace, the little US gadgets may come to symbolize the current medical period in the same way that the stethoscope did in the past. When compared to all other computed tomography, advances in US technology can be applied more easily to the rest of the world. Technological advancements in the United States may have an influence on the sonographer's intermediate position. Automated US evaluation, for example, employing an articulated robotic arm, may become a possibility (Channa et al., 2021).

- **Abdominal MRI:** Innovations in clinical abdominal MRI are expected to focus on workflow and value. More indication-specific treatments will shorten patient time slots from 45-60 minutes to 5-10 minutes. To eliminate any perception of insufficiency, the phrase emphasized on above is favored over shortened. This continuous adjustment will benefit both patient-centered and radiologist workflow challenges linked to increasing picture volume and interpretation time. Customizable MRI procedures are both suitable and important to preserve relevance, minimize expenses, and bring value to our high-volume operations (Pickhardt, 2023). Many early success stories have emerged in focused abdominal MRI protocols, such as quantitative liver evaluation for iron, fat and fibrosis; pancreatic cyst follow-up; active surveillance for renal cell carcinoma; hepatocellular carcinoma screening; adrenal incidentalomas; and prostate cancer evaluation. Focused MRI is also being prescribed to treat liver metastases, adnexal lesions, and deep venous thrombosis. Another developing area of emphasis centers on the environmental sustainability of MRI. Sustainability for MRI encompasses disparate issues such as helium conservation, reduced power consumption, and intelligent design for materials (Canellas et al., 2019). Magnetic field strength advances in abdominal MRI will focus on enhancing picture quality at low field strengths rather than ultrahigh field strengths (7.0 T and above) (0.2–0.5 T). New technology and software advancements are sparking renewed interest in low-field-strength MRI. If the technological obstacles of low-field-strength body MRI are overcome, the logistical advantages are numerous. The advantages of low-field-strength MRI are reduced cost, lower unit weight, less shielding required, less helium, and easier installation (Pickhardt, 2023).

- **Nuclear Medicine and PET Imaging:** Theranostics has the greatest potential for future influence in nuclear medicine and PET imaging. Diagnostic imaging biomarkers are combined with therapeutic medicines that target the same precise target in theranostics. As a result, theranostics offers more precise patient selection for better prediction and assessment of both therapy response and tissue damage. There are several "search and destroy" agents in the works. Prostate-specific membrane antigen imaging, for example, can be tagged with fluorine 18 for diagnostic PET imaging and lutetium 177 for radioligand treatment. Many more theranostic strategies are likely to follow, ushering in an exciting new era in oncology that is closely linked to imaging. Improvements in attenuation correction and image reconstruction using deep learning are also expected. Finally, better image fusion among cross-sectional imaging modalities will aid interpretation and interventions (Vaz et al., 2020). Figure 5 shows the future direction of abdominal imaging.

CONCLUSION

It will be challenging to establish that employing the metaverse has significantly improved healthcare outcomes. This alone will eventually result in the creation of insurance reimbursement, business model and the behavioural changes required for embracing and utilizing a technique that has not previously been employed in patient care. Furthermore, many new technologies in e-healthcare and e-education are emerging. Although these technologies may be complex and difficult to grasp at first, they have the potential to profoundly alter people's lives. To summarize, the metaverse is a relatively new technology that has not yet been thoroughly researched or utilized. The metaverse is a brand-new and excellent training, education, and wellness environment. More specifically, the Metaverse's potential application in medical diagnostics, patient monitoring, healthcare training, surgeries, medical treatments, and theranostics is underlined. In addition, recent and prospective initiatives utilizing blockchain, digital twins, and telemedicine that are important to

Figure 5. Future directions of abdominal imaging

Top Seven Predictions for Abdominal Imaging in the Future

1. X-ray tubes using "cold cathode" technology for medical radiography are feasible and will allow rapid digital operation, low power consumption, and extended durability while maintaining high spatial resolution and small focal spot size.
2. CT has been the single most significant advance in medicine over the past half-century. This imaging revolution will continue with photon-counting CT.
3. Abdominal US technology will evolve along two divergent paths. One path at the cutting edge will serve high-end imaging specialists, including dedicated radiologists and sonographers. The simplified version will expand routine clinical use to serve predominately nonradiology personnel in the trenches.
4. More tailored, indication-specific focused MRI protocols will reduce examination times from 45–60 minutes to as little as 5–10 minutes.
5. The greatest impact of nuclear medicine lies in theranostics, which combines diagnostic imaging biomarkers with therapeutic agents using the same specific target.
6. Rather than replacing us, artificial intelligence algorithms will augment and aid radiologists' diagnostic interpretations and improve our workflow.
7. Opportunistic screening is currently underused, but its ability to stratify risk for a variety of diseases and to detect presymptomatic disease will prove to be cost-effective.

the Metaverse for healthcare are emphasized. The problems and unresolved issues for realizing the full potential of the Metaverse for healthcare are critically examined, and important future scope of directions for confident application of the Metaverse in healthcare are advised. It's an exciting moment to be an abdominal imager, and the future seems even more promising. We should anticipate AI and radiomics to improve our practice through modality-specific improvements and breakthroughs. Rather than replacing us, advances in AI and radiomics will make abdominal imagers even more active and vital in patient care. It is in our best interests to embrace the changes that are coming, or else others will. The Metaverse's evolution will also considerably help remote medical care of patients, altering the current medical treatment style. In the near future, registration, medical consultation, examination, or remote monitoring, Endoscopic therapy can be done entirely in the Metaverse. Despite the fact that the current metaverse is in its infancy, we may nevertheless consider the Metaverse's significance in the field of gastroenterology in the future due to widespread applicability of contemporary Metaverse technologies in the medical profession. I feel that the Metaverse representatives the beginning of a new age for gastroenterology, which will undoubtedly alter the research and The working style of gastroenterologists.

COMPETING INTEREST

The authors declare that there is no conflict of interest among authors.

ACKNOWLEDGMENT

The authors are grateful to the Professor Naveed Akhtar Faculty of Medicine and Allied Health Sciences for the use of their facilities for this study and provided us best facilities to fulfill our academic goal.

REFERENCES

Abouelmehdi, K., Beni-Hessane, A., & Khaloufi, H. (2018). Big healthcare data: Preserving security and privacy. *Journal of Big Data*, 5(1), 1–18. doi:10.118640537-017-0110-7

Adadi, A., & Berrada, M. (2018). Peeking inside the black-box: A survey on explainable artificial intelligence (XAI). *IEEE Access : Practical Innovations, Open Solutions*, 6, 52138–52160. doi:10.1109/ACCESS.2018.2870052

Almarzouqi, A., Aburayya, A., & Salloum, S. A. (2022). Prediction of user's intention to use metaverse system in medical education: A hybrid SEM-ML learning approach. *IEEE Access : Practical Innovations, Open Solutions*, 10, 43421–43434. doi:10.1109/ACCESS.2022.3169285

Athar, A., Ali, S. M., Mozumder, M. A. I., Ali, S., & Kim, H.-C. (2023). Applications and Possible Challenges of Healthcare Metaverse. In *2023 25th International Conference on Advanced Communication Technology (ICACT)*. IEEE.

Bediou, B., Adams, D. M., Mayer, R. E., Tipton, E., Green, C. S., & Bavelier, D. (2018). Meta-analysis of action video game impact on perceptual, attentional, and cognitive skills. *Psychological Bulletin*, 144(1), 77–110. doi:10.1037/bul0000130 PMID:29172564

Bohr, A., & Memarzadeh, K. (2020). The rise of artificial intelligence in healthcare applications. In *Artificial Intelligence in healthcare* (pp. 25–60). Elsevier. doi:10.1016/B978-0-12-818438-7.00002-2

Canellas, R., Rosenkrantz, A. B., Taouli, B., Sala, E., Saini, S., Pedrosa, I., Wang, Z. J., & Sahani, D. V. (2019). Abbreviated MRI protocols for the abdomen. *Radiographics*, *39*(3), 744–758. doi:10.1148/rg.2019180123 PMID:30901285

Cerasa, A., Gaggioli, A., Marino, F., Riva, G., & Pioggia, G. (2022). The promise of the metaverse in mental health: The new era of MEDverse. *Heliyon*, *8*(11), 11762. doi:10.1016/j.heliyon.2022.e11762 PMID:36458297

Chang, L., Zhang, Z., Li, P., Xi, S., Guo, W., Shen, Y., Xiong, Z., Kang, J., Niyato, D., Qiao, X., & Wu, Y. (2022). 6G-enabled edge AI for Metaverse: Challenges, methods, and future research directions. *Journal of Communications and Information Networks*, *7*(2), 107–121. doi:10.23919/JCIN.2022.9815195

Channa, A., Popescu, N., Skibinska, J., & Burget, R. (2021). The rise of wearable devices during the COVID-19 pandemic: A systematic review. *Sensors (Basel)*, *21*(17), 5787. doi:10.339021175787 PMID:34502679

ChenD.ZhangR. (2022). Exploring research trends of emerging technologies in health metaverse: A bibliometric analysis. Available at SSRN 3998068. doi:10.2139/ssrn.3998068

Chengoden, R., Victor, N., Huynh-The, T., Yenduri, G., Jhaveri, R. H., Alazab, M., Bhattacharya, S., Hegde, P., Maddikunta, P. K. R., & Gadekallu, T. R. (2022). *Metaverse for Healthcare: A Survey on Potential Applications, Challenges and Future Directions*. arXiv preprint arXiv:2209.04160.

Chengoden, R., Victor, N., Huynh-The, T., Yenduri, G., Jhaveri, R. H., Alazab, M., Bhattacharya, S., Hegde, P., Maddikunta, P. K. R., & Gadekallu, T. R. (2023). Metaverse for healthcare: A survey on potential applications, challenges and future directions. *IEEE Access : Practical Innovations, Open Solutions*, *11*, 12765–12795. doi:10.1109/ACCESS.2023.3241628

Chimakurthi, V. N. S. S. (2019). Efficacy of Augmented Reality in Medical Education. *Malaysian Journal of Medical and Biological Research*, *6*(2), 135–142. doi:10.18034/mjmbr.v6i2.609

Cornejo, J., Cornejo-Aguilar, J. A., Vargas, M., Helguero, C. G., Milanezi de Andrade, R., Torres-Montoya, S., Asensio-Salazar, J., Rivero Calle, A., Martínez Santos, J., Damon, A., Quiñones-Hinojosa, A., Quintero-Consuegra, M. D., Umaña, J. P., Gallo-Bernal, S., Briceño, M., Tripodi, P., Sebastian, R., Perales-Villarroel, P., De la Cruz-Ku, G., & Russomano, T. (2022). Anatomical Engineering and 3D printing for surgery and medical devices: International review and future exponential innovations. *BioMed Research International, 2022*, 2022. doi:10.1155/2022/6797745 PMID:35372574

Dang, T. H., Nguyen, T. A., Hoang Van, M., Santin, O., Tran, O. M. T., & Schofield, P. (2021). Patient-centered care: Transforming the health care system in Vietnam with support of digital health technology. *Journal of Medical Internet Research, 23*(6), e24601. doi:10.2196/24601 PMID:34085939

Davenport, T., & Kalakota, R. (2019). The potential for artificial intelligence in healthcare. *Future Healthcare Journal, 6*(2), 94–98. doi:10.7861/futurehosp.6-2-94 PMID:31363513

Dutta, P., Bose, M., Sinha, A., Bhardwaj, R., Ray, S., Roy, S., & Prakash, K. B. (2022). *Challenges in metaverse in problem-based learning as a game-changing virtual-physical environment for personalized content development*. Academic Press.

Dwivedi, Y. K., Hughes, L., Baabdullah, A. M., Ribeiro-Navarrete, S., Giannakis, M., Al-Debei, M. M., Dennehy, D., Metri, B., Buhalis, D., Cheung, C. M., Conboy, K., Doyle, R., Dubey, R., Dutot, V., Felix, R., Goyal, D. P., Gustafsson, A., Hinsch, C., Jebabli, I., & Wamba, S. F. (2022). Metaverse beyond the hype: Multidisciplinary perspectives on emerging challenges, opportunities, and agenda for research, practice and policy. *International Journal of Information Management, 66*, 102542. doi:10.1016/j.ijinfomgt.2022.102542

Emmelkamp, P. M., & Meyerbröker, K. (2021). Virtual reality therapy in mental health. *Annual Review of Clinical Psychology, 17*(1), 495–519. doi:10.1146/annurev-clinpsy-081219-115923 PMID:33606946

Ferorelli, D., Nardelli, L., Spagnolo, L., Corradi, S., Silvestre, M., Misceo, F., Marrone, M., Zotti, F., Mandarelli, G., Solarino, B., & Dell'Erba, A. (2020). Medical legal aspects of telemedicine in Italy: Application fields, professional liability and focus on care services during the COVID-19 health emergency. *Journal of Primary Care & Community Health, 11*. doi:10.1177/2150132720985055 PMID:33372570

Galati, R., Simone, M., Barile, G., De Luca, R., Cartanese, C., & Grassi, G. (2020). Experimental setup employed in the operating room based on virtual and mixed reality: Analysis of pros and cons in open abdomen surgery. *Journal of Healthcare Engineering*. doi:10.1155/2020/8851964 PMID:32832048

Győrffy, Z., Radó, N., & Mesko, B. (2020). Digitally engaged physicians about the digital health transition. *PLoS One*, *15*(9), e0238658. doi:10.1371/journal.pone.0238658 PMID:32986733

Hamet, P., & Tremblay, J. (2017). Artificial intelligence in medicine. *Metabolism: Clinical and Experimental*, *69*, S36–S40. doi:10.1016/j.metabol.2017.01.011 PMID:28126242

Hong, J. S., Wasden, C., & Han, D. H. (2021). Introduction of digital therapeutics. *Computer Methods and Programs in Biomedicine*, *209*, 106319. doi:10.1016/j.cmpb.2021.106319 PMID:34364181

Humayun, M. (2020). Role of emerging IoT big data and cloud computing for real time application. *International Journal of Advanced Computer Science and Applications*, *11*(4). Advance online publication. doi:10.14569/IJACSA.2020.0110466

Jabbar, R., Fetais, N., Krichen, M., & Barkaoui, K. (2020). Blockchain technology for healthcare: Enhancing shared electronic health record interoperability and integrity. In *2020 IEEE International Conference on Informatics, IoT, and Enabling Technologies (ICIoT)*. IEEE.

Kaddoura, S., & Al Husseiny, F. (2023). The rising trend of Metaverse in education: Challenges, opportunities, and ethical considerations. *PeerJ. Computer Science*, *9*, e1252. doi:10.7717/peerj-cs.1252 PMID:37346578

Kavanagh, J. M., & Sharpnack, P. (2021). Crisis in Competency: A Defining Moment in Nursing Education. *Online Journal of Issues in Nursing*, *26*(1). doi:10.3912/OJIN.Vol26No01Man02

Kwame, A., & Petrucka, P. M. (2020). Communication in nurse-patient interaction in healthcare settings in sub-Saharan Africa: A scoping review. *International Journal of Africa Nursing Sciences*, *12*, 100198. doi:10.1016/j.ijans.2020.100198

Lee, H., Woo, D., & Yu, S. (2022). Virtual reality metaverse system supplementing remote education methods: Based on aircraft maintenance simulation. *Applied Sciences (Basel, Switzerland)*, *12*(5), 2667. doi:10.3390/app12052667

Lee, L.-H., Braud, T., Zhou, P., Wang, L., Xu, D., Lin, Z., Kumar, A., Bermejo, C., & Hui, P. (2021). *All one needs to know about metaverse: A complete survey on technological singularity, virtual ecosystem, and research agenda.* arXiv preprint arXiv:2110.05352.

Liang, T.-P., & Liu, Y.-H. (2018). Research landscape of business intelligence and big data analytics: A bibliometrics study. *Expert Systems with Applications*, *111*, 2–10. doi:10.1016/j.eswa.2018.05.018

Liu, Q., Luo, D., Haase, J. E., Guo, Q., Wang, X. Q., Liu, S., Xia, L., Liu, Z., Yang, J., & Yang, B. X. (2020). The experiences of health-care providers during the COVID-19 crisis in China: A qualitative study. *The Lancet. Global Health*, *8*(6), e790–e798. doi:10.1016/S2214-109X(20)30204-7 PMID:32573443

López-Ojeda, W., & Hurley, R. A. (2023). The Medical Metaverse, Part 1: Introduction, Definitions, and New Horizons for Neuropsychiatry. *The Journal of Neuropsychiatry and Clinical Neurosciences*, *35*(1), A4–A3. doi:10.1176/appi.neuropsych.20220187 PMID:36633472

McCain, R. S., Diamond, A., Jones, C., & Coleman, H. G. (2018). Current practices and future prospects for the management of gallbladder polyps: A topical review. *World Journal of Gastroenterology*, *24*(26), 2844–2852. doi:10.3748/wjg.v24.i26.2844 PMID:30018479

Miller, R. (2020). *Digital arts based research methods for teenage and young adult (TYA) cancer patients. Goldsmiths*. University of London.

Morrell, A. L. G., Morrell-Junior, A. C., Morrell, A. G., Mendes, J. M. F., Tustumi, F., De-Oliveira-e-Silva, L. G., & Morrell, A. (2021). The history of robotic surgery and its evolution: When illusion becomes reality. *Revista do Colégio Brasileiro de Cirurgiões*, *48*, 48. doi:10.1590/0100-6991e-20202798 PMID:33470371

Mozumder, M. A. I., Sheeraz, M. M., Athar, A., Aich, S., & Kim, H.-C. (2022). Overview: Technology roadmap of the future trend of metaverse based on IoT, blockchain, AI technique, and medical domain metaverse activity. In *2022 24th International Conference on Advanced Communication Technology (ICACT)*. IEEE.

Ning, H., Wang, H., Lin, Y., Wang, W., Dhelim, S., Farha, F., Ding, J., & Daneshmand, M. (2021). *A Survey on Metaverse: the State-of-the-art, Technologies, Applications, and Challenges.* arXiv preprint arXiv:2111.09673.

Oniani, S., Marques, G., Barnovi, S., Pires, I. M., & Bhoi, A. K. (2021). Artificial intelligence for internet of things and enhanced medical systems. *Bio-inspired neurocomputing*, 43-59.

Piacevoli, Q. (2023). Metaverse and Health Care System. *PriMera Scientific Medicine and Public Health, 2*, 06-14.

Pickhardt, P. J. (2023). *Abdominal Imaging in the Coming Decades: Better, Faster, Safer, and Cheaper?* (Vol. 307). Radiological Society of North America.

Pirmoazen, A. M., Khurana, A., El Kaffas, A., & Kamaya, A. (2020). Quantitative ultrasound approaches for diagnosis and monitoring hepatic steatosis in nonalcoholic fatty liver disease. *Theranostics, 10*(9), 4277–4289. doi:10.7150/thno.40249 PMID:32226553

Reardon, C. L., Hainline, B., Aron, C. M., Baron, D., Baum, A. L., Bindra, A., Budgett, R., Campriani, N., Castaldelli-Maia, J. M., Currie, A., Derevensky, J. L., Glick, I. D., Gorczynski, P., Gouttebarge, V., Grandner, M. A., Han, D. H., McDuff, D., Mountjoy, M., Polat, A., & Engebretsen, L. (2019). Mental health in elite athletes: International Olympic Committee consensus statement (2019). *British Journal of Sports Medicine, 53*(11), 667–699. doi:10.1136/bjsports-2019-100715 PMID:31097450

Ren, Y., Yang, Y., Chen, J., Zhou, Y., Li, J., Xia, R., Yang, Y., Wang, Q., & Su, X. (2022). A scoping review of deep learning in cancer nursing combined with augmented reality: The era of intelligent nursing is coming. *Asia-Pacific Journal of Oncology Nursing, 9*(12), 100135. doi:10.1016/j.apjon.2022.100135 PMID:36276884

Schoonjans, L. J. L. M. (2021). *The dominance challenge of European ICT companies against China and the USA*. Academic Press.

Schrodt, P. A. (2019). Artificial intelligence and international relations: An overview. *Artificial Intelligence and International Politics*, 9-31.

Silver, F. H., Deshmukh, T., Kelkar, N., Ritter, K., Ryan, N., & Nadiminti, H. (2021). The "Virtual Biopsy" of Cancerous Lesions in 3D: Non-Invasive Differentiation between Melanoma and Other Lesions Using Vibrational Optical Coherence Tomography. *Dermatopathology (Basel, Switzerland), 8*(4), 539–551. doi:10.3390/dermatopathology8040058 PMID:34940035

Singh, R. P., Hom, G. L., Abramoff, M. D., Campbell, J. P., & Chiang, M. F. (2020). Current challenges and barriers to real-world artificial intelligence adoption for the healthcare system, provider, and the patient. *Translational Vision Science & Technology, 9*(2), 45–45. doi:10.1167/tvst.9.2.45 PMID:32879755

Singh, S., Bhatt, P., Sharma, S. K., & Rabiu, S. (2021). Digital Transformation in Healthcare: Innovation and Technologies. In Blockchain for Healthcare Systems (pp. 61-79). CRC Press.

Slater, M., Gonzalez-Liencres, C., Haggard, P., Vinkers, C., Gregory-Clarke, R., Jelley, S., Watson, Z., Breen, G., Schwarz, R., Steptoe, W., Szostak, D., Halan, S., Fox, D., & Silver, J. (2020). The ethics of realism in virtual and augmented reality. *Frontiers in Virtual Reality*, *1*, 1. doi:10.3389/frvir.2020.00001

Søvold, L. E., Naslund, J. A., Kousoulis, A. A., Saxena, S., Qoronfleh, M. W., Grobler, C., & Münter, L. (2021). Prioritizing the mental health and well-being of healthcare workers: An urgent global public health priority. *Frontiers in Public Health*, *9*, 679397. doi:10.3389/fpubh.2021.679397 PMID:34026720

Starekova, J., & Reeder, S. B. (2020). Liver fat quantification: Where do we stand? *Abdominal Radiology*, *45*(11), 3386–3399. doi:10.100700261-020-02783-1 PMID:33025153

Tyagi, Y., & Saxena, S. (2022). Applications of Artificial Intelligence, Metaverse and Data Science for Intelligent Healthcare. *AAYAM: AKGIM Journal of Management*, *12*(2), 141–149.

Ulhaq, A., Born, J., Khan, A., Gomes, D. P. S., Chakraborty, S., & Paul, M. (2020). COVID-19 control by computer vision approaches: A survey. *IEEE Access : Practical Innovations, Open Solutions*, *8*, 179437–179456. doi:10.1109/ACCESS.2020.3027685 PMID:34812357

Vadalà, G., De Salvatore, S., Ambrosio, L., Russo, F., Papalia, R., & Denaro, V. (2020). Robotic spine surgery and augmented reality systems: A state of the art. *Neurospine*, *17*(1), 88–100. doi:10.14245/ns.2040060.030 PMID:32252158

Vaz, S. C., Oliveira, F., Herrmann, K., & Veit-Haibach, P. (2020). Nuclear medicine and molecular imaging advances in the 21st century. *The British Journal of Radiology*, *93*(1110), 20200095. doi:10.1259/bjr.20200095 PMID:32401541

Wagenius, M. (2021). *Complications and treatment aspects of urological stone surgery*. Lund University.

Wang, G., Badal, A., Jia, X., Maltz, J. S., Mueller, K., Myers, K. J., Niu, C., Vannier, M., Yan, P., & Yu, Z. (2022). Development of metaverse for intelligent healthcare. *Nature Machine Intelligence*, 1–8. PMID:36935774

Wang, Y., Su, Z., Zhang, N., Xing, R., Liu, D., Luan, T. H., & Shen, X. (2022). A survey on metaverse: Fundamentals, security, and privacy. *IEEE Communications Surveys and Tutorials*.

Ward, P. (2018). Trust and communication in a doctor-patient relationship: A literature review. *Archives of Medicine*, *3*(3), 36.

Wong, A., Bhyat, R., Srivastava, S., Lomax, L. B., & Appireddy, R. (2021). Patient care during the COVID-19 pandemic: Use of virtual care. *Journal of Medical Internet Research*, *23*(1), e20621. doi:10.2196/20621 PMID:33326410

Yampolskiy, R. V. (2019). *Unexplainability and incomprehensibility of artificial intelligence.* arXiv preprint arXiv:1907.03869.

Yan, Y., Zhang, J.-W., Zang, G.-Y., & Pu, J. (2019). The primary use of artificial intelligence in cardiovascular diseases: What kind of potential role does artificial intelligence play in future medicine? *Journal of Geriatric Cardiology : JGC*, *16*(8), 585. PMID:31555325

Yang, Y., Siau, K., Xie, W., & Sun, Y. (2022). Smart Health: Intelligent Healthcare Systems in the Metaverse, Artificial Intelligence, and Data Science Era. *Journal of Organizational and End User Computing*, *34*(1), 1–14. doi:10.4018/JOEUC.308814

Chapter 10
The Future of Telemedicine:
Emerging Technologies, Challenges, and Opportunities

Robertas Damaševičius
 https://orcid.org/0000-0001-9990-1084
Vytautas Magnus University, Lithuania

Olusola O. Abayomi-Alli
Kaunas University of Technology, Lithuania

ABSTRACT

Telemedicine, or the delivery of healthcare services via distant communication technology, has grown in importance in recent years. Telemedicine has the ability to alter healthcare delivery and enhance access to treatment for patients in rural and underserved locations. However, there are significant barriers to mainstream telemedicine adoption and implementation, including data privacy and security, funding, and the need for standardization. The authors review telemedicine's current situation and future potential by discussing new technologies that will shape the future of telemedicine, such as 5G networks, augmented and virtual reality, and wearable gadgets. Then the chapter discusses the growing use of telemedicine and its role in improving access to healthcare in rural and underserved areas. In addition to discussing the benefits for telemedicine, the chapter delves into the problems and limits that must be solved before it may achieve its full potential. Finally, it analyzes the future of telemedicine, including prospective uses and interaction with traditional healthcare systems.

DOI: 10.4018/978-1-6684-9823-1.ch010

1. INTRODUCTION

Telemedicine is described as the use of telecommunication and information technology to remotely offer healthcare services (Wootton, 2001). It entails the transmission of medical information and services via the internet, such as video conferencing, remote monitoring, and mobile health applications (Hameed et al., 2021). Telemedicine's major goal is to enhance access to treatment and boost the efficiency of healthcare delivery, especially for patients in distant and under-served regions (Hailey et al., 2002). Prof. Klaus Schwab, who issued a call for smart, efficient, and creative solutions (Roy, 2020), emphasized the significance of technology in driving innovation and improving healthcare delivery through telemedicine. Collaboration and multidisciplinary methods are expected to result in game-changing discoveries and solutions in the healthcare sector.

1.1 The Future of Telemedicine

Telemedicine may take many different forms, such as teleconsultations, remote patient moni-toring, and virtual care (Vanagas et al., 2018; Zaman et al., 2022). A healthcare physician and a patient meet via video conference or phone conversation to discuss medical issues and treatment choices during teleconsultations. Remote patient monitoring entails using wearable gadgets or other medical equipment, as well as ordinary cellphones, to gather and communicate data about a patient's health to a healthcare practitioner for analysis. Virtual care refers to a variety of remote healthcare services, such as teleconsultations, remote patient monitoring, and online health information resources (Rajda and Paz, 2020). Telemedicine is viewed as a critical answer to many difficulties confronting the healthcare sector, including rising healthcare costs and the need to increase access to treatment in rural and disadvantaged areas. Telemedicine can play an increasingly impor-tant role in the delivery of healthcare services in the future, thanks to the fast development of technology (Ekeland et al., 2010).

The COVID-19 pandemic has underlined the crucial role that telemedicine may play in healthcare delivery (Aslan and Ata¸sen, 2021). With the increased requirement for social distance and fewer in-person visits to healthcare institu-tions, telemedicine has become an increasingly significant technique for deliver-ing care to patients while limiting the transmission of the virus (El-Sherif et al., 2022). The telemedicine's impact in the post-COVID-19 world may be observed in many major areas:

- Improving access to care: Telemedicine has assisted in overcoming many of the hurdles to care that existed before to the epidemic, including as distance, time, and expense. Telemedicine has made it simpler for patients to obtain

the treatment they require by allowing them to interact with healthcare practitioners remotely, regardless of their location.
- Telemedicine has played a major impact in decreasing the transmission of COVID-19 and other infectious illnesses, according to (El-Sherif et al., 2022). Telemedicine has helped to reduce the danger of virus infection by eliminat-ing the requirement for in-person visits to healthcare institutions.
- Improving patient outcomes: Telemedicine has been found to enhance pa-tient outcomes in a variety of areas, including chronic disease care and early identification of health concerns. Telemedicine has helped to enhance the quality of care provided to patients by allowing healthcare practitioners to remotely monitor patients and make timely interventions.
- Telemedicine has the potential to considerably lower healthcare delivery costs by eliminating the demand for in-person visits and minimizing the require-ment for hospitalization. This may have a significant influence on the health-care system's sustainability, for example, by utilizing sustainable telehealth business models (Velayati et al., 2022), and help to guarantee that more people have access to high-quality treatment.

In the post-COVID-19 era, telemedicine has become a vital instrument in the delivery of healthcare services. With the continuous advancement of technology and growing awareness of the benefits of telemedicine, it is expected to play an even larger role in the coming years (Ong et al., 2021).

This paper contributes to the subject of healthcare engineering in a unique way by providing an up-to-date and in-depth discussion of the role of telemedicine in the post-COVID-19 era. It is meant to be a useful resource for healthcare prac-titioners, policymakers, researchers, and students interested in investigating the potential of telemedicine to enhance the remote delivery of healthcare services.

2. EMERGING TECHNOLOGIES IN TELEMEDICINE

2.1 Artificial Intelligence and Virtual Assistants (Chatbots) Powered by Large Language Models for Telemedicine

AI and virtual assistants driven by massive language models are developing as important telemedicine tools, since they may assist in automating repetitive chores, providing more accurate and individualized treatment, and improving access to health information (Huq et al., 2022). Large language models, like as OpenAI's GPT-3, have been trained on massive quantities of data and can comprehend and create writing that is human-like. This makes them perfect for powering virtual assistants, who may help patients and healthcare practitioners more effectively access health information and interact. AI-powered chatbots, for example, may help users discover the correct healthcare practitioner, answer basic health queries, and schedule appointments. AI may be used to examine massive volumes of medical data, such as electronic health records and imaging investigations, to help make decisions and enhance diagnosis accuracy Santosh and Gaur (2021b,a). AI systems, for example, may scan medical pictures to detect illness symptoms, as well as forecast patient outcomes and provide indi-vidualized treatment regimens. AI may also assist enhance clinical trial efficiency by automating data collecting and processing and predicting patient outcomes in real time. This can hasten the development of novel medicines and therapies while also improving patient outcomes. By automating repetitive chores, offer-ing more accurate and individualized treatment, and enhancing access to health information, AI and virtual assistants (chatbots) have the potential to signifi-cantly improve telemedicine. As AI technology evolves and matures, it is likely to play an increasingly crucial role in telemedicine and aid enhance patient care delivery.

2.2 5G Networks and Their Impact on Telemedicine

The advent of 5G networks will have a big influence on telemedicine. In com-parison to earlier generations of mobile networks, 5G networks provide quicker and more dependable wireless access. This enhanced speed and dependability is crucial for telemedicine, which depends on the capacity to send massive volumes of data in real-time to facilitate remote diagnosis, treatments, and monitoring (Georgiou et al., 2021). Increased bandwidth and minimal latency are two advan-tages of 5G networks for telemedicine. 5G networks provide substantially better data transmission capacity, allowing telemedicine apps to transport massive vol-umes of data in real-time, such as high-resolution medical photos, videos, and other essential health information. Because 5G networks have minimal latency, the period between transmitting and receiving data is drastically shortened, al-lowing physicians and patients to engage in real time. Increased dependability is another advantage of 5G networks for telemedicine. In comparison to ear-lier generations of mobile networks, 5G networks are meant to be more durable and less sensitive to disturbances. This improved dependability is critical for telemedicine applications that demand a steady and dependable connection to facilitate remote diagnostics and treatments.

5G networks offer novel telemedicine use cases, such as virtual reality (VR) and extended reality (XR)-based telemedicine (Chen et al., 2022), distant telemedicine, and mobile health monitoring (Weinstein et al., 2014). Doctors and patients may communicate through VR-based telemedicine over 5G networks, which gives a more immersive and participatory experience than standard telemedicine (Hameed et al., 2021). Furthermore, 5G networks offer telemedicine in rural places where access to medical treatment may be difficult owing to geographi-cal limitations. Finally, 5G networks enable doctors to remotely monitor patient health via mobile devices, allowing them to keep track of patient health and make diagnoses or administer therapy (Weinstein et al., 2014). The advent of 5G networks will have a big influence on telemedicine. 5G networks give more bandwidth, lower latency, and greater dependability, allowing telemedicine apps to provide more accurate diagnosis, treatments, and monitoring. Furthermore, 5G networks offer novel telemedicine use cases, such as VR-based telemedicine, distant telemedicine, and mobile health monitoring, making telemedicine a more accessible and effective tool for healthcare delivery. Furthermore, there are plans to use forthcoming 6G technology for telemedicine (Srinivasu et al., 2022).

2.3 Augmented and Virtual Reality in Telemedicine

Technologies such as augmented reality (AR) and VR have the potential to trans-form the way healthcare is provided via telemedicine. These technologies allow clinicians and patients to connect in immersive, interactive, and highly visual settings, potentially improving diagnostic accuracy, treatment quality, and pa-tient experience (Yeung et al., 2021). AR technologies superimpose digital data on the actual environment, enabling healthcare practitioners to examine and alter virtual medical models in real time. This can be valuable in telemedicine since it allows healthcare practitioners to examine and alter virtual models of human anatomy and medical disorders, enhancing diagnosis and treatment accu-racy. AR, for example, may be used to display medical scans or other diagnostic pictures, allowing healthcare workers to more easily identify and comprehend medical issues. VR technology have the ability to generate completely virtual settings that may be utilized to imitate real-world scenarios and environments. VR technology may be utilized to construct virtual patient-doctor interactions in which patients can be evaluated, diagnosed, and treated in a virtual setting. This is especially beneficial for patients who live in distant places or have limited mobility, since they may get medical treatment from the comfort of their own homes.

The Metaverse is a fast growing idea that has the potential to alter telemedicine (Musamih et al., 2022). It is a shared virtual area where individuals may commu-nicate and engage in a VR. The Metaverse allows healthcare practitioners and patients to engage virtually, creating an immersive, interactive, and highly visual environment for medical consultations and treatments. This is especially valu-able for complex medical procedures or operations, since healthcare personnel may utilize VR technology to observe and interact with virtual medical mod-els, improving diagnosis and treatment accuracy. AR, VR, and the Metaverse have the potential to transform telemedicine by allowing healthcare practitioners to give more precise diagnosis, treatments, and patient experiences. These tech-nologies produce immersive, interactive, and highly visual environments that can considerably improve both healthcare practitioners' and patients' telemedicine experiences. These technologies are likely to play a significant role in the future of telemedicine as they grow and mature.

2.4 Wearable Devices and Their Potential for Telemedicine

The Internet of Things (IoT) is a network of physical devices, cars, buildings, and other items that are equipped with sensors, software, and connection to gather and share data (Yunana et al., 2021). The Internet of Healthcare Things (IoHT) (Ketu and Mishra, 2021), as well as the related idea of the Internet of Medical Things (IoMT) (Xu et al., 2021), is a fast emerging sector in healthcare that involves the use of IoT devices and systems to enhance healthcare delivery and patient outcomes.

Telemedicine is one use where IoHT can be extremely useful. IoT devices and sensors may be used to remotely gather vital signs and other health-related data, which can then be communicated to healthcare practitioners to aid in the diagnosis and treatment of patients (Issa et al., 2022). Wearable gadgets, such as smartwatches and fitness trackers, can, for example, monitor a patient's heart rate, activity levels, and other health parameters and communicate that data to a telemedicine or assisted living system for analysis (Maskeliunas et al., 2019). Digital twins can be used to create a digital model of a subject using information collected from sensors (Shah et al., 2022; Gaur and Jhanjhi, 2022).

Wearable devices and the Internet of Body Things (IoBT) (Elhayatmy et al., 2017) are quickly developing technologies with the potential to transform telemedicine. These technologies allow for continuous and real-time monitoring of physiological factors including heart rate, body temperature, blood pressure, and activity levels. This data may be wirelessly relayed to healthcare practitioners, who can then utilize it to remotely monitor patients' health. Wearable gadgets exist in a variety of shapes and sizes, including smartwatches, fitness trackers, and smart clothes. These gadgets are outfitted with sensors and other technology that can monitor and communicate real-time data from numerous physiological parame-ters (Tamulis et al., 2022) to healthcare practitioners. Wearable devices can also be combined with other IoBT devices, such as smart home devices, to provide a complete picture of a patient's health. The Internet of Things (IoT) refers to a network of networked medical equipment and wearables that can interact with one another and with healthcare practitioners. This allows healthcare prac-titioners to remotely monitor their patients' health and deliver more accurate diagnosis and treatments. Patients can also utilize wearable gadgets to monitor their own health and communicate this data with healthcare practitioners, al-lowing them to be more actively involved in their own care. Wearables and the IoBT have the potential to significantly improve telemedicine by allowing health-care practitioners to remotely monitor patients' health and deliver more accurate diagnosis and treatments (de-la Fuente-Robles et al., 2022; Kalasin and Surare-ungchai, 2022). These technologies enable continuous and real-time monitoring of many physiological indicators, which can increase diagnostic and treatment accuracy and eliminate the need for in-person visits to healthcare practitioners. Wearable devices and the IoBT are likely to play a significant role in the future of telemedicine as they expand and mature.

2.5 Blockchain and Their Potential for Telemedicine

Blockchain is a distributed ledger system that enables numerous parties to safely and transparently store and exchange data without the need for a central au-thority (Kuo et al., 2017). By offering a safe and decentralized platform for exchanging health data, blockchain technology has the potential to transform telemedicine. Blockchain may be used in the context of telemedicine to securely store and communicate health data, including as medical records, test results, and imaging tests, between healthcare professionals and patients (Ahmad et al., 2021). This removes the need for a centralized database, which is prone to hacks and data breaches. Patients can have control over their own health data by adopting blockchain, since they can give or withdraw access to healthcare pro-fessionals as required. Blockchain can help assure the validity and integrity of health data by securing it with cryptographic techniques and tracking changes over time. This can aid in the prevention of fraud and inaccuracies in medical records, as well as the accuracy of diagnosis and treatments. Blockchain may potentially be used to facilitate decentralized clinical trials, in which patients and healthcare professionals can securely exchange data and cooperate on re-search projects. This can assist to hasten the discovery of novel treatments and therapies while also increasing patient participation in the research process. By offering a safe and decentralized platform for exchanging health data, blockchain technology can improve telemedicine. Blockchain can improve the accuracy of diagnosis and treatments by enabling secure and transparent data interchange, as well as assist avoid fraud and inaccuracies in medical records. As blockchain technology evolves and matures, it is projected to play a significant role in the future of telemedicine (Ahmad et al., 2021).

2.6 Funding of Telemedicine Initiatives

Telemedicine initiatives have gained significant traction in recent years as a transformative approach to healthcare delivery. However, the successful implementation and sustainability of such initiatives necessitate careful consideration

The Future of Telemedicine

of funding models that enable equitable access to telemedicine services while en-suring quality and efficiency Pandya (2007). This analysis delves into three key funding models: public-private partnerships, government grants, and potential reimbursement mechanisms for telemedicine services, examining their merits, challenges, and implications.

Public-private partnerships (PPPs) have emerged as a promising funding model that amalgamates the resources and expertise of both public and private sectors. PPPs leverage the financial strength of private entities while harness-ing the regulatory authority of the government to foster innovative telemedicine solutions. Private stakeholders invest capital and technological prowess, con-tributing to infrastructure development, technological deployment, and service delivery. Simultaneously, the government offers regulatory oversight, policy for-mulation, and infrastructural support, enabling the realization of telemedicine's potential on a broader scale. While PPPs present significant advantages, they are not devoid of challenges. Balancing the interests of public welfare and private profit motives can lead to conflicts, potentially compromising the accessibility and affordability of telemedicine services. Moreover, PPPs require intricate con-tractual agreements and effective governance mechanisms to address disparities and ensure accountability. Navigating these complexities necessitates meticulous structuring, robust legal frameworks, and clear delineation of roles and respon-sibilities between public and private entities.

Government grants represent another vital funding avenue for telemedicine initiatives, driven by the imperative of equitable healthcare access. Government grants provide direct financial support to foster telemedicine projects, enabling the establishment of infrastructure, technology procurement, training, and ca-pacity-building efforts. This funding mechanism aligns with the government's responsibility to ensure healthcare accessibility to all citizens, particularly vul-nerable and underserved populations. However, government grants are often lim-ited by budget constraints and competing healthcare priorities. The allocation of resources necessitates strategic prioritization to maximize the impact of funds while addressing the multifaceted dimensions of telemedicine implementation. Moreover, grant-based funding models may lack the dynamic flexibility required to adapt to evolving technological advancements and changing healthcare needs.

Reimbursement mechanisms for telemedicine services hold significant poten-tial to underpin sustainable initiatives while ensuring high-quality care. Telemedicine reimbursement entails remuneration for healthcare services provided remotely, incentivizing healthcare providers to embrace telemedicine and fostering a robust ecosystem. Government-sponsored insurance programs and private insurers play pivotal roles in reimbursing healthcare providers for telemedicine consultations, creating a financial incentive structure. However, reimbursement mechanisms confront challenges in standardization and regulatory frameworks. Varying re-imbursement rates across different platforms and services, coupled with jurisdic-tional disparities, can create inequities and hinder the seamless integration of telemedicine into mainstream healthcare delivery. Harmonizing reimbursement policies, ensuring fair compensation, and addressing concerns about overutiliza-tion or inappropriate use of telemedicine remain critical aspects that warrant continuous attention.

Funding models for telemedicine initiatives are integral to their successful implementation and long-term viability. Public-private partnerships leverage the strengths of both sectors, government grants prioritize equitable access, and reimbursement mechanisms incentivize healthcare providers. However, each model presents unique challenges requiring strategic mitigation strategies. A comprehensive approach that combines these models, while navigating intricacies of policy, regulation, and accountability, holds the potential to fuel the advance-ment of telemedicine and reshape healthcare delivery paradigms.

Several successful case studies showcase innovative funding approaches for telemedicine initiatives, demonstrating the feasibility and efficacy of diverse mod-els:

Project ECHO (Extension for Community Healthcare Outcomes) based at the University of New Mexico Health Sciences Center, utilizes a novel funding approach Arora et al. (2007). It establishes a hub-and-spoke knowledge-shar-ing network, connecting specialists at academic medical centers with primary care providers in underserved areas. Instead of charging fees for consultations, Project ECHO relies on grants, philanthropic support, and partnerships with healthcare organizations. This collaborative model has enabled rapid knowledge dissemination, reduced healthcare disparities, and garnered substantial financial support through grants and philanthropy.

Aravind Eye Care System focuses on reducing blindness through innovative funding mechanisms Kim et al. (2022). By offering high-quality eye care services to paying patients, Aravind subsidizes free or low-cost treatment for indigent populations. Revenue generated from fee-paying patients cross-subsidizes the cost of care for those who cannot afford it. This sustainable model has enabled Aravind to provide affordable eye care to millions and achieve financial sustain-ability.

Teladoc Health, a telemedicine provider in the United States, leverages a reimbursement-based funding model Miner et al. (2020). By partnering with insurance companies and employers, Teladoc Health enables patients to access vir-tual consultations with healthcare providers and doctors. The reimbursement is typically covered by health insurance or employer-sponsored health plans. This model has led to significant adoption of telemedicine services among patients seeking convenient and cost-effective healthcare.

The Swasthya Slate initiative in India, launched by the nonprofit Swasthya Slate Foundation, employs an innovative approach to funding telemedicine ser-vices Sittig et al. (2013). The initiative offers a handheld diagnostic tool that provides a range of medical tests and sends data to a remote cloud server for analysis. Swasthya Slate generates revenue through nominal fees charged for the diagnostic tests, ensuring sustainability while keeping services affordable for rural and underserved communities.

University of Mississippi Medical Center (UMMC) is an example of how government support and collaboration can drive telemedicine initiatives Goldwater et al. (2023). UMMC's Center for Telehealth, with state funding and support, has established an extensive network of telemedicine services across Mississippi. The state's investment has enabled the development of infrastructure, training programs, and partnerships, leading to improved access to specialized care in underserved regions.

These case studies illustrate diverse funding models for telemedicine initia-tives, highlighting the adaptability and effectiveness of innovative approaches. Whether through grant-based support, cross-subsidization, reimbursement part-nerships, or government investment, these models showcase the potential for sustainable and impactful telemedicine services that address healthcare dispari-ties and enhance patient outcomes.

2.7 Examples of Successful Telemedicine Programs

There are a few diverse telemedicine programs that have made a significant impact on healthcare delivery in rural and underserved regions, along with the challenges they faced during implementation and the strategies employed to overcome them as given in Table 1.

These examples highlight the versatility of telemedicine programs in addressing healthcare disparities. Overcoming challenges often required a combination of technological innovation, infrastructure development, community engagement, and policy advocacy. The success of these programs underscores the importance of tailoring telemedicine solutions to the unique needs and contexts of rural and underserved regions.

3. A FRAMEWORK OF TELEMEDICINE SYSTEM

3.1 Generic Architecture

A telemedicine system framework can include numerous components like as hardware and software, communication networks, and human resources (Chen and Woźniak, 2022). These components function in tandem to enable remote health-care delivery while also ensuring that patients receive high-quality treatment (Ahmad

Table 1. Thelemedicine programs impacting rural underserved region

Program	Impact	Challenges faced	Strategies to Overcome Challenges
Partners in Health (PIH) – Haiti Telemedicine ProgramMcIntyre et al. (2011)	Connects local providers with specialists for remote consultations and diagnostics in Haiti.	Limited internet connectivity, infrastructure, and skilled provider shortages	Established satellite connections, training, and community collaboration
Apollo Telemedicine Networking FoundationGanapathy & Ravindra (2009) – Rural Telehealth Initiative	Provides teleconsultations, diagnostics, and health education in Indian under-served areas	Poor connectivity, cultural barriers, and tech reluctance	Collaborated with NGOs, awareness campaigns, and provider sensitization
UMMC Center for TelehealthGoldwater et al. (2023)	Offers telemedicine services for specialty care in Mississippi's rural areas	Limited broadband, provider resistance, and reimbursement issues	Improved connectivity, privider training, and advocacy for policy changes
Sevamob Khare et al. (2019) – Mobile Clinics and Telehealth in India	Combines mobile clinics with telehealth for primary care and diagnostics in Indian communities	Limited infrastructure, awareness, and affordability issues	Integrated diagnostics, community health worker education, and affordability initiatives
Swinfen Charitable Trust-Global Telemedicare NetworkVassallo et al. (2011)	Connects under-served regions with volunteer specialists worldwide for consultation	Technological berries, language, and volunteer engagement	Technology training, translation services, and partnerships with medical societies

et al., 2022). The service-oriented approach may be used to create the telemedicine system (Blaˇzauskas et al., 2017). A general framework for a telemedicine system is as follows:

- **Hardware and software:** This component comprises all physical and digital telemedicine instruments, such as telemedicine carts, mobile devices, and telemedicine software. The software component, which comprises both client-side and server-side components, is in charge of allowing communication between patients and healthcare professionals, as well as storing and processing medical data.
- **Contact networks:** To transfer medical data and allow real-time contact between patients and healthcare professionals, telemedicine relies on powerful communication networks, which include both wired and wireless technologies such as the Internet, 5G networks, and Wi-Fi (Nawaz et al., 2022).
- **Human resources:** Telemedicine necessitates the availability of healthcare personnel who are educated and equipped to deliver remote treatment. This

component comprises physicians, nurses, and other healthcare professionals who are in charge of providing telemedicine treatment to patients (Kruklitis et al., 2022; Wong et al., 2023).
- **Clinical processes:** Telemedicine systems must be built to support clinical workflows such as patient triage, diagnosis, and therapy. This component contains methods and procedures for ensuring that patients receive timely and adequate care.
- **Data management:** Telemedicine systems must be built to securely handle and retain medical data, such as patient health records, imaging scans, and other information. This component contains both software and hardware for storing and processing medical data, as well as security safeguards to preserve patient privacy (Saleh et al., 2023).

The architecture of the future telemedicine system can be divided into three main components:

- User Interface component is in charge of offering a simple interface for pa-tients, physicians, and other healthcare professionals. It enables patients to use telemedicine services, make appointments, and connect with healthcare providers.
- Data Management component is in charge of storing and maintaining the telemedicine system's data, which includes patient data, appointment information, and medical records. It guarantees that data is safely maintained and that authorized employees may access it.
- Telemedicine Services component provides basic telemedicine services such as teleconsultations, telemonitoring, and telecare. It works in conjunction with the User Interface and Data Management components to deliver a full telemedicine solution.

This architecture may be expanded to include new components like as AI and ML algorithms for illness diagnosis and treatment advice, as well as blockchain technology for safe data management and sharing (Abiodun et al., 2022). Wear-able devices, the internet of things (IoBT), and augmented and VR may all be included into the architecture. Figure 1 depicts the component diagram of a generic future telemedicine system.

The architecture of a telemedicine system consists of four main components: Patient Terminal, Doctors Terminal, Telemedicine Platform, and Virtual Assis-tant.

1. The Patient App and Wearable Devices are part of the Patient Terminal. The Patient App acts as the patient's interaction with the telemedicine platform.

Figure 1. Component diagram of a generic future telemedicine system

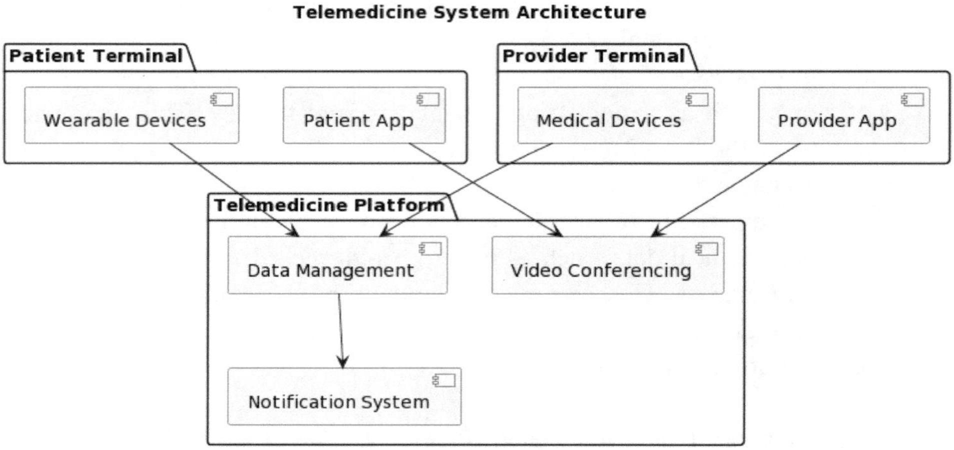

Telemedicine System Architecture

[Patient Terminal: Wearable Devices, Patient App]
[Provider Terminal: Medical Devices, Provider App]
[Telemedicine Platform: Data Management, Video Conferencing, Notification System]

Wearable Devices, such as smartwatches and fitness trackers, can gather and transmit health-related data to the Medical Records System under the Telemedicine Platform component.

2. Doctors Terminal gives access to the Doctors App that functions as a bridge between the doctor and the telemedicine platform. It enables the doctor to view patients' medical records and engage in video consultations with patients via the Telemedicine Platform's Video Conferencing component.
3. The key component of the telemedicine system is the Telemedicine Platform. It is divided into multiple sub-components, including the Medical Records System, Appointments System, Payments System, Video Conferencing component, Notification System, and Blockchain component.
    - The Medical Records System secures and organizes the medical records of patients.
    - The Appointments System allows patients to schedule appointments with doctors and notifies both patients and doctors.
    - The Payments System is in charge of managing money transactions between patients and clinicians.
    - The Video Conferencing component allows patients and doctors to connect via video calls.
    - Notification System notifies patients and physicians about appointments, changes, and other vital information.
    - Blockchain component acts as a secure and decentralized data storage mechanism, assuring data privacy and integrity.

The Future of Telemedicine

4. The Virtual Assistant component offers patients with an AI-powered voice-based interface via which they may engage with the telemedicine system. It is made up of various sub-components, including the User Interface, Voice Recognition, Speech Synthesis, Knowledge Base, NLP Engine, API Connector, AI Engine, and Dialogue Manager.
   - The User Interface is the interface via which patients engage with the Virtual Assistant.
   - The Voice Recognition component transforms voice into text.
   - The NLP Engine uses natural language processing on the incoming text to determine the patient's intent.
   - Dialogue Manager is in charge of managing the communication between the virtual assistant and the users. It determines what information to give to users depending on the questions they ask, and it may also conduct actions based on the instructions they issue. It also controls the flow of communication between the patient and the Virtual Assistant.
   - The AI Engine employs machine learning algorithms to give the patient with individualized replies based on their medical information and past encounters.
   - Knowledge Base has a wealth of information and data, including medical expertise and health and wellness information, that the AI engine may utilize to make educated judgments and offer relevant information to patients and clinicians.
   - The Speech Synthesis component transforms text into speech, allowing the Virtual Assistant to converse with the patient through voice.
   - The API Connector enables the Virtual Assistant to communicate with the other telemedicine system components.

The relationships between the components are as follows:

- The API Connector component connects the Patient App with the Patient Terminal.
- The Wearable Devices of the Telemedicine Platform component deliver data to the Medical Records System.
- The Medical Records System and the Payments System securely store data on the Blockchain component.
- The Video Conferencing component is available in both the Patient App and the Doctors App.
- The Appointments System uses the Notification System component to provide messages to both the Patients App and the Doctors App.

- The NLP Engine component receives data from the Voice Recognition component.

3.2 Examples of Real-Life Working Scenario

To create a seamless and efficient telemedicine experience, the future telemedicine system will bring together many components and technology. The system guar-antees that individuals obtain high-quality healthcare services from the conve-nience of their own homes, from organizing appointments to video consultations to safeguarding medical data and payments. The following is a realistic scenario of how the future telemedicine system may work:

1. A patient with a chronic condition who wishes to see a doctor goes to the patient terminal, where they can use a patient app and wearable gadgets.
2. The patient app allows the patient to make an appointment with a doctor, which is subsequently synced with the telemedicine platform's
3. The wearable devices capture health data such as the patient's heart rate, blood pressure, and other vital indicators, which are subsequently transferred to the telemedicine platform's medical records system.
4. For further protection, the medical records system securely keeps the pa-tient's health data, which is also stored on a blockchain.
5. On the day of the appointment, the patient connects with the doctor using the video conferencing option in the patient app. In addition, the doctor gets access to the video conferencing option in the doctor's app.
6. The doctor may access the patient's medical records and health data, which are kept in the medical records system and on the blockchain, during the video consultation.
7. If a patient has any queries or concerns, they may contact the virtual assis-tant system, which is included within the patient app. The virtual assistant features a user interface, voice recognition, speech synthesis, and a knowledge library that is driven by an NLP engine and an AI engine.
8. The patient can use the virtual assistant to ask inquiries and receive re-sponses created by the AI engine utilizing data from the knowledge base.
9. At the end of the session, the doctor may prescribe medication, which may be filled via the telemedicine platform's payment mechanism. The transaction is safe and transparent since the payment is recorded on the blockchain.
10. The telemedicine platform's notification system will send messages to both the patient and the doctor, reminding them of upcoming visits and keeping them up to speed on the patient's health state.

The Future of Telemedicine

Figure 2. Sequence diagram of telemedicine system use scenario

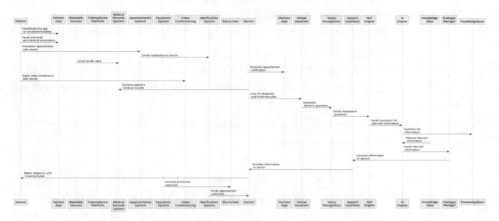

The Sequence diagram of the appointment and consultation scenario is presented in Figure 2. Further we describe how the presented an example of a real-life scenario of the telemedicine system could operate:

1. A patient obtains the "Patient App" on their smartphone or tablet.
2. The patient enters personal and medical information into the app, including data from wearable devices used to monitor their health.
3. The patient makes an appointment with a doctor using the "Appointments System" feature of the "Telemedicine Platform."
4. The "Notification System" notifies the doctor's "Doctors App" of the approaching appointment.
5. The patient initiates a video conference with the doctor on the day of the appointment using the "Video Conferencing" component of the "Telemedicine Platform."
6. The doctor goes over the patient's medical records, which are securely saved in the "Medical Records System" and immutably backed up on the "Blockchain" component.
7. Through the video conference, the doctor asks the patient questions and evaluates their condition.
8. If the doctor believes it is essential, the "Virtual Assistant" component can help with the diagnosis and treatment plan. The virtual assistant interprets the doctor's inquiries using its "Voice Recognition" component, its "NLP Engine" to comprehend the questions, and its "AI Engine" to give appro-priate information from its "Knowledge Base."

9. Through its "Speech Synthesis" component, the virtual assistant speaks with the doctor, speaking the information it has discovered.
10. The doctor develops a diagnostic and treatment plan and communicates it to the patient through video conference.
11. The "Payments System" component of the "Telemedicine Platform" man-ages appointment payment, with the "Blockchain" component securely pro-cessing the transaction.
12. The "Notification System" delivers a summary of the visit and treatment plan to both the doctor and the patient.

This scenario demonstrates how the Telemedicine system, comprising the "Patient Terminal," "Doctors Terminal," "Telemedicine Platform," and "Virtual Assistant" components, might collaborate to offer patients with distant and convenient healthcare services. Figure 3 shows the appointment and consultation scenario's sequence diagram.

3.3 System Deployment

The system's deployment is depicted in Figure 4. The "Patient Terminal" and "Doctors Terminal" components are installed on the patient's smartphone/tablet and the doctor's laptop/desktop, respectively, in this Deployment Diagram. The "Cloud" node represents the cloud, where the "Telemedicine Platform" com-ponent is deployed. The "Virtual Assistant" component is installed on a server that is also cloud-connected. The component "API Connector" links the "Virtual Assistant" to the rest of the system.

3.4 Use Cases and Applications

Telemedicine systems are anticipated to grow more complex in the future, en-abling a wide range of novel use cases and applications. Here are a few prospective telemedicine use cases and applications:

- VR technology will allow patients to connect with healthcare professionals in realistic virtual settings, offering a more engaging and intimate telemedicine experience. VR-powered physical tests, remote operations, and even virtual therapy sessions might be provided to patients (Busnatu et al., 2022).
- Wearable gadgets and other Internet of Body Things (IoBT) devices will be linked into telemedicine systems to give real-time monitoring of patient health data. Patients will be able to watch their vital signs in real time, such

Figure 3. Appointment and consultation scenario using future telemedicine system

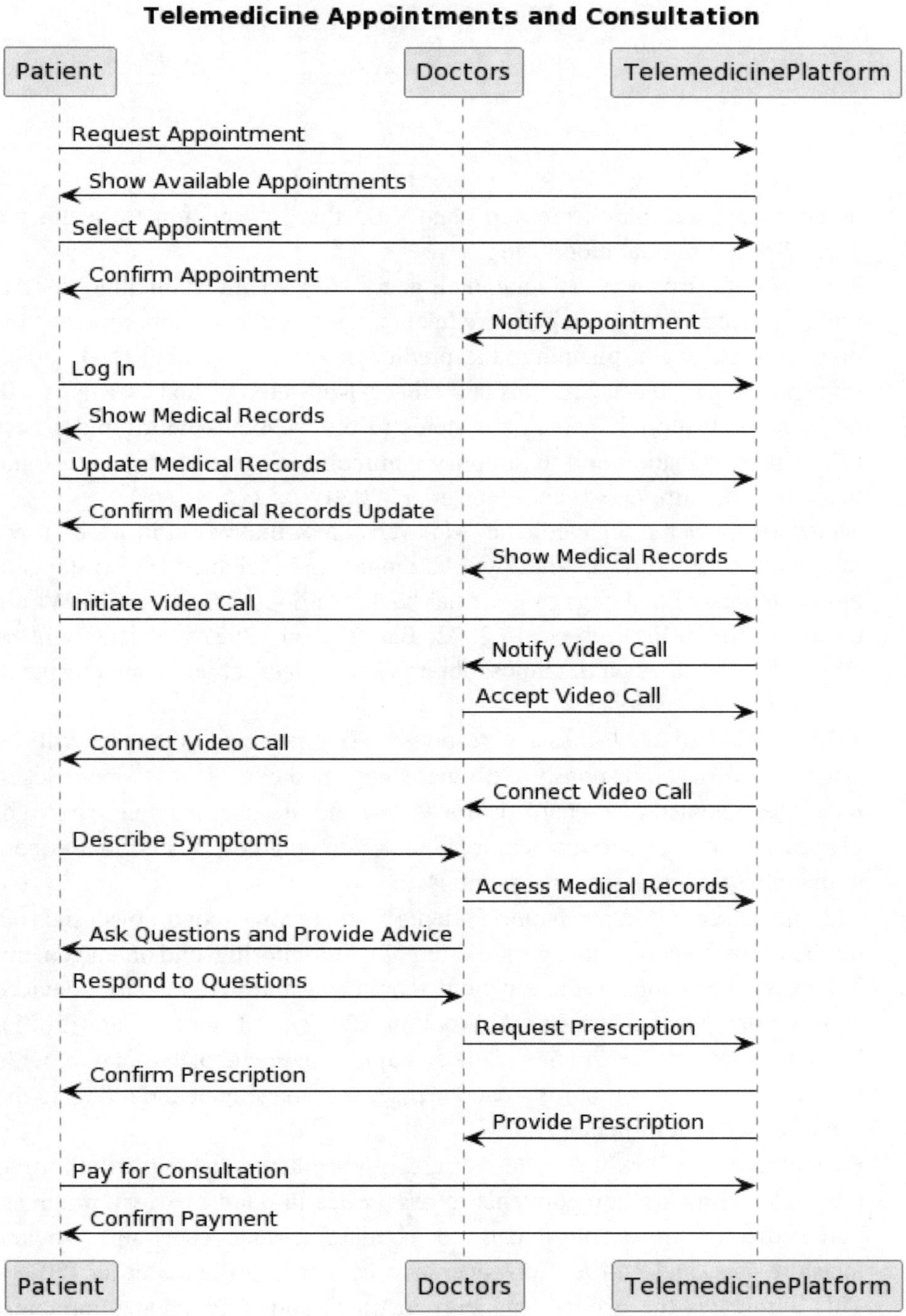

Telemedicine Appointments and Consultation

Patient	Doctors	TelemedicinePlatform

Patient → TelemedicinePlatform: Request Appointment
TelemedicinePlatform → Patient: Show Available Appointments
Patient → TelemedicinePlatform: Select Appointment
TelemedicinePlatform → Patient: Confirm Appointment
TelemedicinePlatform → Doctors: Notify Appointment
Patient → TelemedicinePlatform: Log In
TelemedicinePlatform → Patient: Show Medical Records
Patient → TelemedicinePlatform: Update Medical Records
TelemedicinePlatform → Patient: Confirm Medical Records Update
TelemedicinePlatform → Doctors: Show Medical Records
Patient → TelemedicinePlatform: Initiate Video Call
TelemedicinePlatform → Doctors: Notify Video Call
Doctors → TelemedicinePlatform: Accept Video Call
TelemedicinePlatform → Patient: Connect Video Call
TelemedicinePlatform → Doctors: Connect Video Call
Patient → Doctors: Describe Symptoms
Doctors → TelemedicinePlatform: Access Medical Records
Doctors → Patient: Ask Questions and Provide Advice
Patient → Doctors: Respond to Questions
Doctors → TelemedicinePlatform: Request Prescription
TelemedicinePlatform → Patient: Confirm Prescription
TelemedicinePlatform → Doctors: Provide Prescription
Patient → TelemedicinePlatform: Pay for Consultation
TelemedicinePlatform → Patient: Confirm Payment

Figure 4. Deployment diagram of future telemedicine system

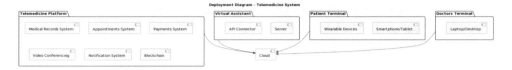

as heart rate and blood pressure, and send this information to healthcare specialists for remote monitoring.
- Telemedicine driven by artificial intelligence (AI): Artificial intelligence (AI) will play a significant role in future telemedicine systems, enabling real-time diagnosis, treatment planning, and predictive analytics (Kakhi et al., 2022; Pap and Oniga, 2022). Chatbots and other AI-powered virtual assistants will be integrated into telemedicine systems to offer patients with rapid access to health information and to simplify communication between patients and healthcare practitioners (Omoregbe et al., 2020).
- Metaverse-powered telemedicine: Metaverse, a virtual world in which users may interact with one another, will be employed in telemedicine systems to build immersive and engaging virtual health settings (Dagli, 2022). Within the metaverse (Musamih et al., 2022; Bansal et al., 2022), patients will be able to visit virtual health clinics, obtain virtual physical tests, and engage in virtual therapy sessions.
- Telemedicine-enabled disaster response: Telemedicine systems will be crucial in disaster response and emergency medicine. In disaster-stricken locations, telemedicine-enabled drones and mobile telemedicine carts will give real-time access to medical treatment, allowing healthcare practitioners to diagnose and treat patients remotely.
- Chronic Disease Management: Patients with chronic conditions, such as dia-betes or hypertension, require ongoing monitoring and management. Telemedicine enables remote patient monitoring through wearable devices and regular vir-tual check-ins Wootton (2012); Alvarez et al. (2021). Physicians can review patients' data, adjust treatment plans, and provide timely guidance, pro-moting proactive disease management and reducing the need for frequent in-person visits.
- Postoperative Follow-up: After surgical procedures, patients often need mul-tiple follow-up appointments to assess healing and recovery progress. Telemedicine allows physicians to conduct virtual check-ups, review incision sites, and ad-dress postoperative concerns Williams et al. (2018). This eliminates the need for patients to travel and wait for appointments, streamlining the follow-up process.

- Mental Health Support: Telemedicine is particularly valuable in mental health services, where consistent support is crucial. Patients can have regular vir-tual therapy sessions with mental health professionals, ensuring ongoing care for conditions like depression or anxiety Barnett and Huskamp (2020). This approach reduces barriers to seeking help and facilitates continuous support without disruptions.
- Elderly Care: Elderly patients may face mobility challenges that make reg-ular clinic visits difficult. Telemedicine enables geriatric patients to consult physicians from their homes, allowing healthcare providers to assess their health, manage medications, and address age-related concerns S¸ahin et al. (2021). It promotes regular check-ins and minimizes stress associated with traveling.
- Specialist Consultations: Patients in rural or remote areas often struggle to access specialist care due to geographical barriers. Telemedicine provides a solution by enabling virtual consultations with specialists, allowing patients to receive expert opinions and treatment recommendations without the need for long journeys Palozzi et al. (2020).
- Prescription Refillsand Medication Management: Telemedicine can facilitate prescription refillsand medication management. Patients can connect with healthcare providers to discuss medication adjustments, side effects, and re-newal of prescriptions. This process streamlines medication management and reduces unnecessary in-person visits Mohiuddin et al. (2021).
- Preoperative Assessments: Before surgery, patients need preoperative assess-ments to ensure they are fitfor the procedure. Telemedicine allows for virtual preoperative evaluations, where healthcare providers review patients' medi-cal histories, conduct necessary tests, and provide guidance remotely Mihalj et al. (2020). This expedites the preoperative process and reduces the time patients spend at the hospital.
- Pediatric Care: For parents of young children, telemedicine can offer con-venience and continuity. Parents can seek advice on common childhood ill-nesses, receive guidance on medication dosages, and discuss developmen-tal concerns with pediatricians via virtual consultations Shah and Badawy (2021).

These are only a handful of the numerous novel applications and use cases for future telemedicine systems. In all these scenarios, telemedicine offers the advantage of timely and accessible care, minimizing disruptions to patients' rou-tines and reducing the burden of in-person visits. By fostering continuity of care, telemedicine not only enhances patient experiences but also contributes to more efficient healthcare processes and resource allocation. As technology advances and healthcare delivery becomes more digital, telemedicine will play an increasingly important role in ensuring that patients receive high-quality treatment regardless of their location.

3.5 Integration With Traditional Healthcare Delivery Systems

To achieve a more effective and efficient healthcare delivery system, future telemedicine technologies must be integrated with existing healthcare delivery systems. This integration will create a consistent and seamless approach to providing health-care services to patients, lowering barriers between patients and healthcare providers (Cobry and Wadwa, 2022). Improved access to healthcare services for patients living in rural and underprivileged locations is one of the key ben-efits of combining telemedicine technologies with traditional healthcare delivery systems (Ayeni et al., 2018; Adeloye et al., 2017). Telemedicine systems can offer virtual consultations, remote monitoring, and real-time contact between patients and healthcare professionals, minimizing the need for patients to travel large distances for medical care. This can dramatically enhance the quality of life for rural people while also lowering healthcare expenditures by minimizing the need for unneeded hospitalization. The capacity to enhance patient outcomes is another advantage of combining telemedicine technology with regular healthcare delivery systems. Telemedicine systems may give more precise and individual-ized diagnosis and treatment plans for patients by using new technology such as artificial intelligence, machine learning, and big data. This can lead to improved health outcomes, fewer hospital readmissions, and more patient satisfaction. In-tegrating telemedicine technologies with traditional healthcare delivery systems can also give healthcare practitioners with new and creative tools to help them provide better treatment. Telemedicine systems, for example, can enable ac-cess to electronic health records (EHRs), real-time patient monitoring, and tele-consultation services, allowing healthcare practitioners to make more educated treatment decisions and deliver better care. The integration of telemedicine with traditional in-person healthcare services is a multifaceted endeavor characterized by both challenges and benefits. The expansion of accessibility, heightened con-venience, potential cost savings, and equitable healthcare provision underscore the promise of integration. Yet, the hurdles of technological readiness, quality assurance, privacy concerns, and patient acceptance warrant proactive strategies for mitigation. By navigating these complexities thoughtfully, healthcare systems can harness the transformative potential of telemedicine integration, ushering in a new era of patient-centric and accessible healthcare delivery.

4. BENEFIS, CHALLENGES, AND LIMITATIONS OF TELEMEDICINE

4.1 Increasing Adoption and Benefits of Telemedicine

Telemedicine is quickly altering the healthcare business, giving patients with new and inventive methods to get medical attention and assistance. Telemedicine is projected to play an increasingly larger role in the future of healthcare delivery as technology advances. Improved access to healthcare services for patients living in rural and underdeveloped locations is one of the key benefits of telemedicine. Telemedicine systems can allow virtual consultations, remote monitoring, and real-time contact between patients and healthcare practitioners by using new technology such as high-speed internet and mobile devices. This has the poten-tial to greatly enhance the quality of life for people in rural regions while also lowering healthcare expenditures by minimizing the need for unneeded hospi-talization. The possibility to enhance patient outcomes is another advantage of telemedicine. Telemedicine systems may give more precise and individualized diagnosis and treatment plans for patients by integrating artificial intelligence, machine learning, and big data. This can lead to improved health outcomes, fewer hospital readmissions, and more patient satisfaction. Telemedicine may also provide healthcare practitioners new and creative tools to help them offer better treatment. Telemedicine systems, for example, can enable access to elec-tronic health records (EHRs), real-time patient monitoring, and teleconsultation services, allowing healthcare practitioners to make more educated treatment de-cisions and deliver better care.

To summarize, telemedicine is a fast emerging industry with enormous poten-tial to enhance patient care delivery. Telemedicine, by harnessing sophisticated technology, can increase access to healthcare services, health outcomes, and pa-tient care. Telemedicine is projected to play an increasingly larger role in the future of healthcare delivery as technology advances.

4.2 Effectiveness of Telemedicine

In ensuring the effective utilization of telemedicine services among diverse pa-tient groups, addressing digital literacy challenges emerges as a critical imper-ative. The ubiquity of digital platforms and the integration of technology in healthcare delivery demand comprehensive strategies that cater to patients' vary-ing levels of familiarity with digital tools. This section discusses practical strate-gies to surmount digital literacy challenges, focusing on designing user-friendly interfaces, offering training sessions, and leveraging community partnerships for optimal telemedicine engagement.

Designing intuitive and user-friendly interfaces is pivotal to accommodate patients of diverse digital literacy levels Aldekhyyel et al. (2021). Employing principles of user-centered design, interfaces should feature clear navigation, minimal complexity, and well-organized content. Visual cues, simplified language, and a logical flow enhance usability, enabling patients to navigate the platform with confidence. Additionally, employing responsive design principles ensures compatibility across various devices, eliminating potential barriers.

Conducting targeted training sessions for patients with varying digital pro-ficiency plays a pivotal role in enhancing their telemedicine experience Adrien et al. (2022). Collaborative efforts between healthcare providers and support personnel can provide personalized guidance to patients, addressing their unique needs and concerns. These sessions encompass interactive tutorials, virtual work-shops, and one-on-one guidance, enabling patients to familiarize themselves with telemedicine tools, from scheduling appointments to participating in virtual con-sultations. Simultaneously, educational resources in multiple formats, such as videos and infographics, can reinforce learning and serve as quick references.

Establishing partnerships with community organizations and local stakehold-ers is instrumental in overcoming digital literacy challenges among underserved patient groups Pak et al. (2008). Collaborations can involve community centers, libraries, senior centers, and non-governmental organizations. These partner-ships facilitate workshops and training programs that directly engage patients within their familiar environments. Such initiatives foster a sense of community and peer support, mitigating hesitancy and apprehensions related to technol-ogy adoption. Furthermore, community partnerships enable the identification of unique challenges specific to the target audience, enabling tailored interventions that resonate with patients' backgrounds and needs.

An overarching strategy involves combining these practical approaches for a comprehensive solution. Creating an integrated ecosystem that includes user-friendly interfaces, targeted training sessions, and community engagement syn-ergistically enhances digital literacy and telemedicine accessibility. Continuous evaluation and iterative improvements, driven by patient feedback, ensure that the implemented strategies remain effective and adaptable to evolving patient needs. Therefore, effective telemedicine adoption mandates proactive measures to address digital literacy challenges among diverse patient groups. By designing intuitive interfaces, providing tailored training sessions, and leveraging commu-nity partnerships, healthcare providers can ensure that all patients, regardless of their digital proficiency, can

The Future of Telemedicine

confidently access and utilize telemedicine services. These strategies contribute to equitable healthcare delivery and to fostering pa-tient empowerment and engagement within the digital healthcare landscape.

4.3 Challenges and Limitations of Telemedicine

Data privacy and security concerns Telemedicine systems are used to gather, store, and communicate sensitive personal health information (PHI). Data privacy and security are crucial considerations for telemedicine's future. Maintaining trust in telemedicine systems and ensuring their effective adoption by patients and healthcare professionals requires ensuring that PHI is secured and not exploited (AlGhamdi et al., 2023). One of the major concerns are data breaches. Because PHI is kept digitally, telemedicine systems are subject to hack-ing and cyberattacks, potentially exposing sensitive information to unauthorized parties. This can have major ramifications, such as identity theft, financial fraud, and a loss of faith in telemedicine systems. Another source of worry is the ab-sence of telemedicine system standardization and regulation. It can be difficult to verify that PHI is secured and that privacy and security standards are main-tained when telemedicine systems operate across many nations and regions. This can lead to disparate approaches to privacy and security, undermining general trust in telemedicine systems. Strong privacy and security measures should be adopted to protect PHI and ensure patient confidence in order to support the effective deployment of telemedicine systems. This involves using encryption, storing and transmitting data securely, and adhering to appropriate privacy and security rules.

Ethical concerns The ethical issues in telemedicine systems are complicated and broad, and they may have a significant influence on underprivileged popu-lations such as persons of color and the LGBT community, such as:

- Access to care: People in marginalized communities may not have access to the technology or internet needed to use telemedicine services. This might result in even more health inequities and uneven access to care.
- Data privacy is a critical topic since telemedicine systems collect and keep vast volumes of personal health information. There is a possibility of data breaches and privacy violations, which might jeopardize patients' personal and health information.
- Care quality: Telemedicine systems may not be able to give the same degree of care as traditional in-person healthcare. This might lead to inaccurate diagnosis, treatments, and other medical blunders, especially for patients with complicated medical problems.

These ethical problems underscore the importance of designing and implementing telemedicine systems with fairness and inclusion in mind. The systems must be accessible, secure, and of high quality, and they must include all pa-tients, regardless of background or geography. They also should be subject to stringent data privacy and security safeguards to protect patients' PHI.

5. CONCLUSION

In the wake of the COVID-19 pandemic, the prominence of telemedicine has grown significantly, emerging as a pivotal component in the landscape of health-care delivery. As technological advancements continue to unfold, the trajectory of telemedicine's evolution and innovation remains poised for further progres-sion. The confluence of 5G networks, wearable devices, the Internet of Things (IoT), blockchain technology, and artificial intelligence (AI) is poised to wield a substantial transformative impact on the future of telemedicine. These techno-logical synergies hold the promise not only of enhancing healthcare delivery but also of ushering in more streamlined and efficacious healthcare solutions.

The integration of these transformative technologies within the domain of telemedicine stands to forge a dynamic landscape. The fusion of 5G networks offers unparalleled connectivity, enabling real-time interactions and high-quality video conferencing that underpins seamless telemedical consultations. Wearable devices and IoT-enabled sensors empower patients to monitor their health re-motely, furnishing healthcare professionals with a comprehensive picture of pa-tients' well-being. Blockchain technology, recognized for its security and trans-parency, lends credibility to medical records, ensuring data integrity and privacy. Furthermore, AI-driven innovations, including virtual assistants and predictive analytics, hold the potential to augment diagnostic accuracy and personalized treatment recommendations.

Foreseeing the confluence of telemedicine with established healthcare delivery systems, the scope of healthcare accessibility is poised for substantial expansion.

Particularly significant is the potential for underserved populations, who have historically encountered barriers to healthcare access, to gain entry to these es-sential services. This aligns with the overarching goal of promoting healthcare equity and inclusivity, thereby addressing long-standing healthcare disparities.

Nonetheless, the proliferation of future telemedicine endeavors is not devoid of challenges. It gives rise to pressing concerns related to privacy, data secu-rity, and ethical considerations. The transmission and storage of sensitive med-ical information in digital landscapes necessitate rigorous safeguards to thwart potential breaches and unauthorized access. Addressing these concerns man-dates comprehensive strategies encompassing encryption, authentication proto-cols, and adherence to stringent data protection regulations.

In the face of these challenges, the undeniable benefits of telemedicine re-main poised to propel its sustained expansion and adoption. Augmented patient outcomes, reduced healthcare costs, and the capacity to circumvent geographical barriers underscore its potential to redefine healthcare paradigms. As the health-care sector progressively embraces these transformative technologies, stakehold-ers must navigate the complex terrain of regulation, privacy concerns, and ethical considerations to harness the full potential of future telemedicine systems. In do-ing so, they pave the way for a healthcare landscape characterized by innovation, accessibility, and enhanced patient-centric care.

REFERENCES

Abiodun, T. N., Okunbor, D., & Osamor, V. C. (2022). Remote health moni-toring in clinical trial using machine learning techniques: A conceptual frame-work. *Health and Technology*, *12*(2), 359–364. doi:10.100712553-022-00652-z PMID:35308032

Adeloye, D., Adigun, T., Misra, S., & Omoregbe, N. (2017). Assessing the coverage of e-health services in sub-saharan africa: A systematic review and analysis. *Methods of Information in Medicine*, *56*(3), 189–199. doi:10.3414/ME16-05-0012 PMID:28244548

Adrien, T. V., Kim, H. J., Cray, H. V., & Vahia, I. V. (2022). Training older adults to use telemedicine for mental health may have limited impact. *The American Journal of Geriatric Psychiatry*, *30*(2), 262–263. doi:10.1016/j.jagp.2021.05.017 PMID:34176731

Ahmad, I., Asghar, Z., Kumar, T., Li, G., Manzoor, A., Mikhaylov, K., Shah, S. A., Hoyhtya, M., Reponen, J., Huusko, J., & Harjula, E. (2022). Emerging technologies for next generation remote health care and assisted living. *IEEE Access : Practical Innovations, Open Solutions*, *10*, 56094–56132. doi:10.1109/ACCESS.2022.3177278

Ahmad, R. W., Salah, K., Jayaraman, R., Yaqoob, I., Ellahham, S., & Omar, M. (2021). The role of blockchain technology in telehealth and telemedicine. *International Journal of Medical Informatics*, *148*, 104399. doi:10.1016/j.ijmedinf.2021.104399 PMID:33540131

Aldekhyyel, R. N., Almulhem, J. A., & Binkheder, S. (2021). Usability of telemedicine mobile applications during covid-19 in saudi arabia: A heuristic evaluation of patient user interfaces. In Healthcare (Vol. 9, p. 1574). MDPI. doi: 10.3390/healthcare9111574

AlGhamdi, R., Alassafi, M. O., Alshdadi, A. A., Dessouky, M. M., Ramdan, R. A., & Aboshosha, B. W. (2023). Developing trusted iot healthcare information-based ai and blockchain. *Processes (Basel, Switzerland)*, *11*(1), 34. doi:10.3390/pr11010034

Alvarez, P., Sianis, A., Brown, J., Ali, A., & Briasoulis, A. (2021). Chronic disease management in heart failure: Focus on telemedicine and remote moni-toring. *Reviews in Cardiovascular Medicine*, *22*(2), 403–413. doi:10.31083/j.rcm2202046 PMID:34258907

Arora, S., Thornton, K., Jenkusky, S. M., Parish, B., & Scaletti, J. V. (2007). Project echo: Linking university specialists with rural and prison-based clini-cians to improve care for people with chronic hepatitis c in new mexico. *Public Health Reports*, *122*(2_suppl, SUPPL. 2), 74–77. doi:10.1177/00333549071220S214 PMID:17542458

Aslan, B., & Ata‚sen, K. (2021). Covid-19 information sharing with blockchain. *Information Technology and Control*, *50*(4), 674–685. doi:10.5755/j01.itc.50.4.29064

Ayeni, F., Omogbadegun, Z., Omoregbe, N., Misra, S., and Garg, L. (2018). Overcoming barriers to healthcare access and delivery. *EAI Endorsed Trans-actions on Pervasive Health and Technology, 4*(15). doi: 10.4108/eai.24-7-2018.156515

Bansal, G., Rajgopal, K., Chamola, V., Xiong, Z., & Niyato, D. (2022). Healthcare in metaverse: A survey on current metaverse applications in healthcare. *IEEE Access : Practical Innovations, Open Solutions*, *10*, 119914–119946. doi:10.1109/ACCESS.2022.3219845

Barnett, M. L., & Huskamp, H. A. (2020). Telemedicine for mental health in the united states: Making progress, still a long way to go. *Psychiatric Services (Washington, D.C.)*, *71*(2), 197–198. doi:10.1176/appi.ps.201900555 PMID:31847735

Blažauskas, T., Muliuolis, A., Bikulčienė, L., and Butkevičiūtė, E. (2017). Service-oriented architecture solution for ecg signal processing. *Information Technology and Control*, *46*(4), 445–458. doi: 10.5755/j01.itc.46.4.18470

Busnatu, S., Niculescu, A., Bolocan, A., Andronic, O., Pantea Stoian, A. M., Scafa-Udriște, A., Stănescu, A. M. A., Păduraru, D. N., Nicolescu, M. I., Grumezescu, A. M., & Jinga, V. (2022). A review of digital health and biotelemetry: Modern approaches towards personalized medicine and remote health assessment. *Journal of Personalized Medicine*, *12*(10), 1656. doi:10.3390/jpm12101656 PMID:36294795

Chen, H., & Wo'zniak, M. (2022). Mathematical model simulation of detailed classification of telemedicine sensing data. *Mobile Networks and Applications*. doi:10.100711036-022-02025-2

Chen, Y., Zhou, Z., Cao, M., Liu, M., Lin, Z., Yang, W., Yang, X., Dhaidhai, D., & Xiong, P. (2022). Extended reality (xr) and telehealth interventions for children or adolescents with autism spectrum disorder: Systematic review of qualitative and quantitative studies. *Neuroscience and Biobehavioral Reviews*, *138*, 138. doi:10.1016/j.neubiorev.2022.104683 PMID:35523302

Cobry, E. C., & Wadwa, R. P. (2022). The future of telehealth in type 1 diabetes. *Current Opinion in Endocrinology, Diabetes, and Obesity*, *29*(4), 397–402. doi:10.1097/MED.0000000000000745 PMID:35777972

Dagli, N. (2022). Advancement in telemedicine and teledentistry with virtual reality and metaverse. Journal of International Oral Health, 14(6), 529–530.

Ekeland, A. G., Bowes, A., & Flottorp, S. (2010). Effectiveness of telemedicine: A systematic review of reviews. *International Journal of Medical Informatics*, *79*(11), 736–771. doi:10.1016/j.ijmedinf.2010.08.006 PMID:20884286

El-Sherif, D. M., Abouzid, M., Elzarif, M. T., Ahmed, A. A., Albakri, A., & Alshehri, M. M. (2022). Telehealth and artificial intelligence insights into healthcare during the covid-19 pandemic. *Health Care*, *10*(2). PMID:35206998

Elhayatmy, G., Dey, N., & Ashour, A. S. (2017). Internet of things based wireless body area network in healthcare. In Studies in Big Data, 3–20.

Ganapathy, K., & Ravindra, A. (2009). Telemedicine in india: The apollo story. *Telemedicine Journal and e-Health*, *15*(6), 576–585. doi:10.1089/tmj.2009.0066 PMID:19659414

Gaur, L. and Jhanjhi, N. (2022). *Digital twins and healthcare: Trends, techniques, and challenges.* doi: 10.4018/978-1-6684-5925-6

Georgiou, K. E., Georgiou, E., & Satava, R. M. (2021). 5g use in healthcare: The future is present. *JSLS: Journal of the Society of Laparoscopic & Robotic Surgeons*, *25*(4), e2021.00064.

Goldwater, J. C., Zhang, Y., Harris, Y., Saurabh, C., & Summers, R. L. (2023). A new frontier in telehealth research: A national telehealth data warehouse. *Telemedicine Journal and e-Health*, *29*(9), 1426–1429. doi:10.1089/tmj.2022.0422 PMID:36799938

Hailey, D., Roine, R., & Ohinmaa, A. (2002). Systematic review of evidence for the benefits of telemedicine. *Journal of Telemedicine and Telecare*, *8*(1_suppl, Suppl 1), 1–30. doi:10.1258/1357633021937604 PMID:12020415

Hameed, K., Bajwa, I. S., Sarwar, N., Anwar, W., Mushtaq, Z., & Rashid, T. (2021). Integration of 5g and block-chain technologies in smart telemedicine using iot. *Journal of Healthcare Engineering, 2021*, 2021. doi:10.1155/2021/8814364 PMID:33824715

Huq, S. M., Maskeliūnas, R., & Damaševičius, R. (2022). Dialogue agents for artificial intelligence-based conversational systems for cognitively disabled: A systematic review. *Disability and Rehabilitation. Assistive Technology*, 1–20. doi: 10.1080/17483107.2022.2146768 PMID:36413423

Issa, M. E., Helm, A. M., Al-Qaness, M. A. A., Dahou, A., Elaziz, M. A., & Damaševičius, R. (2022). Human activity recognition based on embedded sensor data fusion for the internet of healthcare things. *Health Care, 10*(6). PMID:35742136

Kakhi, K., Alizadehsani, R., Kabir, H. M. D., Khosravi, A., Nahavandi, S., & Acharya, U. R. (2022). The internet of medical things and artificial intelli-gence: Trends, challenges, and opportunities. *Biocybernetics and Biomedical Engineering, 42*(3), 749–771. doi:10.1016/j.bbe.2022.05.008

Kalasin, S., & Surareungchai, W. (2022). Challenges of emerging wearable sen-sors for remote monitoring toward telemedicine healthcare. *Analytical Chemistry*. doi: 10.1021/acs.analchem.2c02642

Ketu, S., & Mishra, P. K. (2021). Internet of healthcare things: A contemporary survey. *Journal of Network and Computer Applications, 192*, 192. doi:10.1016/j.jnca.2021.103179

Khare, V., Agrawal, A., Gupta, P., & Saxena, S. (2019). Artificial intelli-gence based afb microscopy for pulmonary tuberculosis in north india: A pilot study. [IJSRP]. *International Journal of Scientific and Research Publications, 9*(12), 9669. doi:10.29322/IJSRP.9.12.2019.p9669

Kim, R., Mishra, C., & Sen, S. (2022). The use of teleconsultation and technol-ogy by the aravind eye care system, india. *Community Eye Health, 35*(114), 10. PMID:36035096

Kruklitis, R., Miller, M., Valeriano, L., Shine, S., Opstbaum, N., and Chestnut, V. (2022). Applications of remote patient monitoring. *Primary Care - Clinics in Office Practice, 49*(4), 543–555.

Kuo, T., Kim, H., & Ohno-Machado, L. (2017). Blockchain distributed ledger technologies for biomedical and health care applications. *Journal of the American Medical Informatics Association, 24*(6), 1211–1220. doi:10.1093/jamia/ocx068 PMID:29016974

Maskeliunas, R., Damaševicius, R., and Segal, S. (2019). A review of internet of things technologies for ambient assisted living environments. *Future Internet, 11*(12). doi: 10.3390/fi11120259

McIntyre, T., Hughes, C. D., Pauyo, T., Sullivan, S. R., Rogers, S. O. Jr, Ray-monville, M., & Meara, J. G. (2011). Emergency surgical care delivery in post-earthquake haiti: Partners in health and zanmi lasante experience. *World Journal of Surgery, 35*(4), 745–750. doi:10.100700268-011-0961-6 PMID:21249359

Mihalj, M., Carrel, T., Gregoric, I. D., Andereggen, L., Zinn, P. O., Doll, D., Stueber, F., Gabriel, R. A., Urman, R. D., & Luedi, M. M. (2020). Telemedicine for preoperative assessment during a covid-19 pandemic: Rec-ommendations for clinical care. *Best Practice & Research. Clinical Anaesthesiology, 34*(2), 345–351. doi:10.1016/j.bpa.2020.05.001 PMID:32711839

Miner, H., Koenig, K., & Bozic, K. J. (2020). Value-based healthcare: Not going anywhere—why orthopaedic surgeons will continue using tele-health in a post-covid-19 world. *Clinical Orthopaedics and Related Research, 478*(12), 2717–2719. doi:10.1097/CORR.0000000000001561 PMID:33165045

Mohiuddin, S. I., Thorakkattil, S. A., Abushoumi, F., Nemr, H. S., Jabbour, R., & Al-Ghamdi, F. (2021). Implementation of pharmacist-led tele medica-tion management clinic in ambulatory care settings: A patient-centered care model in covid-19 era. *Exploratory Research in Clinical and Social Pharmacy, 4*, 100083. doi:10.1016/j.rcsop.2021.100083 PMID:34723240

Musamih, A., Yaqoob, I., Salah, K., Jayaraman, R., Al-Hammadi, Y., Omar, M., & Ellahham, S. (2022). Metaverse in healthcare:applications, challenges,and future directions. IEEE Consumer Electronics Magazine, vol. 12, no. 4, pp. 33-46, 1 July 2023, doi: 10.1109/MCE.2022.3223522..

Nawaz, N. A., Abid, A., Rasheed, S., Farooq, M. S., Shahzadi, A., & Mubarik, I. (2022). Impact of telecommunication network on future of telemedicine in healthcare: A systematic literature review. *International Journal of Advanced and Applied Sciences, 9*(7), 122–138. doi:10.21833/ijaas.2022.07.013

Omoregbe, N. A. I., Ndaman, I. O., Misra, S., Abayomi-Alli, O. O., & Damaševičius, R. (2020). Text messaging-based medical diagnosis using nat-ural language processing and fuzzy logic. *Journal of Healthcare Engineering*, 2020. doi: 10.1155/2020/8839524

Pak, H. S., Brown-Connolly, N. E., Bloch, C., Clarke, M., Clyburn, C., Doarn, C. R., Llewellyn, C., Merrell, R. C., Montgomery, K., Rasche, J., & Sullivan, B. (2008). Global forum on telemedicine: Connecting the world through partnerships. *Telemedicine Journal and e-Health*, *14*(4), 389–395. doi:10.1089/tmj.2008.0030 PMID:18570571

Palozzi, G., Schettini, I., & Chirico, A. (2020). Enhancing the sustainable goal of access to healthcare: Findings from a literature review on telemedicine employment in rural areas. *Sustainability*, *12*(8), 3318. doi:10.3390u12083318

Pandya, S. (2007). *Telemedicine, telehealth and e-health: An emerging role in private industry and international health policy.*

Pap, I. A., & Oniga, S. (2022). A review of converging technologies in ehealth pertaining to artificial intelligence. *International Journal of Environmental Research and Public Health*, *19*(18), 11413. doi:10.3390/ijerph191811413 PMID:36141685

Rajda, J., & Paz, H. L. (2020). The future of virtual care services: A payor's perspective. *Telemedicine Journal and e-Health*, *26*(3), 267–269. doi:10.1089/tmj.2019.0020 PMID:31058584

Roy, A. (2020). The fourth industrial revolution. *Journal of International Consumer Marketing*, *32*(3), 268–270. doi:10.1080/08961530.2020.1727164

S¸ahin, E., Yavuz Veizi, B. G., and Naharci, M. I. (2021). Telemedicine inter-ventions for older adults: a systematic review. *Journal of telemedicine and telecare*. doi: 10.1177/1357633X21105834

Saleh, S., Cherradi, B., Gannour, O. E., Gouiza, N., & Bouattane, O. (2023). Healthcare monitoring system for automatic database management using mo-bile application in iot environment. *Bulletin of Electrical Engineering and Informatics*, *12*(2), 1055–1068. doi:10.11591/eei.v12i2.4282

Santosh, K., & Gaur, L. (2021a). *Ai in precision medicine*. SpringerBriefs in Applied Sciences and Technology. doi:10.1007/978-981-16-6768-8_5

Santosh, K., & Gaur, L. (2021b). *Ai solutions to public health issues*. Springer-Briefs in Applied Sciences and Technology. doi:10.1007/978-981-16-6768-8_3

Shah, A. C. & Badawy, S. M. (2021). Telemedicine in pediatrics: system-atic review of randomized controlled trials. *JMIR pediatrics and parenting, 4*(1), e22696.

Shah, I., Sial, Q., Jhanjhi, N., and Gaur, L. (2022). *The role of the IoT and digital twin in the healthcare digitalization process: IoT and digital twin in the healthcare digitalization process*. In Digital Twins and Healthcare: Trends, Techniques, and Challenges. doi: 10.4018/978-1-6684-5925-6.ch002

Sittig, D. F., Kahol, K., & Singh, H. (2013). Sociotechnical evaluation of the safety and effectiveness of point-of-care mobile computing devices: a case study conducted in india. *Electronic Health Records: Challenges in Design and Implementation, 115*.

Srinivasu, P. N., Ijaz, M. F., Shafi, J., Wozniak, M., & Sujatha, R. (2022). 6g driven fast computational networking framework for healthcare applications. *IEEE Access: Practical Innovations, Open Solutions*, 10, 94235–94248. doi:10.1109/ACCESS.2022.3203061

Tamulis, Vasiljevas, M., Damaševičius, R., Maskeliunas, R., & Misra, S. (2022). Affective Computing for eHealth Using Low-Cost Remote Internet of Things-Based EMG Platform. *Internet of Things*. doi: 10.1007/978-3-030-81473-1_3

Vanagas, G., Engelbrecht, R., Damaševičius, R., Suomi, R., & Solanas, A. (2018). Ehealth solutions for the integrated healthcare. *Journal of Healthcare Engineering*, 2018.doi: 10.1155/2018/3846892 PMID:30123441

Vassallo, D., Swinfen, P., Swinfen, R., & Wootton, R. (2001). Experience with a low-cost telemedicine system in three developing countries. *Journal of Telemedicine and Telecare*, 7(1, Suppl), 56–58. doi:10.1177/1357633X010070S123 PMID:11576493

Velayati, F., Ayatollahi, H., Hemmat, M., & Dehghan, R. (2022). Telehealth business models and their components: Systematic review. *Journal of Medical Internet Research*, 24(3), e33128. doi:10.2196/33128 PMID:35348471

Weinstein, R. S., Lopez, A. M., Joseph, B. A., Erps, K. A., Holcomb, M., Barker, G. P., & Krupinski, E. A. (2014). Telemedicine, telehealth, and mobile health applications that work: Opportunities and barriers. *The American Journal of Medicine*, 127(3), 183–187. doi:10.1016/j.amjmed.2013.09.032 PMID:24384059

Williams, A. M., Bhatti, U. F., Alam, H. B., & Nikolian, V. C. (2018). The role of telemedicine in postoperative care. *mHealth*, 4, 4. doi:10.21037/mhealth.2018.04.03 PMID:29963556

Wong, D. H., Bolton, R. E., Sitter, K. E., & Vimalananda, V. G. (2023). Endocrinologists' experiences with telehealth: A qualitative study with impli-cations for promoting sustained use. *Endocrine Practice*, 29(2), 104–109. doi:10.1016/j.eprac.2022.11.003 PMID:36370984

Wootton, R. (2001). Telemedicine. British medical journal, 323(7312), 557–560.

Xu, Y., Holanda, G., Souza, L. F. D. F., Silva, H., Gomes, A., Silva, I., Fer-reira, M., Jia, C., Han, T., De Albuquerque, V. H. C., & Filho, P. P. R. (2021). Deep learning-enhanced internet of medical things to analyze brain ct scans of hemorrhagic stroke patients: A new approach. *IEEE Sensors Journal*, *21*(22), 24941–24951. doi:10.1109/JSEN.2020.3032897

Yeung, A. W. K., Tosevska, A., Klager, E., Eibensteiner, F., Laxar, D., Stoyanov, J., Glisic, M., Zeiner, S., Kulnik, S. T., Crutzen, R., Kimberger, O., Kletecka-Pulker, M., Atanasov, A. G., & Willschke, H. (2021). Virtual and augmented reality applications in medicine: Analysis of the scientific literature. *Journal of Medical Internet Research*, *23*(2), e25499. doi:10.2196/25499 PMID:33565986

Yunana, K., Alfa, A. A., Misra, S., Damasevicius, R., Maskeliunas, R., & Olu-ranti, J. (2021). Internet of Things: Applications, Adoptions and Components. In: Hybrid Intelligent Systems. doi: 10.1007/978-3-030-73050-5_50

Zaman, N., Gaur, L., and Humayun, M. (2022). *Approaches and applications of deep learning in virtual medical care*. IGI Global. doi: 10.4018/978-1-7998-8929-8.

Compilation of References

Karthikeyan, M. V. & Manickam, M. (2017). Security Issues in Wireless Body Area Networks: In Bio-signal Input Fuzzy Security. *Research Journal of Pharmaceutical, Biological and Chemical Sciences,. 7*(6), 1755-1773.

Karthikeyan, M. V. & Manickam, M. (2017). A novel fast chaff point generation method using bio-inspired flower pollination algorithm for fuzzy vault systems with physiological signal for wireless body area sensor networks. *Artificial Intelligent Techniques for Bio-Medical Signal Processing*. Biomedical Research.

Upadhye, A. (2021). A survey on machine learning algorithms for applications in cognitive radio networks. *2021 IEEE International Conference on Electronics, Computing and Communication Technologies (CONECCT)*. IEEE. 10.1109/CONECCT52877.2021.9622610

Tian, J., Cheng, P., Chen, Z., Li, M., Hu, H., Li, Y., & Vucetic, B. (2019). A machine learning-enabled spectrum sensing method for ofdm systems. *IEEE Trans. Veh. Technol., 68*(11).

Zheng, S., Chen, S., Qi, P., Zhou, H., & Yang, X. (2020, February). Spectrum sensing based on deep learning classification for cognitive radios. *China Communications, 17*(2), 138–148. doi:10.23919/JCC.2020.02.012

Sarikhani, R., & Keynia, F. (2020, July). Cooperative spectrum sensing meets machine learning: Deep reinforcement learning approach. *IEEE Communications Letters, 24*(7), 1459–1462. doi:10.1109/LCOMM.2020.2984430

Shawel, B. S., Woldegebreal, D. H., & Pollin, S. (2019). Convolutional lstmbased long-term spectrum prediction for dynamic spectrum access. *Proceedings of the ... European Signal Processing Conference (EUSIPCO). EUSIPCO (Conference)*, (Sep), 1–5.

Xu, Y., Cheng, P., Chen, Z., Li, Y., & Vucetic, B. (2018, November). Mobile collaborative spectrum sensing for heterogeneous networks: A bayesian machine learning approach. *IEEE Transactions on Signal Processing, 66*(21), 5634–5647. doi:10.1109/TSP.2018.2870379

Zhao F., & Tang, Q. (2018). A knn learning algorithm for collusion-resistant spectrum auction in small cell networks. *IEEE Access, 6*, 796–4.

Agarwal, A., Dubey, S., Khan, M. A., Gangopadhyay, R., & Debnath, S. (2016). Learning based primary user activity prediction in cognitive radio networks for efficient dynamic spectrum access. *Proc. International Conference on Signal Processing and Communications (SPCOM)*, (pp. 1–5). IEEE. 10.1109/SPCOM.2016.7746632

Bourouis, A., Feham, M., & Bouchachia, A. (2011). Ubiquitous Mobile Health Monitoring System for Elderly (UMHMSE). *International Journal of Computer Science and Information Technologies*, *3*(3), 74–82. doi:10.5121/ijcsit.2011.3306

Munivel, K. V., Samraj, T., Kandasamy, V., & Chilamkurti, N. (2020). Improving the Lifetime of an Out-Patient Implanted Medical Device Using a Novel Flower Pollination-Based Optimization Algorithm in WBAN Systems. M. V. Karthikeyan, Advances in Mathematical Methods for Machine Learning Algorithms for Computer Aided Diagnostic Systems. mathematics. *Mathematics*, *8*(12), 2189. doi:10.3390/math8122189

Li, H., Ding, X., Yang, Y., Huang, X., & Zhang, G. (2019). Spectrum occupancy prediction for internet of things via long short-term memory. *Proc. IEEE International Conference on Consumer Electronics - Taiwan (ICCE-TW)*. IEEE. 10.1109/ICCE-TW46550.2019.8991968

Yu, L., Chen, J., Zhang, Y., Zhou, H., & Sun, J. (2018, September). Deep spectrum prediction in high frequency communication based on temporal-spectral residual network. *China Communications*, *15*(9), 25–34. doi:10.1109/CC.2018.8456449

Karthikeyan, M. V. & Manickam, M. (2017). A 128-Bit Secret Key Generation Using Unique Ecg Bio-Signal for Medical Data Cryptography in Lightweight Wireless Body Area Networks. *Journal of Pakistan journal of Biotechnology, 14*(2), 257-264.

Tumuluru, V. K., Wang, P., & Niyato, D. (2010). A neural network based spectrum prediction scheme for cognitive radio. *Proc. IEEE International Conference on Communications*. IEEE. 10.1109/ICC.2010.5502348

Mohanakurup, V., Baghela, V. S., Kumar, S., Srivastava, P. K., Doohan, N. V., Soni, M., & Awal, H. (2022). 5G Cognitive Radio Networks Using Reliable Hybrid Deep Learning Based on Spectrum Sensing. Wireless Communications and Mobile Computing. doi:10.1155/2022/1830497

Shi, Y., Erpek, T., Sagduyu, Y. E., & Li, J. H. (2018). Spectrum Data Poisoning with Adversarial Deep Learning. *MILCOM IEEE Military Communications Conference*, Los Angeles, CA. 10.1109/MILCOM.2018.8599832

Shalev-Shwartz, S., Livni, R., & Shamir, O. (2014). On the computational efficiency of training neural networks. *Proceedings of the 27th International Conference on Neural Information Processing Systems*, (pp. 855-863). IEEE.

Sarmah, R., Taggu, A., & Marchang, N. (2020). Detecting Byzantine attack in cognitive radio networks using machine learning. *Wireless Networks*, *26*(8), 5939–5950. doi:10.100711276-020-02398-w

Compilation of References

Gul, N., Khan, M. S., Kim, S. M., Kim, J., Elahi, A., & Khalil, Z. (2020). Boosted trees algorithm as reliable spectrum sensing scheme in the presence of malicious users. *Electronics (Basel)*, *9*(6), 1–23. doi:10.3390/electronics9061038

Ullah, S., & Khan, P. (2009). NiamatUllah, Shahnaz Saleem, Henry Higgins, Kyung Sup Kwak. *International Journal of Communications, Network and Systems Sciences*, 797–803. doi:10.4236/ijcns.2009.28093

Liu, H., Zhu, X., & Fujii, T. (2019). Ensemble deep learning based cooperative spectrum sensing with semi-soft stacking fusion center. In *Proceedings of the 2019 IEEE Wireless Communications and Networking Conference (WCNC)*, Marrakesh, Morocco. 10.1109/WCNC.2019.8885866

Karthikeyan, M. V. & Manickam, M. (2017). Three Tire Proxy Re-Encryption Secret Key (PRESK) Generation for Secure Transmission of Biosignals in Wireless Body Area Sensor Networks. *Journal of Chemical and Pharmaceutical Sciences*.

Karthikeyan, M. V. & Manickam, M. (2017). Secret Key Generation Of 128-Bits Using Patient ECG Signal and Secret Transmission For IMDs Authentication. *International Journal of Pure and Applied Mathematics*.

Timcenko, V., & Gajin, S. (2017). Ensemble classifiers for supervised anomaly based network intrusion detection. *Proceedings of the 13th IEEE International Conference on Intelligent Computer Communication and Processing (ICCP)*, Cluj-Napoca, Romania. 10.1109/ICCP.2017.8116977

Muñoz, E. C., Luis, F. P. M., & Jorge, E. O. T. (2020). Detection of Malicious Primary User Emulation Based on a Support Vector Machine for a Mobile Cognitive Radio Network Using Software-Defined Radio. *Electronics, MDPI*, *9*, 1–17.

Tephillah, S., & Martin Leo Manickam, J. (2020). An SETM Algorithm for Combating SSDF Attack in Cognitive Radio Networks. Wireless Communications and Mobile Computing. doi:10.1155/2020/9047809

Arjoune, Y., & Kaabouch, N. (2019). On Spectrum Sensing, a Machine Learning Method for Cognitive Radio Systems. *2019 IEEE International Conference on Electro Information Technology (EIT)*, (pp. 333-338). IEEE. 10.1109/EIT.2019.8834099

Umar R. & Sheikh, A. (2012). A Comparative Study of Spectrum Awareness Techniques for Cognitive Radio Oriented Wireless Networks. *Physical Communication*.

Madushan, K., Kae, T., Choi, W., Saquib, N., & Hossain, E. (2013). Machine Learning Techniques for Cooperative Spectrum Sensing in Cognitive Radio Networks. *IEEE Journal on Selected Areas in Communications*, *31*(11), 2209–2221. doi:10.1109/JSAC.2013.131120

Khalfi, B., Zaid, A., & Hamdaoui, B. (2017). When Machine Learning Meets Compressive Sampling for Wideband Spectrum Sensing. *Wireless Communications and Mobile Computing Conference*, (pp. 1120-1125). IEEE. 10.1109/IWCMC.2017.7986442

Zhang, H., Poon, C., & Zhang, Y. (2011). *ISNR Communication and Networking*.

Lu, Y., Zhu, P., Wang, D., & Fattouche, M. (2016). Machine Learning Techniques with Probability Vector for Cooperative Spectrum Sensing in Cognitive Radio Networks. *IEEE Wireless Communications and Networking Conference*, (pp. 1-6). IEEE. 10.1109/WCNC.2016.7564840

Santosh, K. C., Gaur, L., Santosh, K. C., & Gaur, L. (2021). *AI in Sustainable Public Healthcare. Artificial Intelligence and Machine Learning in Public Healthcare: Opportunities and Societal Impact*, (pp. 33-40). IGI Global.

Santosh, K. C., Gaur, L., Santosh, K. C., & Gaur, L. (2021). Case Studies—AI for Infectious Disease. *Artificial Intelligence and Machine Learning in Public Healthcare: Opportunities and Societal Impact,* (pp. 55-63). IGI Global.

Chaudhary, M., Gaur, L., Chakrabarti, A., & Jhanjhi, N. Z. (2023). Unravelling the Barriers of Human Resource Analytics: Multi-Criteria Decision-Making Approach. *Journal of Survey in Fisheries Sciences*, 306-321.

Crosby, G., Ghosh, T., Murimi, R., & Chin, C. (2012). Wireless Body Area Networks for Healthcare: A Survey. *International Journal of Ad hoc, Sensor & Ubiquitous Computing, 3.*

Mohanavalli, S.S. & Anand, S. (2011). International Journal of Ad hoc [IJASUC]. *Sensor & Ubiquitous Computing, 2*(1), 60–69. doi:10.5121/ijasuc.2011.2106

Karthikeyan, M. V. (2021). Raspberry Pi implemented with MATLAB simulation and communication of Physiological Signal based fast Chaff point (RPSC) generation algorithm for WBAN systems. *Biomedical Engineering/Biomedizinische Technik, 66*(2). . doi:10.1515/bmt-2019-0336

Karthikeyan, M. V. & Manickam, M. (2017). An enhanced flower pollination algorithm based chaff point generation method with hardware implementation in WBAN. *International Journal of Communication Systems*. Wiley. . doi:10.1002/dac.4447

Karthikeyan, M. V. (2019ECG-Signal Based Secret Key Generation (ESKG) Scheme for WBAN and Hardware Implementation. *J. Martin Leo Manickam, Wireless Personal Communications, Springer, 106*(4), 2037–2052. doi:10.100711277-018-5924-x

Karthikeyan, M. V. & Manickam, M. (2017). Efficient Bio-Signal Feature Based Secure Secret Key Generation Scheme a Simplified Model for Wireless Body Area Network (EFSKG Scheme). *Journal of Medical Imaging and Health Informatics, American Scientific Publishers, 8*(5). . doi:10.1166/jmihi.2018.2415

Abdusatarov, J. (2023, April 26). *Issues That Need To Be Resolved When Developing The Legal Framework Of International Private Law Relations In Metaverse.* Scholar Express. https://www.scholarexpress.net/index.php/wbml/article/view/2626

Abe, T. K., Beamon, B. M., Storch, R. L., & Agus, J. (2016). Operations research applications in hospital operations: Part II. *IIE Transactions on Healthcare Systems Engineering, 6*(2), 96–109. doi:10.1080/19488300.2016.1162880

Compilation of References

Abiodun, T. N., Okunbor, D., & Osamor, V. C. (2022). Remote health moni-toring in clinical trial using machine learning techniques: A conceptual frame-work. *Health and Technology*, *12*(2), 359–364. doi:10.100712553-022-00652-z PMID:35308032

Abouelmehdi, K., Beni-Hessane, A., & Khaloufi, H. (2018). Big healthcare data: Preserving security and privacy. *Journal of Big Data*, *5*(1), 1–18. doi:10.118640537-017-0110-7

AbuKhousa, E., El-Tahawy, M. S., & Atif, Y. (2023). Envisioning architecture of Metaverse Intensive Learning Experience (MILEX): Career readiness in the 21st century and collective intelligence development scenario. *Future Internet*, *15*(2), 53. doi:10.3390/fi15020053

Adadi, A., & Berrada, M. (2018). Peeking inside the black-box: A survey on explainable artificial intelligence (XAI). *IEEE Access : Practical Innovations, Open Solutions*, *6*, 52138–52160. doi:10.1109/ACCESS.2018.2870052

Adam, Ng, E. Y. K., Oh, S. L., Heng, M. L., Hagiwara, Y., Tan, J. H., Tong, J. W. K., & Acharya, U. R. (2018, August). Automated detection of diabetic foot with and without neuropathy using double density-dual tree-complex wavelet transform on foot thermograms. *Infrared Physics & Technology*, *92*, 270–279. doi:10.1016/j.infrared.2018.06.010

Adam, S., Sohail, I., & Phuong, L. N. (2023). Meditation, Geomedicine, and Anticipatory Cities: Emerging Issues and Visions of Futures without Non Communicable Diseases. *Journal of Futures Studies*, *27*(3), 121–136. doi:10.6531/JFS.202303_27(3).0009

Adams, J., Mauldin, T., Yates, K., Zumwalt, C., Ashe, T., Cervantes, D., & Tao, M.-H. (2022). Factors related to the accurate application of NHSN surveillance definitions for CAUTI and CLABSI in Texas hospitals: A cross-sectional survey. *American Journal of Infection Control*, *50*(1), 111–113. doi:10.1016/j.ajic.2021.07.007 PMID:34303723

Adeloye, D., Adigun, T., Misra, S., & Omoregbe, N. (2017). Assessing the coverage of e-health services in sub-saharan africa: A systematic review and analysis. *Methods of Information in Medicine*, *56*(3), 189–199. doi:10.3414/ME16-05-0012 PMID:28244548

Adrian, D., Frances, D., & Burns, A. (2023). *An Examination of the Virtual Event Experience of Cyclists Competing on Zwift*. Ingenta Connect., doi:10.3727/152599523X16907613842110

Adrien, T. V., Kim, H. J., Cray, H. V., & Vahia, I. V. (2022). Training older adults to use telemedicine for mental health may have limited impact. *The American Journal of Geriatric Psychiatry*, *30*(2), 262–263. doi:10.1016/j.jagp.2021.05.017 PMID:34176731

Afaq, A., Gaur, L., & Singh, G. (2022). A Latent Dirichlet allocation Technique for Opinion Mining of Online Reviews of Global Chain Hotels. *2022 3rd International Conference on Intelligent Engineering and Management (ICIEM)*, (pp. 201–206). IEEE. 10.1109/ICIEM54221.2022.9853114

Afaq, A., & Gaur, L. (2021). The Rise of Robots to Help Combat Covid-19. *2021 International Conference on Technological Advancements and Innovations (ICTAI)*, (pp. 69–74). IEEE. 10.1109/ICTAI53825.2021.9673256

Afaq, A., Gaur, L., & Singh, G. (2023a). Social CRM: Linking the dots of customer service and customer loyalty during COVID-19 in the hotel industry. *International Journal of Contemporary Hospitality Management, Emerald Publishing Limited*, *35*(3), 992–1009. doi:10.1108/IJCHM-04-2022-0428

Afaq, A., Gaur, L., & Singh, G. (2023b). A trip down memory lane to travellers' food experiences. *British Food Journal, Emerald Publishing Limited*, *125*(4), 1390–1403. doi:10.1108/BFJ-01-2022-0063

Afaq, A., Gaur, L., Singh, G., & Dhir, A. (2021). *COVID-19: transforming air passengers' behaviour and reshaping their expectations towards the airline industry. Tourism Recreation Research*. Routledge. doi:10.1080/02508281.2021.2008211

Afsar, M. M., Saqib, S., Alarfaj, M., Alatiyyah, M. H., Alnowaiser, K., Aljuaid, H., Jalal, A., & Park, J. (2023). Body-Worn sensors for recognizing physical sports activities in exergaming via deep learning model. *IEEE Access : Practical Innovations, Open Solutions*, *11*, 12460–12473. doi:10.1109/ACCESS.2023.3239692

Agac, G., Sevim, F., Celik, O., Bostan, S., Erdem, R. and Yalcin, Y.I. (2023). Research hotspots, trends and opportunities on the metaverse in health education: a bibliometric analysis. *Library Hi Tech*. Emerald Publishing Limited. doi:. doi:10.1108/LHT-04-2023-0168

Agarwal, A. and Alathur, S. (2023). Metaverse revolution and the digital transformation: intersectional analysis of Industry 5.0. *Transforming Government: People, Process and Policy*. Emerald Publishing Limited. . doi:10.1108/TG-03-2023-0036

Ahmad, I., Asghar, Z., Kumar, T., Li, G., Manzoor, A., Mikhaylov, K., Shah, S. A., Hoyhtya, M., Reponen, J., Huusko, J., & Harjula, E. (2022). Emerging technologies for next generation remote health care and assisted living. *IEEE Access : Practical Innovations, Open Solutions*, *10*, 56094–56132. doi:10.1109/ACCESS.2022.3177278

Ahmad, R. W., Salah, K., Jayaraman, R., Yaqoob, I., Ellahham, S., & Omar, M. (2021). The role of blockchain technology in telehealth and telemedicine. *International Journal of Medical Informatics*, *148*, 104399. doi:10.1016/j.ijmedinf.2021.104399 PMID:33540131

Ahmed, A. S. R. a. S. H. S. H. T. T. (2023, July 7). *Find out the innovative techniques of data sharing using cryptography by systematic literature review*. Turcomat. https://www.turcomat.org/index.php/turkbilmat/article/view/13953

Ahmed, S., Biswas, M., Hasanuzzaman, M., Mahi, M. J. N., Islam, M. A., Chaki, S., & Gaur, L. (2022). A Secured Peer-to-Peer Messaging System Based on Blockchain. *2022 3rd International Conference on Intelligent Engineering and Management (ICIEM)*, (pp. 332–337). IEEE. 10.1109/ICIEM54221.2022.9853040

Ahmed, S., Shaharier, M. M., Roy, S., Lima, A. A., Biswas, M., Mahi, M. J. N., & Chaki, S. (2022), "An Intelligent and Multi-Functional Stick for Blind People Using IoT. *2022 3rd International Conference on Intelligent Engineering and Management (ICIEM)*, (pp. 326–331). IEEE. 10.1109/ICIEM54221.2022.9853012

Compilation of References

Ahuja, A. S., Polascik, B. W., Doddapaneni, D., Byrnes, E. S., & Sridhar, J. (2023). The digital metaverse: Applications in artificial intelligence, medical education, and integrative health. *Integrative Medicine Research*, *12*(1), 100917. doi:10.1016/j.imr.2022.100917 PMID:36691642

Aladem M. & Rawashdeh, S. (2019). *A Multi-Cluster Tracking Algorithm with an Event Camera*. IEEE. . doi:10.1109/NAECON46414.2019.9058204

Aldekhyyel, R. N., Almulhem, J. A., & Binkheder, S. (2021). Usability of telemedicine mobile applications during covid-19 in saudi arabia: A heuristic evaluation of patient user interfaces. In Healthcare (Vol. 9, p. 1574). MDPI. doi: 10.3390/healthcare9111574

Alenizi, B. A., Humayun, M., & Jhanjhi, N. Z. (2021). Security and privacy issues in cloud computing. *Journal of Physics: Conference Series*, *1979*(1), 012038. doi:10.1088/1742-6596/1979/1/012038

AlGhamdi, R., Alassafi, M. O., Alshdadi, A. A., Dessouky, M. M., Ramdan, R. A., & Aboshosha, B. W. (2023). Developing trusted iot healthcare information-based ai and blockchain. *Processes (Basel, Switzerland)*, *11*(1), 34. doi:10.3390/pr11010034

Ali, S. G., Wang, X., Li, P., Jung, Y., Bi, L., Kim, J., Chen, Y., Feng, D. D., Thalmann, N. M., Wang, J., & Sheng, B. (2023). A systematic review: Virtual-reality-based techniques for human exercises and health improvement. *Frontiers in Public Health*, *11*, 1143947. doi:10.3389/fpubh.2023.1143947 PMID:37033028

Ali, S., Abdullah, N., Armand, T. P. T., Athar, A., Hussain, A., Ali, M., Muhammad, Y., Joo, M., & Kim, H. C. (2023). Metaverse in Healthcare Integrated with Explainable AI and Blockchain: Enabling Immersiveness, Ensuring Trust, and Providing Patient Data Security. *Sensors (Basel)*, *23*(2), 565. doi:10.339023020565 PMID:36679361

Aljanabi, M. (2023). Metaverse: open possibilities. *ESJournal*. journal.esj.edu.iq. doi:10.52866/ijcsm.2023.02.03.007

Almarzouqi, A., Aburayya, A., & Salloum, S. A. (2022). Prediction of user's intention to use metaverse system in medical education: A hybrid SEM-ML learning approach. *IEEE Access : Practical Innovations, Open Solutions*, *10*, 43421–43434. doi:10.1109/ACCESS.2022.3169285

Al-Masri, S. (2021). Deep learning for diabetic foot ulcer image analysis: A comprehensive review. Journal of Healthcare Engineering, 1–17. doi:10.1155/2021/8891321

Almeida, L. G. G. (2023). *Innovating Industrial Training with Immersive Metaverses: A Method for Developing Cross-Platform Virtual Reality Environments*. MDPI., doi:10.3390/app13158915

Almusaylim, Z. A., Jhanjhi, N. Z., & Jung, L. T. (2018). Proposing A Data Privacy Aware Protocol for Roadside Accident Video Reporting Service Using 5G In Vehicular Cloud Networks Environment. *2018 4th International Conference on Computer and Information Sciences (ICCOINS)*. doi:10.1109/iccoins.2018.8510588

Almusaylim, Z. A., Jhanjhi, N. Z., & Jung, L. T. (2018). Proposing A Data Privacy Aware Protocol for Roadside Accident Video Reporting Service Using 5G In *Vehicular Cloud Networks Environment. 2018 4th International Conference on Computer and Information Sciences (ICCOINS).* IEEE. 10.1109/ICCOINS.2018.8510588

Almusaylim, Z. A., & Jhanjhi, N. Z. (2019). Comprehensive Review: Privacy Protection of User in Location-Aware Services of Mobile Cloud Computing. *Wireless Personal Communications, 111*(1), 541–564. doi:10.100711277-019-06872-3

Alotaibi, Y. K., & Federico, F. (2017). The impact of health information technology on patient safety. *Saudi Medical Journal, 38*(12), 1173–1180. doi:10.15537mj.2017.12.20631 PMID:29209664

Alsem, S. C., Van Dijk, A., Verhulp, E., Dekkers, T. J., & De Castro, B. O. (2023). Treating children's aggressive behavior problems using cognitive behavior therapy with virtual reality: A multicenter randomized controlled trial. *Child Development*, cdev.13966. Advance online publication. doi:10.1111/cdev.13966 PMID:37459452

Alvarez, P., Sianis, A., Brown, J., Ali, A., & Briasoulis, A. (2021). Chronic disease management in heart failure: Focus on telemedicine and remote moni-toring. *Reviews in Cardiovascular Medicine, 22*(2), 403–413. doi:10.31083/j.rcm2202046 PMID:34258907

Alzubaidi, L., Fadhel, M. A., Al-Shamma, O., & Zhang, J. (2020). Towards a better understanding of transfer learning for medical imaging: A case study. *Applied Sciences (Basel, Switzerland), 10*(13), 4523. doi:10.3390/app10134523

Alzubaidi, L., Fadhel, M. A., Al-Shamma, O., & Zhang, J. (2021). Robust application of new deep learning tools: An experimental study in medical imaging. *Multimedia Tools and Applications*, 1–29.

Ameta, D., Garg, A., Kumar, P., & Dutt, V. (2023). *Evaluating the Effectiveness of Mantra Meditation in a 360 Virtual Reality Environment.* ResearchGate. doi:10.1145/3594806.3596587

An, N. (2023, May 2). *Toward learning societies for digital aging.* arXiv.org. https://arxiv.org/abs/2305.01137

Anderson, F. C., Rabello Casali, K., Cunha, S. T., & Matheus, C. M. (2023). *Automatic Classification of Emotions Based on Cardiac Signals: A Systematic Literature Review.* Spinger Link. https://link.springer.com/article/10.1007/s10439-023-03341-8

Angelos, E. (n.d.). *Mindfulness Misconceptions in Counselor Education and Supervision: Mitigating Vicarious Trauma among Counselors-in-Training.* DigitalCommons@SHU. https://digitalcommons.sacredheart.edu/jcps/vol17/iss2/10/

Anshari, M., Syafrudin, M., & Alfian, G. (2023). *Metaverse applications for new business models and disruptive innovation.* IGI Global. doi:10.4018/978-1-6684-6097-9

Anshari, M., Syafrudin, M., Fitriyani, N. L., & Razzaq, A. (2022). Ethical Responsibility and Sustainability (ERS) Development in a Metaverse Business Model. *Sustainability MDPI, 14*(23), 15805. doi:10.3390u142315805

Compilation of References

Anshu, K., & Gaur, L. (2018). Managing Customers Online Recovery – An Insight for E-Retailers Using Conjoint Analysis. *2018 4th International Conference on Computational Intelligence & Communication Technology (CICT)*, (pp. 1–7). IEEE. 10.1109/CIACT.2018.8480207

Apicella, A., Barbato, S., Chacón, L. B., D'Errico, G., De Paolis, L. T., Maffei, L., Massaro, P., Mastrati, G., Moccaldi, N., Pollastro, A., & Wriessenegger, S. C. (2023). Electroencephalography correlates of fear of heights in a virtual reality environment. *Acta IMEKO*, *12*(2), 1–7. doi:10.21014/actaimeko.v12i2.1457

Armstrong, D. G., Swerdlow, M. A., Armstrong, A. A., Conte, M. S., Padula, W. V., & Bus, S. A. (2020, March). Five year mortality and direct costs of care for people with diabetic foot complications are comparable to cancer. *Journal of Foot and Ankle Research*, *13*(1), 16. doi:10.118613047-020-00383-2 PMID:32209136

Arora, S., Thornton, K., Jenkusky, S. M., Parish, B., & Scaletti, J. V. (2007). Project echo: Linking university specialists with rural and prison-based clini-cians to improve care for people with chronic hepatitis c in new mexico. *Public Health Reports*, *122*(2_suppl, SUPPL. 2), 74–77. doi:10.1177/00333549071220S214 PMID:17542458

Arpaci, I., & Bahari, M. (2023). Investigating the role of psychological needs in predicting the educational sustainability of Metaverse using a deep learning-based hybrid SEM-ANN technique. *Interactive Learning Environments*, 1–13. doi:10.1080/10494820.2022.2164313

Arul, P., & Tahir, M. (2023). The effect of social media on customer relationship management: A case of airline industry customers. *International Journal of Management & Entrepreneurship Research*, *5*(6), 360–372. doi:10.51594/ijmer.v5i6.496

Arya, V., Sambyal, R., Sharma, A., & Dwivedi, Y. K. (2023). Brands are calling your AVATAR in Metaverse–A study to explore XR-based gamification marketing activities & consumer-based brand equity in virtual world. *Journal of Consumer Behaviour*, cb.2214. doi:10.1002/cb.2214

Aslan, B., & Ata¸sen, K. (2021). Covid-19 information sharing with blockchain. *Information Technology and Control*, *50*(4), 674–685. doi:10.5755/j01.itc.50.4.29064

Athar, A., Ali, S. M., Mozumder, M. A. I., Ali, S., & Kim, H.-C. (2023). Applications and Possible Challenges of Healthcare Metaverse. *2023 25th International Conference on Advanced Communication Technology (ICACT)*, (pp. 328–332). IEEE. 10.23919/ICACT56868.2023.10079314

Athar, A., Ali, S. M., Mozumder, M. A. I., Ali, S., & Kim, H.-C. (2023). Applications and Possible Challenges of Healthcare Metaverse. In *2023 25th International Conference on Advanced Communication Technology (ICACT)*. IEEE.

Atud, V. (2023). *Reclaiming Focus In The Age Of Ai: Strategies For Deep Thinking In A Distracted Culture*. Sunburst Markets.

Aung, Y. M., & Al-Jumaily, A. (2017). *Augmented reality-based RehaBio system for shoulder rehabilitation.* In *2017 International Conference on Electrical and Electronic Engineering (ICEEE),* Istanbul. doi: 10.1109/ICEEE2.2017.8338852

Ayeni, F., Omogbadegun, Z., Omoregbe, N., Misra, S., and Garg, L. (2018). Overcoming barriers to healthcare access and delivery. *EAI Endorsed Trans-actions on Pervasive Health and Technology, 4*(15). doi: 10.4108/eai.24-7-2018.156515

Bahir, O. (2023). Online Training in Present-Day Conditions: Opportunities and Prospects. In Arts, research, innovation and society (pp. 193–212). doi:10.1007/978-3-031-24101-7_11

Bai, P. (2023). Application and mechanisms of Internet-Based Cognitive Behavioral Therapy (ICBT) in improving psychological state in cancer patients. *Journal of Cancer, 14*(11), 1981–2000. doi:10.7150/jca.82632 PMID:37497400

Baker, J., Nam, K., & Dutt, C. (2023). *A user experience perspective on heritage tourism in the metaverse: Empirical evidence and design dilemmas for VR.* Spinger. https://link.springer.com/article/10.1007/s40558-023-00256-x

Bandyopadhyay, A., Ghosh, S., Bose, M., Kessi, L., & Gaur, L. (2023). Supervised Neural Networks for Fruit Identification. In K. C. Santosh, A. Goyal, D. Aouada, A. Makkar, Y.-Y. Chiang, & S. K. Singh (Eds.), *Recent Trends in Image Processing and Pattern Recognition* (pp. 220–230). Springer Nature Switzerland. doi:10.1007/978-3-031-23599-3_16

Banerji, S. (2023). Future of Well-being- The Metaverse Era. *OCAD University Open Research Repository.* https://openresearch.ocadu.ca/id/eprint/4103

Bannell, D. J., France-Ratcliffe, M., Buckley, B. J. R., Crozier, A., Davies, A., Hesketh, K., Jones, H., Cocks, M., & Sprung, V. S. (2023). Adherence to unsupervised exercise in sedentary individuals: A randomised feasibility trial of two mobile health interventions. *Digital Health, 9,* 20552076231183552. doi:10.1177/20552076231183552 PMID:37426588

Bansal, G., Rajgopal, K., Chamola, V., Xiong, Z., & Niyato, D. (2022). Healthcare in Metaverse: A Survey on Current Metaverse Applications in Healthcare. *IEEE Access : Practical Innovations, Open Solutions, 10,* 119914–119946. doi:10.1109/ACCESS.2022.3219845

BarberaS. (2023). Navigating the Virtual Frontier: The Convergence of Decentralized Finance and the Metaverse. *Preprint.org.* doi:10.20944/preprints202307.1734.v1

Barnett, M. L., & Huskamp, H. A. (2020). Telemedicine for mental health in the united states: Making progress, still a long way to go. *Psychiatric Services (Washington, D.C.), 71*(2), 197–198. doi:10.1176/appi.ps.201900555 PMID:31847735

Batrakoulis, A., Veiga, O. L., Franco, S., Thomas, E., Alexopoulos, A., Torrente, M. V., Santos-Rocha, R., Ramalho, F., Di Credico, A., Vitucci, D., Ramos, L., Simões, V., Romero-Caballero, A., Vieira, I., Mancini, A., & Bianco, A. (2023). Health and fitness trends in Southern Europe for 2023: A cross-sectional survey. *AIMS Public Health, 10*(2), 378–408. doi:10.3934/publichealth.2023028 PMID:37304589

Compilation of References

Bays, H., Fitch, A., Cuda, S., Rickey, E., Hablutzel, J., Coy, R., & Censani, M. (2023). Artificial intelligence and obesity management: An Obesity Medicine Association (OMA) Clinical Practice Statement (CPS) 2023. *Obesity Pillars*, *6*, 100065. doi:10.1016/j.obpill.2023.100065

Bediou, B., Adams, D. M., Mayer, R. E., Tipton, E., Green, C. S., & Bavelier, D. (2018). Meta-analysis of action video game impact on perceptual, attentional, and cognitive skills. *Psychological Bulletin*, *144*(1), 77–110. doi:10.1037/bul0000130 PMID:29172564

Belt, E. S., & Lowenthal, P. R. (2022). Synchronous video-based communication and online learning: An exploration of instructors' perceptions and experiences. *Education and Information Technologies*, *28*(5), 4941–4964. doi:10.100710639-022-11360-6 PMID:36320822

Beng, C. O., Gang, C., Shou, Z. M., Tan, K.-L., Tung, A., Xiao, X., James, W. L. Y., Bingxue, Z., & Meihui, Z. (2023). The Metaverse Data Deluge: What Can We Do About It? In *2023 IEEE 39th International Conference on Data Engineering (ICDE)*. IEEE. 10.1109/ICDE55515.2023.00296

Benjamins, R., Rubio Viñuela, Y., & Alonso, C. (2023). Social and ethical challenges of the metaverse. *AI and Ethics*, *3*(3), 689–697. doi:10.100743681-023-00278-5

BentiB. S. (2023). Sports and eSports: A structural comparison based on the B|Orders in Motion Framework. opus4.kobv.de. doi:10.11584/opus4-1293

Berggren, N. (2023). *Unlocking the Fashion Metaverse: Exploring the impact of external factors on innovation diffusion in the metaverse fashion industry*. DIVA. https://www.diva-portal.org/smash/record.jsf?pid=diva2%3A1761437&dswid=-6051

Beristain-Colorado, M. P., Ambros-Antemate, J. F., Vargas-Treviño, M., Gutierrez-Gutierrez, J., Moreno-Rodriguez, A., Hernandez-Cruz, P. A., Gallegos-Velasco, I. B., & Torres-Rosas, R. (2020). Standardizing the Development of Serious Games for Physical Rehabilitation: Conceptual Framework Proposal. *IEEE Access : Practical Innovations, Open Solutions*, *8*, 26119–26130. doi:10.1109/ACCESS.2020.2971707

Bhandari, M., Parajuli, P., Chapagain, P., & Gaur, L. (2022). Evaluating Performance of Adam Optimization by Proposing Energy Index. In K. C. Santosh, R. Hegadi, & U. Pal (Eds.), *Recent Trends in Image Processing and Pattern Recognition* (pp. 156–168). Springer International Publishing. doi:10.1007/978-3-031-07005-1_15

Bhattacharya, S., & Hofmann, S. G. (2023). Mindfulness-based interventions for anxiety and depression. *Clinics in Integrated Care*, *16*, 100138. doi:10.1016/j.intcar.2023.100138

Bhumika, N., Kaur, A., & Datta, P. (2023). Happiness through Metaverse: Health and Innovation Relationship. *2023 IEEE 12th International Conference on Communication Systems and Network Technologies (CSNT)*. doi:10.1109/csnt57126.2023.10134713

Bi, Q., Goodman, K. E., Kaminsky, J., & Lessler, J. (2019). What is machine learning? A primer for the epidemiologist. *American Journal of Epidemiology*, *188*, 2222–2239. doi:10.1093/aje/kwz189 PMID:31509183

Biswas, M. (2023). *Light Convolutional Neural Network to Detect Eye Diseases from Retinal Images.* ResearchGate. https://www.researchgate.net/publication/371101233_Light_Convolutional_Neural_Network_to_Detect_Eye_Diseases_from_Retinal_Images_Diabetic_Retinopathy_and_Glaucoma

Biswas, M., Chaki, S., Ahammed, F., Anis, A., Ferdous, J., Siddika, A. M., & Shila, D. A. (2022). Prototype Development of an Assistive Smart-Stick for the Visually Challenged Persons. *2022 2nd International Conference on Innovative Practices in Technology and Management (ICIPTM).* IEEE. 10.1109/ICIPTM54933.2022.9754183

Biswas, M., Chaki, S., Mallik, S., Gaur, L., & Ray, K. (2023). Light Convolutional Neural Network to Detect Eye Diseases from Retinal Images: Diabetic Retinopathy and Glaucoma. in M.S. Kaiser, S. Waheed, A. Bandyopadhyay, M. Mahmud, & K. Ray (Eds.), *Proceedings of the Fourth International Conference on Trends in Computational and Cognitive Engineering.* Springer Nature Singapore, Singapore. 10.1007/978-981-19-9483-8_7

Blažauskas, T., Muliuolis, A., Bikulčienė, L., and Butkevičiūtė, E. (2017). Service-oriented architecture solution for ecg signal processing. *Information Technology and Control*, *46*(4), 445–458. doi: 10.5755/j01.itc.46.4.18470

Blowers, M., Jaimes, N., & Williams, J. (2023). *Benefits and challenges of a military metaverse.* SPIE. doi:10.1117/12.2663772

Bohr, A., & Memarzadeh, K. (2020). The rise of artificial intelligence in healthcare applications. In *Artificial Intelligence in healthcare* (pp. 25–60). Elsevier. doi:10.1016/B978-0-12-818438-7.00002-2

Brayshaw, M., Gordon, N., Kambili-Mzembe, F., & Jaber, T. A. (2023). Why the Educational Metaverse Is Not All About Virtual Reality Apps. In Lecture Notes in Computer Science (pp. 22–32). doi:10.1007/978-3-031-34550-0_2

Brewer, L. C., Abraham, H., Kaihoi, B., Leth, S., Egginton, J. S., Slusser, J. P., Scott, R. J., Penheiter, S. G., Albertie, M., Squires, R. W., Thomas, R. J., Scales, R., Trejo-Gutiérrez, J. F., & Kopecky, S. L. (2022). A Community-Informed Virtual World-Based cardiac rehabilitation program as an extension of Center-Based cardiac rehabilitation. *Journal of Cardiopulmonary Rehabilitation and Prevention*, *43*(1), 22–30. doi:10.1097/HCR.0000000000000705 PMID:35881503

Brown, L. (n.d.). *From Coffee Houses to Internet Speech: Civility and Moderation within The Contemporary Public Sphere.* Works. https://works.swarthmore.edu/theses/323/

Browning, M. H., Shin, S., Drong, G., McAnirlin, O., Gagnon, R. J., Ranganathan, S., Sindelar, K., Hoptman, D., Bratman, G. N., Yuan, S., Prabhu, V. G., & Heller, W. (2023). Daily exposure to virtual nature reduces symptoms of anxiety in college students. *Scientific Reports*, *13*(1), 1239. doi:10.103841598-023-28070-9 PMID:36690698

Bubenek, S. I. (2021). *Incendiu la Institutul Matei Bals, Societatea Romana de Anestezie si Terapie Intensiva, [Fire at the Matei Bals Institute, Romanian Society of Anesthesia and Intensive Care].* SRATI. https://www.srati.ro/noutati/comunicat-de-presa-incendiu-institutul-matei-bals

Compilation of References

Buhalis, D., Leung, D., & Lin, M. (2023). Metaverse as a disruptive technology revolutionising tourism management and marketing. *Tourism Management*, *97*, 104724. doi:10.1016/j.tourman.2023.104724

Busnatu, S., Niculescu, A., Bolocan, A., Andronic, O., Pantea Stoian, A. M., Scafa-Udriște, A., Stănescu, A. M. A., Păduraru, D. N., Nicolescu, M. I., Grumezescu, A. M., & Jinga, V. (2022). A review of digital health and biotelemetry: Modern approaches towards personalized medicine and remote health assessment. *Journal of Personalized Medicine*, *12*(10), 1656. doi:10.3390/jpm12101656 PMID:36294795

Calabrò, R. S., Cerasa, A., Ciancarelli, I., Pignolo, L., Tonin, P., Iosa, M., & Morone, G. (2022). The Arrival of the Metaverse in Neurorehabilitation: Fact, Fake or Vision? *Biomedicines*, *10*(10), 2602. doi:10.3390/biomedicines10102602 PMID:36289862

Cameron, L., & Ride, J. (2023). The role of mental health in online gambling decisions: A discrete choice experiment. *Social Science & Medicine*, *326*, 115885. doi:10.1016/j.socscimed.2023.115885 PMID:37087972

Camilleri, M.A. (2023). Metaverse applications in education: a systematic review and a cost-benefit analysis. *Interactive Technology and Smart Education*, Emerald Publishing Limited. doi:. doi:10.1108/ITSE-01-2023-0017

Campbell, A. H., Barta, K., Sawtelle, M., & Walters, A. (2023). Progressive muscle relaxation, meditation, and mental practice-based interventions for the treatment of tremor after traumatic brain injury. *Physiotherapy Theory and Practice*, 1–17. doi:10.1080/09593985.2023.2243504 PMID:37551705

Canellas, R., Rosenkrantz, A. B., Taouli, B., Sala, E., Saini, S., Pedrosa, I., Wang, Z. J., & Sahani, D. V. (2019). Abbreviated MRI protocols for the abdomen. *Radiographics*, *39*(3), 744–758. doi:10.1148/rg.2019180123 PMID:30901285

Carrión, C. (2023). Research streams and open challenges in the metaverse. *The Journal of Supercomputing*. doi:10.100711227-023-05544-1

Carr, K., & England, R. (2023). *Simulated And Virtual Realities: Elements Of Perception*. CRC Press.

Cassidy, B. (2021). The DFUC 2020 Dataset: Analysis Towards Diabetic Foot Ulcer Detection. *TouchEndocrinology*. https://www.touchendocrinology.com/diabetes/journal-articles/the-dfuc-2020-dataset-analysis-towards-diabetic-foot-ulcer-detection/ (accessed Jan. 29, 2023).

Cennamo, C., Dagnino, G. B., & Zhu, F. (2023). *Research Handbook on Digital Strategy*. Edward Elgar Publishing. doi:10.4337/9781800378902

Cerasa, A., Gaggioli, A., Marino, F., Riva, G., & Pioggia, G. (2022). The promise of the metaverse in mental health: The new era of MEDverse. *Heliyon*, *8*(11), 11762. doi:10.1016/j.heliyon.2022.e11762 PMID:36458297

Chae, H. L., & Seul, C. L. (2023). *The Effects of Degrees of Freedom and Field of View on Motion Sickness in a Virtual Reality Context*. Taylors Ad Francis. doi:10.1080/10447318.2023.2241620

Chakraborty, D., Patre, S., & Tiwari, D. (2023). Metaverse mingle: Discovering dating intentions in metaverse. *Journal of Retailing and Consumer Services*, *75*, 103509. Advance online publication. doi:10.1016/j.jretconser.2023.103509

Champion, E. (2022). Mixed histories, augmented pasts. In Human-computer interaction series (pp. 163–184). doi:10.1007/978-3-031-10932-4_7

Chang, L., Zhang, Z., Li, P., Xi, S., Guo, W., Shen, Y., Xiong, Z., Kang, J., Niyato, D., Qiao, X., & Wu, Y. (2022). 6G-enabled edge AI for Metaverse: Challenges, methods, and future research directions. *Journal of Communications and Information Networks*, *7*(2), 107–121. doi:10.23919/JCIN.2022.9815195

Channa, A., Popescu, N., Skibinska, J., & Burget, R. (2021). The rise of wearable devices during the COVID-19 pandemic: A systematic review. *Sensors (Basel)*, *21*(17), 5787. doi:10.339021175787 PMID:34502679

Chatrati, S. P., Hossain, G., Goyal, A., Bhan, A., Bhattacharya, S., Gaurav, D., & Tiwari, S. (2022). Smart home health monitoring system for predicting type 2 diabetes and hypertension. *Journal of King Saud University - Computer and Information Sciences*, *34*(3), 862–870. doi:10.1016/j.jksuci.2020.01.010

Chaudhary, M., Gaur, L., & Chakrabarti, A. (2022a). Comparative Analysis of Entropy Weight Method and C5 Classifier for Predicting Employee Churn. *2022 3rd International Conference on Intelligent Engineering and Management (ICIEM)*, (pp. 232–236). IEEE. 10.1109/ICIEM54221.2022.9853181

Chaudhary, M., Gaur, L., & Chakrabarti, A. (2022b). Detecting the Employee Satisfaction in Retail: A Latent Dirichlet allocation and Machine Learning approach. *2022 3rd International Conference on Computation, Automation and Knowledge Management (ICCAKM)*, (pp. 1–6). IEEE. 10.1109/ICCAKM54721.2022.9990186

Chaudhary, M., Gaur, L., Jhanjhi, N. Z., Masud, M., & Aljahdali, S. (2022). Envisaging Employee Churn Using MCDM and Machine Learning. Intelligent Automation & Soft Computing, 33(2). doi:10.32604/iasc.2022.023417

Chauhan, M., & Agarwal, R. (2023). Impact of screens on how users think. *IEEE Conference P2023 3rd International Conference on Intelligent Technologies (CONIT)Ublication*. IEEE Xplore. 10.1109/CONIT59222.2023.10205565

ChenD.ZhangR. (2022). Exploring research trends of emerging technologies in health metaverse: A bibliometric analysis. Available at SSRN 3998068. doi:10.2139/ssrn.3998068

Chen, G., Peachey, J. W., & Stodolska, M. (2023). Sense of community among virtual race participants: The case of the Illinois Marathon. *Managing Sport and Leisure*, 1–23. doi:10.1080/23750472.2023.2239246

Compilation of References

Chengoden, R., Victor, N., Huynh-The, T., Yenduri, G., Jhaveri, R. H., Alazab, M., Bhattacharya, S., Hegde, P., Maddikunta, P. K. R., & Gadekallu, T. R. (2022). *Metaverse for Healthcare: A Survey on Potential Applications, Challenges and Future Directions.* arXiv preprint arXiv:2209.04160.

Chengoden, R., Victor, N., Huynh-The, T., Yenduri, G., Jhaveri, R. H., Alazab, M., Bhattacharya, S., Hegde, P., Maddikunta, P. K. R., & Gadekallu, T. R. (2023). Metaverse for Healthcare: A survey on potential applications, challenges and future directions. *IEEE Access : Practical Innovations, Open Solutions, 11*, 12765–12795. doi:10.1109/ACCESS.2023.3241628

Chen, H., & Wo'zniak, M. (2022). Mathematical model simulation of detailed classification of telemedicine sensing data. *Mobile Networks and Applications*. doi:10.100711036-022-02025-2

Chen, W., Guo, H., & Tsui, K.-L. (2019). A new medical staff allocation via simulation optimization for an emergency department in Hong Kong. *International Journal of Production Research, 58*, 1–20.

Chen, X., Zou, D., Xie, H., & Wang, F. L. (2023). Metaverse in Education: Contributors, cooperations, and research themes. *IEEE Transactions on Learning Technologies*, 1–18. doi:10.1109/TLT.2023.3277952

Chen, Y., He, H., & Yang, Y. (2023). Effects of Social Support on Professional Identity of Secondary Vocational Students major in Preschool Nursery Teacher Program: A Chain Mediating Model of Psychological Adjustment and School Belonging. *Sustainability, 15*(6), 5134. doi:10.3390u15065134

Chen, Y., Zhou, Z., Cao, M., Liu, M., Lin, Z., Yang, W., Yang, X., Dhaidhai, D., & Xiong, P. (2022). Extended reality (xr) and telehealth interventions for children or adolescents with autism spectrum disorder: Systematic review of qualitative and quantitative studies. *Neuroscience and Biobehavioral Reviews, 138*, 138. doi:10.1016/j.neubiorev.2022.104683 PMID:35523302

Chimakurthi, V. N. S. S. (2019). Efficacy of Augmented Reality in Medical Education. *Malaysian Journal of Medical and Biological Research, 6*(2), 135–142. doi:10.18034/mjmbr.v6i2.609

Cho, K.-H., Park, J.-B., & Kang, A. (2023). Metaverse for Exercise Rehabilitation: Possibilities and Limitations. *International Journal of Environmental Research and Public Health, 20*(8), 5483. doi:10.3390/ijerph20085483 PMID:37107765

Chopra, R. (2023). *Online Religion*, 521–535. Wiley. doi:10.1002/9781119671619.ch33

Cho, Y., Park, M., & Kim, J. (2023). XAVE: Cross-platform based Asymmetric Virtual Environment for Immersive Content. *IEEE Access : Practical Innovations, Open Solutions, 1*, 71890–71904. doi:10.1109/ACCESS.2023.3294390

Chuanhua, Y. (2023). Using Cognitive Therapy to Explore the Potential Application of Traditional Therapy and Metaverse Therapy from a Cognitive Perspective. *SHS Web of Conferences, 171*, 01030. doi:10.1051hsconf/202317101030

Claisse, C., & Durrant, A. (2023). *'Keeping our Faith Alive': Investigating Buddhism Practice during COVID-19 to Inform Design for the Online Community Practice of Faith*. ACM. doi:10.1145/3544548.3581177

Cobry, E. C., & Wadwa, R. P. (2022). The future of telehealth in type 1 diabetes. *Current Opinion in Endocrinology, Diabetes, and Obesity*, *29*(4), 397–402. doi:10.1097/MED.0000000000000745 PMID:35777972

Cooper, R. A., Ohnabe, H., & Hobson, D. A. (2006). *An Introduction to Rehabilitation Engineering*. CRC Press. doi:10.1201/9781420012491

Cornejo, J., Cornejo-Aguilar, J. A., Vargas, M., Helguero, C. G., Milanezi de Andrade, R., Torres-Montoya, S., Asensio-Salazar, J., Rivero Calle, A., Martínez Santos, J., Damon, A., Quiñones-Hinojosa, A., Quintero-Consuegra, M. D., Umaña, J. P., Gallo-Bernal, S., Briceño, M., Tripodi, P., Sebastian, R., Perales-Villarroel, P., De la Cruz-Ku, G., & Russomano, T. (2022). Anatomical Engineering and 3D printing for surgery and medical devices: International review and future exponential innovations. *BioMed Research International*, *2022*, 2022. doi:10.1155/2022/6797745 PMID:35372574

Coulter, J. S. (1947). History and development of physical medicine. *Archives of Physical Medicine and Rehabilitation*, *28*(9), 600–602. PMID:20262280

Covaci, A., Alhasan, K., Loonker, M., Farrell, B., Tabbaa, L., Ppali, S., & Ang, C. S. (2023). *No Pie in the (Digital) Sky: Co-Imagining the Food Metaverse*. ACM. doi:10.1145/3544548.3581305

Crawford, T. (2023). *Sonic Urban Exploration: Connections between disused urban environments and electroacoustic music composition*. SES. https://ses.library.usyd.edu.au/handle/2123/31519

Crew, E. (2023, April 20). How can virtual reality sports training help athletes? *4Experience*. https://4experience.co/how-virtual-reality-sports-training-helps-athletes/

Czegledy, P. K. (2023). Crystal Ball Gazing: The future of sports betting. *Gaming Law Review*, *27*(2), 65–70. doi:10.1089/glr2.2022.0046

Da Silva Schlickmann, D., Molz, P., Uebel, G. C., Santos, C. D., Brand, C., Colombelli, R. W., Da Silva, T. G., Steffens, J. P., Da Silva Limberger Castilhos, E., Benito, P. J., Rieger, A., & Franke, S. I. R. (2023). The moderating role of macronutrient intake in relation to body composition and genotoxicity: A study with gym users. *Mutation Research*, *503660*, 503660. doi:10.1016/j.mrgentox.2023.503660 PMID:37567647

Dagli, N. (2022). Advancement in telemedicine and teledentistry with virtual reality and metaverse. Journal of International Oral Health, 14(6), 529–530.

Damaris, A. (2023, July 4). *The Effect of Physical Activity on Mental Well-being among College Students*. Cari Journals. https://carijournals.org/journals/index.php/ijars/article/view/1336

Compilation of References

Dang, T. H., Nguyen, T. A., Hoang Van, M., Santin, O., Tran, O. M. T., & Schofield, P. (2021). Patient-centered care: Transforming the health care system in Vietnam with support of digital health technology. *Journal of Medical Internet Research*, *23*(6), e24601. doi:10.2196/24601 PMID:34085939

Dash, S., Shakyawar, S. K., Sharma, M., & Kaushik, S. (2019). Big data in healthcare: Management, analysis and future prospects. *Journal of Big Data*, *6*(54), 54. doi:10.118640537-019-0217-0

Davenport, T., & Kalakota, R. (2019). The potential for artificial intelligence in healthcare. *Future Healthcare Journal*, *6*(2), 94–98. doi:10.7861/futurehosp.6-2-94 PMID:31363513

Davis, J., Finlay-Jones, A., Bear, N., Prescott, S. L., Silva, D., & Ohan, J. L. (2023). Time-out for well-being: A mixed methods evaluation of attitudes and likelihood to engage in different types of online emotional well-being programmes in the perinatal period. *Women's Health (London, England)*, *19*. doi:10.1177/17455057231184507 PMID:37431205

De Engenharia, F. (2023, July 25). *Instrument Position In Immersive Audio: A Study On Good Practices And Comparison With Stereo Approaches*. https://repositorio-aberto.up.pt/handle/10216/152055

De Felice, F., Rehman, M., Petrillo, A., & Baffo, I. (2023). A metaworld: Implications, opportunities and risks of the metaverse. *IET Collaborative Intelligent Manufacturing*, *The Institution of Engineering and Technology*, *5*(3), e12079.

De Villiers Bosman, I., Buruk, O. T., Jørgensen, K., & Hamari, J. (2023). The effect of audio on the experience in virtual reality: A scoping review. *Behaviour & Information Technology*, 1–35. doi:10.1080/0144929X.2022.2158371

Degenhard, S. M. (n.d.). *Mobile phone mindfulness: Effects of app-based meditation intervention on stress and HRV of undergraduate students*. UTC Scholar. https://scholar.utc.edu/mps/vol29/iss1/1/

DeGuzman, K. (2021b). What is Virtual Reality — Games, Movies & Storytelling. *StudioBinder*. https://www.studiobinder.com/blog/what-is-virtual-reality/

Delloite (2022). *The hospital of the future; How digital technologies can change hospitals globally*. Deloitte. https://www2.deloitte.com/content/dam/Deloitte/global/Documents/Life-Sciences-Health-Care/us-lshc-hospital-of-the-future.pdf

Demeco, A., Zola, L., Frizziero, A., Martini, C., Palumbo, A., Foresti, R., Buccino, G., & Cipolla, C. (2023). Immersive Virtual Reality in Post-Stroke Rehabilitation: A Systematic Review. *Sensors (Basel)*, *23*(3), 1712. doi:10.339023031712 PMID:36772757

Denecke, K. (2019). Ethical issues of using artificial intelligence in medicine. *Digital Health*, *5*, 1–11. doi:10.1177/2055207619877208

Deng, J., Tajuddin, R. B. M., Chen, Z., Ren, B., & Shariff, S. M. (2023). *The impact of virtual presence on the behavior of live E-Commerce consumers*. Atlantis Press. doi:10.2991/978-94-6463-210-1_47

Desai, K., Bahirat, K., Ramalingam, S., Prabhakaran, B., Annaswamy, T., & Makris, U. E. (2019). Augmented reality-based exergames for rehabilitation. *Journal of Medical Systems*, *43*(10), 316. doi:10.100710916-019-1489-2 PMID:31506773

Desbordes, M. (2023). Analysis of the sport ecosystem and its value chain, What lessons in an uncertain world? In Sports economics, management and policy (pp. 109–142). doi:10.1007/978-981-19-7010-8_6

Dhiman, D. B. (2023, March 10). *Key issues and New Challenges in New Media Technology in 2023: A Critical review.* https://papers.ssrn.com/sol3/papers.cfm?abstract_id=4387353

DhimanB. (2023). Ethical Issues and Challenges in social Media: A current scenario. *Social Science Research Network*. doi:10.2139/ssrn.4406610

DiasS. B.JelinekH. F.HadjileontiadisL. (2023). Wearable Neurofeedback Acceptance Model: An Investigation within Academic Settings to Explore a Multimodal Framework for Student Stress and Anxiety Management. SSRN. doi:10.2139/ssrn.4485826

Diaz-Lopez, D. M., Lopez-Valencia, N. A., Gonzalez-Neira, E. M., Barrera, D., Suarez, D. R., Caro-Gutierrez, M. P., & Sefair, C. (2018). A simulation-optimization approach for the surgery scheduling problem: A case study considering stochastic surgical times. *International Journal of Industrial Engineering Computations*, *9*(4), 409–422. doi:10.5267/j.ijiec.2018.1.002

Dionísio Corrêa, A. G., Ficheman, I. K., do Nascimento, M., & de Deus Lopes, R. (2012). *Contributions of an Augmented Reality Musical System for the Stimulation of Motor Skills in Music Therapy Sessions.* Learning Disabilities. 10.5772/30142

Dirin, A., Nieminen, M., Laine, T. H., Nieminen, L., & Ghalabani, L. (2023). Emotional contagion in Collaborative Virtual Reality Learning Experiences: An eSports approach. *Education and Information Technologies*. doi:10.100710639-023-11769-7

Dogheim, G. M. (2023, June 5). *Patient Care through AI-driven Remote Monitoring: Analyzing the Role of Predictive Models and Intelligent Alerts in Preventive Medicine.* DL Press. https://publications.dlpress.org/index.php/jcha/article/view/20

Dogra, V., Verma, S., Kavita, K., Jhanjhi, N. Z., Ghosh, U., & Le, D. (2022). A comparative analysis of machine learning models for banking news extraction by multiclass classification with imbalanced datasets of financial news: Challenges and solutions. *International Journal of Interactive Multimedia and Artificial Intelligence*, *7*(3), 35. doi:10.9781/ijimai.2022.02.002

Doronzo, F., Nardacchione, G., & Di Muro, E. (2023). Processi neuroplastici associati all'adozione della realtà virtuale: Una revisione sistematica verso un nuovo approccio del trattamento dei disturbi mentali. *IUL Research*, *4*(7), 126–147. doi:10.57568/iulresearch.v4i7.411

Doskarayev, B., Omarov, N., Omarov, B., Ismagulova, Z., Kozhamkulova, Z., Nurlybaeva, E., & Kasimova, G. (2023). Development of computer vision-enabled augmented reality games to increase motivation for sports. *International Journal of Advanced Computer Science and Applications*, *14*(4). doi:10.14569/IJACSA.2023.0140428

Compilation of References

Dosovitskiy, A. (2020). An Image is Worth 16x16 Words: Transformers for Image Recognition at Scale. *Proceedings of the Conference on Neural Information Processing Systems (NeurIPS)*. IEEE.

Dreher, F., & Ströbel, T. (2023). How gamified online loyalty programs enable and facilitate value co-creation: A case study within a sports-related service context. *Journal of Service Theory and Practice*, *33*(5), 671–696. doi:10.1108/JSTP-10-2022-0229

Dreisoerner, A., Ferrandina, C., Schulz, A. P., Nater, U. M., & Junker, N. M. (2023). *Using group-based interactive video teleconferencing to make self-compassion more accessible: A randomized controlled trial*. ScienceDirect. doi:10.1016/j.jcbs.2023.08.001

Dutta, P., Bose, M., Sinha, A., Bhardwaj, R., Ray, S., Roy, S., & Prakash, K. B. (2022). *Challenges in metaverse in problem-based learning as a game-changing virtual-physical environment for personalized content development*. Academic Press.

Dwivedi, Y. K., Hughes, L., Baabdullah, A. M., Ribeiro-Navarrete, S., Giannakis, M., Al-Debei, M. M., Dennehy, D., Metri, B., Buhalis, D., Cheung, C. M., Conboy, K., Doyle, R., Dubey, R., Dutot, V., Felix, R., Goyal, D. P., Gustafsson, A., Hinsch, C., Jebabli, I., & Wamba, S. F. (2022). Metaverse beyond the hype: Multidisciplinary perspectives on emerging challenges, opportunities, and agenda for research, practice and policy. *International Journal of Information Management*, *66*, 102542. doi:10.1016/j.ijinfomgt.2022.102542

Dwivedi, Y. K., Kshetri, N., Hughes, L., Rana, N. P., Baabdullah, A. M., Kar, A. K., Koohang, A., Ribeiro-Navarrete, S., Belei, N., Balakrishnan, J., Basu, S., Behl, A., Davies, G. H., Dutot, V., Dwivedi, R., Evans, L., Felix, R., Foster-Fletcher, R., Giannakis, M., & Yan, M. (2023). Exploring the Darkverse: A Multi-Perspective Analysis of the negative societal impacts of the Metaverse. *Information Systems Frontiers*, *25*(5), 2071–2114. doi:10.100710796-023-10400-x PMID:37361890

Dwivedi, Y.K., Hughes, L., Wang, Y., Alalwan, A.A., & Ahn, S.J., Balakrishnan, J., & Barta, S. (2023). Metaverse marketing: How the metaverse will shape the future of consumer research and practice. *Psychology & Marketing*. John Wiley & Sons.

Ebner, J. T., Hill, R. C., & O'Connor, T. F. (2021, October). Deep learning for automated wound segmentation and measurement in clinical images. *Journal of Wound Care*, *30*(10), 750–757. doi:10.12968/jowc.2021.30.10.750

Ekandjo, T. (2023). *Human-ai collaboration in everyday work-life practices: a coregulation perspective*. AIS Electronic Library (AISeL). https://aisel.aisnet.org/ecis2023_rp/213/

Ekeland, A. G., Bowes, A., & Flottorp, S. (2010). Effectiveness of telemedicine: A systematic review of reviews. *International Journal of Medical Informatics*, *79*(11), 736–771. doi:10.1016/j.ijmedinf.2010.08.006 PMID:20884286

Elhayatmy, G., Dey, N., & Ashour, A. S. (2017). Internet of things based wireless body area network in healthcare. In Studies in Big Data, 3–20.

Elor, A., & Kurniawan, S. (2019). The Ultimate Display for Physical Rehabilitation: A Bridging Review on Immersive Virtual Reality. *Journal of interactive technology and pedagogy*, (15). doi:10.21985/jitp.v0i15.1285

El-Sherif, D. M., Abouzid, M., Elzarif, M. T., Ahmed, A. A., Albakri, A., & Alshehri, M. M. (2022). Telehealth and artificial intelligence insights into healthcare during the covid-19 pandemic. *Health Care, 10*(2). PMID:35206998

Emmelkamp, P. M., & Meyerbröker, K. (2021). Virtual reality therapy in mental health. *Annual Review of Clinical Psychology, 17*(1), 495–519. doi:10.1146/annurev-clinpsy-081219-115923 PMID:33606946

Eom, S., Kim, S., Jiang, Y., Chen, R. J., Roghanizad, A. R., Rosenthal, M. Z., Dunn, J., & Gorlatova, M. (2023). Investigation of Thermal Perception and Emotional Response in Augmented Reality using Digital Biomarkers: A Pilot Study. In *2023 IEEE Conference on Virtual Reality and 3D User Interfaces Abstracts and Workshops (VRW)*. IEEE. 10.1109/VRW58643.2023.00042

EScholarship. (n.d.). One shot learning of simple visual concepts. *eScholarship*. https://escholarship.org/content/qt4ht821jx/qt4ht821jx.pdf

Etehadtavakol, E. Y. K. N., & Kaabouch, N. (2017, November). Automatic segmentation of thermal images of diabetic-at-risk feet using the snakes algorithm. *Infrared Physics & Technology, 86*, 66–76. doi:10.1016/j.infrared.2017.08.022

Evans, R. S. (2016). Electronic health records: Then, now, and in the future. *Yearbook of Medical Informatics, 25*(S 01. Suppl 1), S48–S61. doi:10.15265/IYS-2016-s006 PMID:27199197

Ezawa, I. D., Hollon, S. D., & Robinson, N. J. (2023). Examining Predictors of Depression and Anxiety Symptom change in Cognitive Behavioral Immersion: Observational study. *JMIR Mental Health, 10*, e42377. doi:10.2196/42377 PMID:37450322

Facciola, A. (2019). The role of the hospital environment in the health-care associated infections: A general review of the literature. *European Review for Medical and Pharmacological Sciences, 23*, 1266–1278. PMID:30779096

Fan, X., Wang, H., & Wang, L. (2023). P-2.8: Metaverse: Origin, Current Applications and Prospects for Future Development. *SID Symposium Digest of Technical Papers*, John Wiley & Sons, Ltd. 10.1002dtp.16342

Fazia, T., Bubbico, F., Nova, A., Bruno, S., Iozzi, D., Calgan, B., Caimi, G., Terzaghi, M., Manni, R., & Bernardinelli, L. (2023). Beneficial Effects of an Online Mindfulness-Based Intervention on Sleep Quality in Italian Poor Sleepers during the COVID-19 Pandemic: A Randomized Trial. *International Journal of Environmental Research and Public Health, 20*(3), 2724. doi:10.3390/ijerph20032724 PMID:36768089

Compilation of References

Fazia, T., Bubbico, F., Nova, A., Buizza, C., Cela, H., Iozzi, D., Calgan, B., Maggi, F., Floris, V., Sutti, I., Bruno, S., Ghilardi, A., & Bernardinelli, L. (2023). Improving stress management, anxiety, and mental well-being in medical students through an online Mindfulness-Based Intervention: A randomized study. *Scientific Reports*, *13*(1), 8214. doi:10.103841598-023-35483-z PMID:37217666

Feng, H., Li, C., Liu, J., Wang, L., Ma, J., Li, G., Gan, L., Shang, X., & Wu, Z. (2019). Virtual reality rehabilitation versus conventional physical therapy for improving balance and gait in Parkinson's disease patients: A randomized controlled trial. *Medical Science Monitor*, *25*, 4186–4192. doi:10.12659/MSM.916455 PMID:31165721

Fernandes, F. A., & Werner, C. M. L. (2023). A Scoping review of the metaverse for Software Engineering Education: Overview, Challenges, and opportunities. *Presence (Cambridge, Mass.)*, 1–40. doi:10.1162/pres_a_00371

Fernandez, C. B., & Hui, P. (2022). Life, the Metaverse and Everything: An Overview of Privacy, Ethics, and Governance in Metaverse. *2022 IEEE 42nd International Conference on Distributed Computing Systems Workshops (ICDCSW)*, (pp. 272–277). IEEE. 10.1109/ICDCSW56584.2022.00058

Ferorelli, D., Nardelli, L., Spagnolo, L., Corradi, S., Silvestre, M., Misceo, F., Marrone, M., Zotti, F., Mandarelli, G., Solarino, B., & Dell'Erba, A. (2020). Medical legal aspects of telemedicine in Italy: Application fields, professional liability and focus on care services during the COVID-19 health emergency. *Journal of Primary Care & Community Health*, *11*. doi:10.1177/2150132720985055 PMID:33372570

Ferraro, C., Hemsley, A., & Sands, S. (2022). Embracing diversity, equity, and inclusion (DEI): Considerations and opportunities for brand managers. *Business Horizons*. doi:10.1016/j.bushor.2022.09.005

Ferreira, M. S. L., Antão, J., Pereira, R., Bianchi, I. S., Tovma, N., & Shurenov, N. (2023). Improving real estate CRM user experience and satisfaction: A user-centered design approach. *Journal of Open Innovation*, *9*(2), 100076. doi:10.1016/j.joitmc.2023.100076

Fiske, J. (2023, June 1). *Identity Assurance in an era of Digital Disruption: Planning a Controlled transition*. Harvard Press. https://dash.harvard.edu/handle/1/37376453

Frykberg, G., Gordon, I. L., Reyzelman, A. M., Cazzell, S. M., Fitzgerald, R. H., Rothenberg, G. M., Bloom, J. D., Petersen, B. J., Linders, D. R., Nouvong, A., & Najafi, B. (2017, May). Feasibility and Efficacy of a Smart Mat Technology to Predict Development of Diabetic Plantar Ulcers. *Diabetes Care*, *40*(7), 973–980. doi:10.2337/dc16-2294 PMID:28465454

Furht, B. (2011). *Handbook of Augmented Reality*. Springer Science & Business Media. doi:10.1007/978-1-4614-0064-6

Gaertner, R. J., Kossmann, K. E., Benz, A., Bentele, U. U., Meier, M., Denk, B., Klink, E. S. C., Dimitroff, S. J., & Pruessner, J. C. (2023). Relaxing effects of virtual environments on the autonomic nervous system indicated by heart rate variability: A systematic review. *Journal of Environmental Psychology, 88*, 102035. doi:10.1016/j.jenvp.2023.102035

Gagliardi, E., Bernardini, G., Quagliarini, E., Schumacher, M., & Calvaresi, D. (2023). Characterization and future perspectives of Virtual Reality Evacuation Drills for safe built environments: A Systematic Literature Review. *Safety Science, 163*, 106141. doi:10.1016/j.ssci.2023.106141

Galati, R., Simone, M., Barile, G., De Luca, R., Cartanese, C., & Grassi, G. (2020). Experimental setup employed in the operating room based on virtual and mixed reality: Analysis of pros and cons in open abdomen surgery. *Journal of Healthcare Engineering.* doi:10.1155/2020/8851964 PMID:32832048

Ganapathy, K., & Ravindra, A. (2009). Telemedicine in india: The apollo story. *Telemedicine Journal and e-Health, 15*(6), 576–585. doi:10.1089/tmj.2009.0066 PMID:19659414

Gao, Q., & Zhang, L. (2023). Brief mindfulness meditation intervention improves attentional control of athletes in virtual reality shooting competition: Evidence from fNIRS and eye tracking. *Psychology of Sport and Exercise, 102477.* doi:10.1016/j.psychsport.2023.102477 PMID:37665918

Garfin, D. R., Amador, A., Osorio, J., Ruivivar, K. S., Torres, A., & Nyamathi, A. (2023). Adaptation of a mindfulness-based intervention for trauma-exposed, unhoused women with substance use disorder. *Psychological Trauma: Theory, Research, Practice, and Policy.* doi:10.1037/tra0001486 PMID:37307346

Gasmet. (2022). *Emission Monitoring Book.* GT500 Terra, gasmet.com.

Gaur, L. and Jhanjhi, N. (2022). *Digital twins and healthcare: Trends, techniques, and challenges.* doi: 10.4018/978-1-6684-5925-6

Gaur, L., Jhanjhi, N. Z., Bakshi, S., & Gupta, P. (2022). Analyzing Consequences of Artificial Intelligence on Jobs using Topic Modeling and Keyword Extraction. *2022 2nd International Conference on Innovative Practices in Technology and Management (ICIPTM),* (pp. 435–440). IEEE. 10.1109/ICIPTM54933.2022.9754064

Gaur, L., & Afaq, A. (2020). Metamorphosis of CRM: incorporation of social media to customer relationship management in the hospitality industry. In *Handbook of Research on Engineering Innovations and Technology Management in Organizations* (pp. 1–23). IGI Global. doi:10.4018/978-1-7998-2772-6.ch001

Gaur, L., Afaq, A., Arora, G. K., & Khan, N. (2023). Artificial intelligence for carbon emissions using system of systems theory. *Ecological Informatics, 76*, 102165. doi:10.1016/j.ecoinf.2023.102165

Compilation of References

Gaur, L., Afaq, A., Singh, G., & Dwivedi, Y. K. (2021). Role of artificial intelligence and robotics to foster the touchless travel during a pandemic: A review and research agenda. *International Journal of Contemporary Hospitality Management, Emerald Publishing Limited, 33*(11), 4079–4098. doi:10.1108/IJCHM-11-2020-1246

Gaur, L., Afaq, A., Solanki, A., Singh, G., Sharma, S., Jhanjhi, N. Z., My, H. T., & Le, D.-N. (2021). Capitalizing on big data and revolutionary 5G technology: Extracting and visualizing ratings and reviews of global chain hotels. *Computers & Electrical Engineering, 95*, 107374. doi:10.1016/j.compeleceng.2021.107374

Gaur, L., Bhatia, U., Jhanjhi, N. Z., Muhammad, G., & Masud, M. (2021). Medical image-based detection of COVID-19 using Deep Convolution Neural Networks. *Multimedia Systems*. doi:10.100700530-021-00794-6 PMID:33935377

Gaur, L., & Garg, P. K. (2023). *Emerging Trends, Techniques, and Applications in Geospatial Data Science*. IGI Global. doi:10.4018/978-1-6684-7319-1

Gaur, L., & Jhanjhi, N. Z. (2023). *Metaverse Applications for Intelligent Healthcare*. IGI Global.

Gaur, L., Rana, J., & Jhanjhi, N. Z. (2023). *Digital Twin and Healthcare: Trends, Techniques, and Challenges*. IGI Global. doi:10.4018/978-1-6684-5925-6

Gaur, L., & Sahoo, B. M. (2022). Explainable AI in ITS: Ethical Concerns. In *Explainable Artificial Intelligence for Intelligent Transportation Systems: Ethics and Applications* (pp. 79–90). Springer. doi:10.1007/978-3-031-09644-0_5

Gaur, L., Singh, G., & Agarwal, V. (2021). Leveraging Artificial Intelligence Tools to Combat the COVID-19 Crisis. In P. K. Singh, G. Veselov, V. Vyatkin, A. Pljonkin, J. M. Dodero, & Y. Kumar (Eds.), *Futuristic Trends in Network and Communication Technologies* (pp. 321–328). doi:10.1007/978-981-16-1480-4_28

Gaur, L., Singh, G., Hinchey, M., Singh, G., & Jain, V. (2022). Applications of computational intelligence techniques to software engineering problems. *Innovations in Systems and Software Engineering, 18*(2), 231–232. doi:10.100711334-021-00394-7

Gaur, L., Solanki, A., Wamba, S. F., & Jhanjhi, N. Z. (Eds.). (2021). *Advanced AI Techniques and Applications in Bioinformatics*. CRC Press. doi:10.1201/9781003126164

Georgiou, K. E., Georgiou, E., & Satava, R. M. (2021). 5g use in healthcare: The future is present. *JSLS: Journal of the Society of Laparoscopic & Robotic Surgeons, 25*(4), e2021.00064.

Ghose, A., Acharjee, U., & Sharmin, S. (2022). Deep viewing for the identification of Covid-19 infection status from chest X-Ray image using CNN based architecture. *Intelligent systems with applications, 16*, 200130–200130. . doi:10.1016/j.iswa.2022.200130

Ghose, P., Uddin, A., Manzurul M., Islam, M., & Acharjee, U. (2022). *A Breast Cancer Detection Model using a Tuned SVM Classifier*. IEEE. . doi:10.1109/ICCIT57492.2022.10055054

Ghose, P., Biswas, M., & Gaur, L. (2023). BrainSegNeT: A Lightweight Brain Tumor Segmentation Model Based on U-Net and Progressive Neuron Expansion. In F. Liu, Y. Zhang, H. Kuai, E. P. Stephen, & H. Wang (Eds.), *Brain Informatics* (pp. 249–260). Springer Nature Switzerland. doi:10.1007/978-3-031-43075-6_22

Ghose, P., Sharmin, S., Gaur, L., & Zhao, Z. (2022). Grid-Search Integrated Optimized Support Vector Machine Model for Breast Cancer Detection. *2022 IEEE International Conference on Bioinformatics and Biomedicine (BIBM)*, (pp. 2846–2852). IEEE. 10.1109/BIBM55620.2022.9995703

Gill, S. H., Razzaq, M. A., Ahmad, M., Almansour, F. M., Haq, I. U., Jhanjhi, N. Z., Alam, M. Z., & Masud, M. (2022). Security and privacy aspects of cloud Computing: A Smart Campus case study. *Intelligent Automation and Soft Computing*, *31*(1), 117–128. doi:10.32604/iasc.2022.016597

Glen, S. (2023). History of the metaverse in one picture. *Data Science Central*. https://www.datasciencecentral.com/history-of-the-metaverse-in-one-picture/

Goel, R., Baral, S. K., Mishra, T., & Jain, V. (2023). *Augmented and Virtual Reality in Industry 5.0*. Walter de Gruyter GmbH & Co KG. doi:10.1515/9783110790146

Goldsworthy, A., Chawla, J., Birta, J., Baumanna, O., & Gough, S. (2023). Use of extended reality in sleep health, medicine, and research: A scoping review. *Sleep (Basel)*, zsad201. doi:10.1093leep/zsad201 PMID:37498981

Goldwater, J. C., Zhang, Y., Harris, Y., Saurabh, C., & Summers, R. L. (2023). A new frontier in telehealth research: A national telehealth data warehouse. *Telemedicine Journal and e-Health*, *29*(9), 1426–1429. doi:10.1089/tmj.2022.0422 PMID:36799938

Goodfellow, I., Pouget-Abadie, J., Mirza, M., Xu, B., Warde-Farley, D., Ozair, S., Courville, A., & Bengio, Y. (2014). Generative Adversarial Nets. Advances in Neural Information Processing Systems (NIPS), (pp. 2672-2680).

Goyal, M. (2020). *Robust Methods for Real-time Diabetic Foot Ulcer, Detection and Localization on Mobile Devices*. IEEE.

Goyal, M., Reeves, N. D., Rajbhandari, S., Ahmad, N., Wang, C., & Yap, M. H. (2020, February). Recognition of ischaemia and infection in diabetic foot ulcers: Dataset and techniques. *Computers in Biology and Medicine*, *117*, 103616. doi:10.1016/j.compbiomed.2020.103616 PMID:32072964

Grech, A., Mehnen, J., & Wodehouse, A. (2023). An extended AI-Experience: Industry 5.0 in Creative Product innovation. *Sensors (Basel)*, *23*(6), 3009. doi:10.339023063009 PMID:36991718

Greenhalgh, G. P., & Goebert, C. (2023). From Gearshifts to Gigabytes: An analysis of how NASCAR used iRacing to engage fans during the COVID-19 shutdown. *International Journal of Sport Communication*, 1–15. doi:10.1123/ijsc.2023-0145

Gulick, W. (2023). Polanyi, zen and non-linguistic knowledge. In Comparative philosophy of religion (pp. 91–106). doi:10.1007/978-3-031-18013-2_7

Compilation of References

Gupta, N. S., & Kumar, P. (2023). Perspective of artificial intelligence in healthcare data management: A journey towards precision medicine. *Computers in Biology and Medicine*, *162*, 107051. doi:10.1016/j.compbiomed.2023.107051 PMID:37271113

Győrffy, Z., Radó, N., & Mesko, B. (2020). Digitally engaged physicians about the digital health transition. *PLoS One*, *15*(9), e0238658. doi:10.1371/journal.pone.0238658 PMID:32986733

Hadi, R., Melumad, S., & Park, E. S. (2023). The Metaverse: A new digital frontier for consumer behavior. *Journal of Consumer Psychology*, jcpy.1356. doi:10.1002/jcpy.1356

Hailey, D., Roine, R., & Ohinmaa, A. (2002). Systematic review of evidence for the benefits of telemedicine. *Journal of Telemedicine and Telecare*, *8*(1_suppl, Suppl 1), 1–30. doi:10.1258/1357633021937604 PMID:12020415

Haley, A. C., Thorpe, D., Pelletier, A., Yarosh, S., & Keefe, D. F. (2023). Inward VR: Toward a qualitative method for investigating interoceptive awareness in VR. *IEEE Transactions on Visualization and Computer Graphics*, *29*(5), 2557–2566. doi:10.1109/TVCG.2023.3247074 PMID:37027715

Hall, J. F. (2007). The History of Rehabilitation Medicine: A Brief Overview. *The Journal of the American Osteopathic Association*, *107*(9), 385–390.

Hameed, K., Bajwa, I. S., Sarwar, N., Anwar, W., Mushtaq, Z., & Rashid, T. (2021). Integration of 5g and block-chain technologies in smart telemedicine using iot. *Journal of Healthcare Engineering*, *2021*, 2021. doi:10.1155/2021/8814364 PMID:33824715

Hamet, P., & Tremblay, J. (2017). Artificial intelligence in medicine. *Metabolism: Clinical and Experimental*, *69*, S36–S40. doi:10.1016/j.metabol.2017.01.011 PMID:28126242

Hamid, B., Jhanjhi, N. Z., Humayun, M., Khan, A. F., & Alsayat, A. (2019). Cyber Security Issues and Challenges for Smart Cities: A survey. *2019 13th International Conference on Mathematics, Actuarial Science, Computer Science and Statistics (MACS)*. 10.1109/macs48846.2019.9024768

Hamid, B., Jhanjhi, N. Z., Humayun, M., Khan, A. F., & Alsayat, A. (2019). Cyber Security Issues and Challenges for Smart Cities: A survey. In *2019 13th International Conference on Mathematics, Actuarial Science, Computer Science and Statistics (MACS)*. ACM. 10.1109/MACS48846.2019.9024768

Han, E., Miller, M. R., DeVeaux, C., Jun, H., Nowak, K. L., Hancock, J. T., Ram, N., & Bailenson, J. N. (2023). People, places, and time: A large-scale, longitudinal study of transformed avatars and environmental context in group interaction in the metaverse. *Journal of Computer-Mediated Communication*, *28*(2), zmac031. doi:10.1093/jcmc/zmac031

Hang, Y. (2023). Research on the problems and countermeasures in the In-Person Fitness industry in the post-pandemic era. *Highlights in Business, Economics and Management*, *13*, 29–38. doi:10.54097/hbem.v13i.8618

Harutyunyan, M. (2023). Exploring the Rich Tapestry of Gardens and Parks: A Journey through History, Education, and Artistic Expressions. *Harutyunyan | Indonesian Journal of Multidiciplinary Research*. doi:10.17509/ijomr.v3i2.60561

Hasapeehko, A. (2023). *Marketing determinants of consumer behaviour change in the food market*. SUM DU. https://essuir.sumdu.edu.ua/handle/123456789/92038

Hasson, H., Rundgren, E. H., & Schwarz, U. V. T. (2023). *The adaptation and fidelity tool to support social service practitioners in balancing fidelity and adaptations: Longitudinal, mixed-method evaluation study*. SIRC. doi:10.1177/26334895231189198

Hawajri, O., Lindberg, J., & Suominen, S. (2023). Virtual Reality Exposure Therapy as a Treatment Method Against Anxiety Disorders and Depression-A Structured Literature Review. *Issues in Mental Health Nursing*, 1–25. 10.1080/01612840.2023.2190051

He, K., Zhang, X., Ren, S., & Sun, J. (2016). *Identity Mappings in Deep Residual Networks*. arXiv.org. https://arxiv.org/abs/1603.05027 doi:10.1007/978-3-319-46493-0_38

Heinrich, D., & O'Connell, K. A. (2023). The effects of mindfulness meditation on nursing students' stress and anxiety levels. *Nursing Education Perspectives*. doi:10.1097/01.NEP.0000000000001159 PMID:37404039

Hensher, D. A., Mulley, C., & Nelson, J. D. (2023). What is an ideal (Utopian) mobility as a service (MaaS) framework? A communication note. *Transportation Research Part A, Policy and Practice*, *172*, 103675. doi:10.1016/j.tra.2023.103675

Hillebrand, K., Hornuf, L., Müller, B., & Vrankar, D. (2023). The social dilemma of big data: Donating personal data to promote social welfare. *Information and Organization*, *33*(1), 100452. doi:10.1016/j.infoandorg.2023.100452

Høeg, E. R., Andersen, N. B., Malmkjær, N., Vaaben, A. H., & Uth, J. (2023). Hospitalized older adults' experiences of virtual reality-based group exercise therapy with cycle ergometers: An early feasibility study. *Computers in Human Behavior Reports*, *11*, 100301. doi:10.1016/j.chbr.2023.100301

Hollensen, S., Kotler, P., & Opresnik, M. O. (2023). Metaverse – the new marketing universe. *Journal of Business Strategy, Emerald Publishing Limited*, *44*(3), 119–125. doi:10.1108/JBS-01-2022-0014

Holley, R., Moldow, E., Chaudhary, S., Gaumond, G., Hacker, R. L., Kahn, P., Boeldt, D., & Hubley, S. (2022). A qualitative study of virtual reality and mindfulness for substance use disorders. *Journal of Technology in Behavioral Science*, *8*(1), 36–46. doi:10.100741347-022-00284-0

Höner, O., Dugandzic, D., Hauser, T., Stügelmaier, M., Willig, N., & Schultz, F. (2023). Do you have a good all-around view? Evaluation of a decision-making skills diagnostic tool using 360° videos and head-mounted displays in elite youth soccer. *Frontiers in Sports and Active Living*, *5*, 1171262. doi:10.3389/fspor.2023.1171262 PMID:37342613

Compilation of References

Hong, J. S., Wasden, C., & Han, D. H. (2021). Introduction of digital therapeutics. *Computer Methods and Programs in Biomedicine*, *209*, 106319. doi:10.1016/j.cmpb.2021.106319 PMID:34364181

Hopkins, J. L., & Bardoel, A. (2023). The future is hybrid: How organisations are designing and supporting sustainable hybrid work models in Post-Pandemic Australia. *Sustainability*, *15*(4), 3086. doi:10.3390u15043086

Huang, H., Li, Y., & Cai, S. (2023). Best Practices for Integrating 360 VR Videos into Psychology Teaching. *2023 9th International Conference on Virtual Reality (ICVR)*. 10.1109/icvr57957.2023.10169358

Huang, L. (2020). Deep learning-based prediction of diabetic foot ulcer healing potential: A prospective multicenter study. *Wound Repair and Regeneration*, *28*(2), 251–258. doi:10.1111/wrr.12801

Hughes, J., Martin, T., Gladwell, T. D., Akiyode, O., Purnell, M. C., Shahid, M., Moultry, A. M., Rapp, K. I., & Unonu, J. (2023). Lessons from a cross-institutional online professional development pilot. *Currents in Pharmacy Teaching & Learning*, *15*(5), 534–540. doi:10.1016/j.cptl.2023.05.004 PMID:37202331

Humayun, M. (2020). Role of emerging IoT big data and cloud computing for real time application. *International Journal of Advanced Computer Science and Applications*, *11*(4). Advance online publication. doi:10.14569/IJACSA.2020.0110466

Humayun, M., Jhanjhi, N. Z., Alruwaili, M., Amalathas, S. S., Balasubramanian, V., & Selvaraj, B. (2020). Privacy protection and energy optimization for 5G-Aided industrial internet of things. *IEEE Access : Practical Innovations, Open Solutions*, *8*, 183665–183677. doi:10.1109/ACCESS.2020.3028764

Humayun, M., Niazi, M., Jhanjhi, N. Z., Alshayeb, M., & Mahmood, S. (2020b). Cyber Security Threats and Vulnerabilities: A Systematic Mapping study. *Arabian Journal for Science and Engineering*, *45*(4), 3171–3189. doi:10.100713369-019-04319-2

Huq, S. M., Maskeliūnas, R., & Damaševičius, R. (2022). Dialogue agents for artificial intelligence-based conversational systems for cognitively disabled: A systematic review. *Disability and Rehabilitation. Assistive Technology*, 1–20. doi:10.1080/17483107.2022.2146768 PMID:36413423

Hutson, J. (n.d.). *Life, death, and AI: Exploring digital necromancy in popular culture—Ethical considerations, technological limitations, and the pet cemetery conundrum*. Digital Commons@ Lindenwood University. https://digitalcommons.lindenwood.edu/faculty-research-papers/478/

Huynh-The, T., Pham, Q., Pham, X., Nguyen, T., Han, Z., & Kim, D. (2023). Artificial intelligence for the metaverse: A survey. *Engineering Applications of Artificial Intelligence*, *117*, 105581. doi:10.1016/j.engappai.2022.105581

Hwang, G.-J., & Chien, S.-Y. (2022). Definition, roles, and potential research issues of the metaverse in education: An artificial intelligence perspective. *Computers and Education: Artificial Intelligence*, *3*, 100082. doi:10.1016/j.caeai.2022.100082

Ibanez Valdes, L. F., Joseph, S. S., & Sibat, H. F. (2023). Rituximab in Refractory Myasthenia Gravis: A Systematic Review. *Clinical Schizophrenia & Related Psychoses*, *17*(1), 1–8.

Iloudi, M., Lindner, P., Ali, L., Wallström, S., Thunström, A. O., Ioannou, M., Anving, N., Johansson, V., Hamilton, W., Falk, Ö., & Steingrimsson, S. (2022). Physical Versus Virtual Reality-based Calm Rooms for Psychiatric Inpatients: A Quasi-randomized Trial (Preprint). *Journal of Medical Internet Research*. doi:10.2196/42365

Inceoglu, M. M., & Ciloglugil, B. (2022). Use of Metaverse in Education. In O. Gervasi, B. Murgante, S. Misra, A. M. A. C. Rocha, & C. Garau (Eds.), *Computational Science and Its Applications – ICCSA 2022 Workshops* (pp. 171–184). Springer International Publishing. doi:10.1007/978-3-031-10536-4_12

Ingendoh, R. M., Posny, E. S., & Heine, A. (2023). Binaural beats to entrain the brain? A systematic review of the effects of binaural beat stimulation on brain oscillatory activity, and the implications for psychological research and intervention. *PLoS One*, *18*(5), e0286023. doi:10.1371/journal.pone.0286023 PMID:37205669

Inwood, H. (2022). Towards Sinophone Game Studies. *Apollo (London. 1925)*, *12*(2), 1–10. doi:10.51661/bjocs.v12i2.219

Issa, M. E., Helm, A. M., Al-Qaness, M. A. A., Dahou, A., Elaziz, M. A., & Damaševičius, R. (2022). Human activity recognition based on embedded sensor data fusion for the internet of healthcare things. *Health Care*, *10*(6). PMID:35742136

Iwanaga, J., Muo, E. C., Tabira, Y., Watanabe, K., Tubbs, S. J., D'Antoni, A. V., & Rajaram-Gilkes, M. (2023). Who really needs a Metaverse in anatomy education? A review with preliminary survey results. *Clinical Anatomy*. John Wiley & Sons. doi:10.1002/ca.23949 PMID:36087277

Jaap, J. van Netten, D., Lazzarini, P., & Janda, M. (2020). The validity and reliability of remote diabetic foot ulcer assessment using mobile phone images. Springer. link.springer.com/content/pdf/10.1038/s41598-017-09828-4.pdf

Jabbar, R., Fetais, N., Krichen, M., & Barkaoui, K. (2020). Blockchain technology for healthcare: Enhancing shared electronic health record interoperability and integrity. In *2020 IEEE International Conference on Informatics, IoT, and Enabling Technologies (ICIoT)*. IEEE.

Jain, M., Singh, G., & Gaur, L. (2021). Green Internet of Things: Next-Generation Intelligence for Sustainable Development. In P. K. Kapur, G. Singh, & S. Panwar (Eds.), *Advances in Interdisciplinary Research in Engineering and Business Management* (pp. 359–367). doi:10.1007/978-981-16-0037-1_28

JAMA. (2023). *Home*. JAMA: The Latest Medical Research, Reviews, and Guidelines. https://jamanetwork.com/journals/jama

Jamshidi, M. (2023). *The Meta-Metaverse: Ideation and future Directions*. MDPI., doi:10.3390/fi15080252

Compilation of References

Javed, N., Ahmed, T., Faisal, M., Sadia, H., & Sidaine-Daumiller, E. Z. J. (2023). Workplace cyberbullying in the Remote-Work era. In *Advances in human and social aspects of technology book series* (pp. 166–177). doi:10.4018/978-1-6684-8133-2.ch009

Jee, Y.-S. (2023). Application of metaverse technology to exercise rehabilitation: Present and future. *Journal of Exercise Rehabilitation*, *19*(2), 93–94. doi:10.12965/jer.2346050.025 PMID:37163182

Jerath R. Syam M. Ahmed S. Z. (2023). *The Future of Stress Management: Integration Smartwatches and HRV Technology*. doi:10.20944/preprints202307.1283.v2

Jhanjhi, N. Z., Humayun, M., & Almuayqil, S. N. (2021). Cyber security and privacy issues in industrial internet of things. *Computer Systems Science and Engineering*, *37*(3), 361–380. doi:10.32604/csse.2021.015206

Jhuang, Y., Yan, Y., & Horng, G. (2023). GDPR Personal Privacy Security Mechanism for smart home system. *Electronics (Basel)*, *12*(4), 831. doi:10.3390/electronics12040831

Jiang, X., Deng, N., & Zheng, S. (2023). Understanding the core technological features of virtual and augmented reality in tourism: A qualitative and quantitative review. *Current Issues in Tourism*, 1–21. doi:10.1080/13683500.2023.2198118

Jin, N., Wu, Y., Park, J., Qin, Z., & Li, Z. (2023). Brain-Metaverse Interaction for Anxiety Regulation. *2023 9th International Conference on Virtual Reality (ICVR)*. 10.1109/icvr57957.2023.10169785

Jo, H. (2023). Tourism in the digital frontier: a study on user continuance intention in the metaverse. *Springer Link*. https://link.springer.com/article/10.1007/s40558-023-00257-w

Jo, H., Seidel, L., Pahud, M., Sinclair, M., & Bianchi, A. (2023). *FlowAR: How Different Augmented Reality Visualizations of Online Fitness Videos Support Flow for At-Home Yoga Exercises*. ACM. doi:10.1145/3544548.3580897

Jonathan, N. T., Bachri, M. R., Wijaya, E., Ramdhan, D., & Chowanda, A. (2023). The efficacy of virtual reality exposure therapy (VRET) with extra intervention for treating PTSD symptoms. *Procedia Computer Science*, *216*, 252–259. doi:10.1016/j.procs.2022.12.134

Jones, L., Lee, M., & Gomes, R. S. M. (2023). Remote rehabilitation (telerehabilitation) in the sight loss sector: Reflections on challenges and opportunities from service providers in the United Kingdom. *British Journal of Visual Impairment*, 02646196231188634. doi:10.1177/02646196231188634

Joshi, J. (2023, August 5). *PhysioKit: open-source, low-cost physiological computing toolkit for single and multi-user studies*. https://arxiv.org/abs/2308.02756

Kaaria, A. G., & Mwaruta, S. S. (2023). Mental Health Ingenuities and the Role of computer Technology on Employees' Mental Health: A Systematic review. *East African Journal of Health & Science*, *6*(1), 219–231. doi:10.37284/eajhs.6.1.1268

Kaddoura, S., & Al Husseiny, F. (2023). The rising trend of Metaverse in education: Challenges, opportunities, and ethical considerations. *PeerJ Computer Science*, *9*, e1252. PMID:37346578

Kaddoura, S., & Husseiny, F. A. (2023). The rising trend of Metaverse in education: Challenges, opportunities, and ethical considerations. *PeerJ*, *9*, e1252. doi:10.7717/peerj-cs.1252 PMID:37346578

Kahlmann, V., Moor, C. C., Van Helmondt, S. J., Mostard, R. L. M., Van Der Lee, M., Grutters, J. C., Wijsenbeek, M., & Veltkamp, M. (2023). Online mindfulness-based cognitive therapy for fatigue in patients with sarcoidosis (TIRED): A randomised controlled trial. *The Lancet. Respiratory Medicine*, *11*(3), 265–272. doi:10.1016/S2213-2600(22)00387-3 PMID:36427515

Kaihua, N. (2023, June 1). *Disruptive Innovation in Finnish hospitality: An analysis and mapping of incumbent perceptions*. Osuva. https://osuva.uwasa.fi/handle/10024/15987

Kaiser, M. (2023). *Proceedings of the Fourth International Conference on Trends in Computational and Cognitive Engineering*. Springer. https://doi.org/. doi:10.1007-978-981-19-9483-8

Kakhi, K., Alizadehsani, R., Kabir, H. M. D., Khosravi, A., Nahavandi, S., & Acharya, U. R. (2022). The internet of medical things and artificial intelli-gence: Trends, challenges, and opportunities. *Biocybernetics and Biomedical Engineering*, *42*(3), 749–771. doi:10.1016/j.bbe.2022.05.008

Kalasin, S., & Surareungchai, W. (2022). Challenges of emerging wearable sen-sors for remote monitoring toward telemedicine healthcare. *Analytical Chemistry*. doi: 10.1021/acs.analchem.2c02642

Kaleva, I., & Riches, S. (2023). Stepping inside the whispers and tingles: Multisensory virtual reality for enhanced relaxation and wellbeing. *Frontiers in Digital Health*, *5*, 1212586. doi:10.3389/fdgth.2023.1212586 PMID:37534028

Kamaruddin, I. K., Ma'rof, A. M., Nazan, A. I. N. M., & Jalil, H. A. (2023). A systematic review and meta-analysis of interventions to decrease cyberbullying perpetration and victimization: An in-depth analysis within the Asia Pacific region. *Frontiers in Psychiatry*, *14*, 1014258. doi:10.3389/fpsyt.2023.1014258 PMID:36778634

Kanwal, N., Janssen, E. M., & Engan, K. (2023). *Balancing privacy and progress in artificial intelligence: Anonymization in histopathology for biomedical research and education*. Cornell University. doi:10.48550/arxiv.2307.09426

Karamizadeh, S. (2021). A machine learning approach for the prediction of diabetic foot ulceration: Development and validation of a clinical decision support system. *Journal of Medical Internet Research*, *23*(1), e17544. doi:10.2196/17544

Karthi, M., Alsager, M., Metha, R., & Nash, N. F. (2023). Digital Solution: Breaking the barriers to address stigma of mental health. In *IEEE EUROCON 2023 - 20th International Conference on Smart Technologies*. IEEE. 10.1109/EUROCON56442.2023.10198879

Kaswan, K. S., Gaur, L., Dhatterwal, J. S., & Kumar, R. (2021). AI-based natural language processing for the generation of meaningful information electronic health record (EHR) data. In L. Gaur, A. Solanki, S. F. Wamba, & N. Z. Jhanjhi (Eds.), *Advanced AI Techniques and Applications in Bioinformatics* (pp. 46–86). CRC Press. doi:10.1201/9781003126164-3

Compilation of References

Kato, N. (2023). *Comparison of Smoothness, Movement Speed and Trajectory during Reaching Movements in Real and Virtual Spaces Using a Head-Mounted Display*. MDPI. doi:10.3390/life13081618

Kavakiotis, I., Tsave, O., Salifoglou, A., Maglaveras, N., Vlahavas, I., & Chuvarada, I. (2017). Machine Learning and Data Mining Methods in Diabetes Research. *Computational and Structural Biotechnology Journal, 15*, 104–116. doi:10.1016/j.csbj.2016.12.005 PMID:28138367

Kavanagh, J. M., & Sharpnack, P. (2021). Crisis in Competency: A Defining Moment in Nursing Education. *Online Journal of Issues in Nursing, 26*(1). doi:10.3912/OJIN.Vol26No01Man02

Kępińska, A., & Wiśniewski, R. (2023). Metaverse and its creative potential for visual arts. *Acta Universitatis Lodziensis, 85*(85), 57–75. doi:10.18778/0208-600X.85.04

Kesavan, D., & N, M. A. (2023). *Emerging insights on the relationship between cryptocurrencies and decentralized economic models*. IGI Global.

Ketu, S., & Mishra, P. K. (2021). Internet of healthcare things: A contemporary survey. *Journal of Network and Computer Applications, 192*, 192. doi:10.1016/j.jnca.2021.103179

Khalifa, A., Mesbah, A., & El-Metwally, A. (2021). Deep Learning-Based Prediction of Diabetic Foot Ulcers: A Review. *IEEE Access: Practical Innovations, Open Solutions, 9*, 8576–8597. doi:10.1109/ACCESS.2021.3044089

Khandakar, Chowdhury, M. E. H., Ibne Reaz, M. B., Md Ali, S. H., Hasan, M. A., Kiranyaz, S., Rahman, T., Alfkey, R., Bakar, A. A. A., & Malik, R. A. (2021, October). A machine learning model for early detection of diabetic foot using thermogram images. *Computers in Biology and Medicine, 137*, 104838. doi:10.1016/j.compbiomed.2021.104838 PMID:34534794

Khan, S., Kannapiran, T., Muthiah, A., & Shetty, S. (2023). *Exergaming intervention for children, adolescents, and elderly people*. IGI Global. doi:10.4018/978-1-6684-6320-8

Khare, V., Agrawal, A., Gupta, P., & Saxena, S. (2019). Artificial intelli-gence based afb microscopy for pulmonary tuberculosis in north india: A pilot study. [IJSRP]. *International Journal of Scientific and Research Publications, 9*(12), 9669. doi:10.29322/IJSRP.9.12.2019.p9669

Khemchandani, V., Goswani, K., Teotia, M. P., Chandra, S., & Wadalkar, N. M. (2023). Virtual Reality Based Attention Simulator using EEG Signals. In *2023 2nd Edition of IEEE Delhi Section Flagship Conference (DELCON)*. IEEE. 10.1109/delcon57910.2023.10127358

Kim, D. Y., & Kim, S. Y. (2023). Investigating the effect of customer-generated content on performance in online platform-based experience goods market. *Journal of Retailing and Consumer Services, 74*, 103409. doi:10.1016/j.jretconser.2023.103409

Kim, E. J., & Kim, J. (2023). The Metaverse for Healthcare: Trends, applications, and future directions of digital therapeutics for Urology. *International Neurourology Journal, 27*(Suppl 1), S3–S12. doi:10.5213/inj.2346108.054 PMID:37280754

Kim, K. B., & Baek, H. J. (2023). Photoplethysmography in Wearable Devices: A comprehensive review of technological advances, current challenges, and future directions. *Electronics (Basel)*, *12*(13), 2923. doi:10.3390/electronics12132923

Kim, R., Mishra, C., & Sen, S. (2022). The use of teleconsultation and technol-ogy by the aravind eye care system, india. *Community Eye Health*, *35*(114), 10. PMID:36035096

King, J., Halversen, A., Richards, O., John, K. K., & Strong, B. (2023). Anxiety and physiological responses to virtual reality and audio meditation in racial and ethnic minorities. *Journal of Technology in Behavioral Science*. doi:10.1007/s41347-023-00330-5

Knoll, T., Liaqat, A., & Monroy-Hernández, A. (2023). *ARctic Escape: Promoting Social Connection, Teamwork, and Collaboration Using a Co-Located Augmented Reality Escape Room*. ACM Digital Library. doi:10.1145/3544549.3585841

Koizumi, Y., Suzuki, Y., Kojima, M., & Sujikai, H. (2019). *Evaluation of Prototype Transmitter and Receiver with 64APSK Coded Modulation in Non-Linear Channel*. IEEE. . doi:10.1109/ICCE.2019.8662070

Koleck, T. A., Dreisbach, C., Bourne, P. E., & Bakken, S. (2019). Natural language processing of symptoms documented in free-text narratives of electronic health records: A systematic review. *Journal of the American Medical Informatics Association*, *26*(4), 364–379. doi:10.1093/jamia/ocy173 PMID:30726935

Koohang, A., Nord, J. H., Ooi, K., Tan, G. W., Al-Emran, M., Aw, E. C., Baabdullah, A. M., Buhalis, D., Cham, T., Dennis, C., Dutot, V., Dwivedi, Y. K., Hughes, L., Mogaji, E., Pandey, N., Phau, I., Raman, R., Sharma, A., Sigala, M., & Wong, L. (2023). Shaping the Metaverse into Reality: A Holistic Multidisciplinary Understanding of Opportunities, Challenges, and Avenues for Future Investigation. *Journal of Computer Information Systems*, *63*(3), 735–765. doi:10.1080/08874417.2023.2165197

Korzynski, P., Koźmiński, A. K., & Baczyńska, A. (2023). Navigating leadership challenges with technology: Uncovering the potential of ChatGPT, virtual reality, human capital management systems, robotic process automation, and social media. *Przedsiębiorczość Międzynarodowa*, *9*(2), 7–18. doi:10.15678/IER.2023.0902.01

Krueger, J. (2022). *Affordances and spatial agency in psychopathology*. Taylors and Francis Online. doi:10.1080/09515089.2023.2243975

Kruja. (2017). *Editor of the European Journal of Neurology*. Research Gate. https://www.researchgate.net/publication/318653536_Editor_of_the_European_Journal_of_Neurology_Volume_24_Supplement_1_June_2017

Kruklitis, R., Miller, M., Valeriano, L., Shine, S., Opstbaum, N., and Chestnut, V. (2022). Applications of remote patient monitoring. *Primary Care - Clinics in Office Practice, 49*(4), 543–555.

Compilation of References

Kshetri, N. (2022). Policy, Ethical, Social, and Environmental Considerations of Web3 and the Metaverse. *IT Professional*, *24*(3), 4–8. doi:10.1109/MITP.2022.3178509

Kulkarni A. & Deshmukh, S. (2020). *Efficiency Intensification of a Solar Structure and Comparison of PI Controller Based Converter Topologies using MATLAB SIMULINK*. IEEE. . doi:10.1109/INOCON50539.2020.9298440

KumarP. T.MohamedJ. S.PadmajaR. (2023). *Contrasting virtual reality and augmented reality in the health care system - Briefing*. Zenodo. doi:10.5281/zenodo.8068117

Kuo, T., Kim, H., & Ohno-Machado, L. (2017). Blockchain distributed ledger technologies for biomedical and health care applications. *Journal of the American Medical Informatics Association*, *24*(6), 1211–1220. doi:10.1093/jamia/ocx068 PMID:29016974

Kwame, A., & Petrucka, P. M. (2020). Communication in nurse-patient interaction in healthcare settings in sub-Saharan Africa: A scoping review. *International Journal of Africa Nursing Sciences*, *12*, 100198. doi:10.1016/j.ijans.2020.100198

Kwon, H., An, S., Lee, H.-Y., Cha, W. C., Kim, S., Cho, M., & Kong, H.-J. (2022). Review of Smart Hospital Services in Real Healthcare Environments. *Healthcare Informatics Research*, *28*(1), 3–15. doi:10.4258/hir.2022.28.1.3 PMID:35172086

Kwon, S., Park, J. K., & Koh, Y. H. (2023). A systematic review and meta-analysis on the effect of virtual reality-based rehabilitation for people with Parkinson's disease. *Journal of Neuroengineering and Rehabilitation*, *20*(1), 94. doi:10.118612984-023-01219-3 PMID:37475014

Kyi, L., Shivakumar, S. A., Santos, C., Roesner, F., Zufall, F., & Biega, A. J. (2023). *Investigating Deceptive Design in GDPR's Legitimate Interest*. ACM. doi:10.1145/3544548.3580637

Labbaf, S., Abbasian, M., Azimi, I., Dutt, N., & Rahmani, A. M. (2023). *ZotCare: a flexible, personalizable, and affordable MHealth service provider*. https://doi.org//arxiv.2307.01905 doi:10.48550

Lan, L., Sikov, J., Lejeune, J., Ji, C., Brown, H., Bullock, K., & Spencer, A. E. (2023). A Systematic Review of using Virtual and Augmented Reality for the Diagnosis and Treatment of Psychotic Disorders. *Current Treatment Options in Psychiatry*, *10*(2), 87–107. doi:10.100740501-023-00287-5 PMID:37360960

Laver, K. E. (2017). Virtual reality for stroke rehabilitation. *Cochrane Database of Systematic Reviews*, *11*(2). doi:10.1002/14651858.CD008349.pub4 PMID:29156493

Lee, L.-H., Braud, T., Zhou, P., Wang, L., Xu, D., Lin, Z., Kumar, A., Bermejo, C., & Hui, P. (2021). *All one needs to know about metaverse: A complete survey on technological singularity, virtual ecosystem, and research agenda.* arXiv preprint arXiv:2110.05352.

Lee, H., Woo, D., & Yu, S. (2022). Virtual reality metaverse system supplementing remote education methods: Based on aircraft maintenance simulation. *Applied Sciences (Basel, Switzerland)*, *12*(5), 2667. doi:10.3390/app12052667

Lee, J. C., & Lin, R. (2023). The continuous usage of artificial intelligence (AI)-powered mobile fitness applications: The goal-setting theory perspective. *Industrial Management & Data Systems*, *123*(6), 1840–1860. doi:10.1108/IMDS-10-2022-0602

Lee, S. (2023). *Sustainable Vocational Preparation for Adults with Disabilities: A Metaverse-Based Approach*. MDPI. doi:10.3390u151512000

Leite, R. (2023). *The effects of Virtual Reality-Based Mindfulness Meditation on cognition*. STARS. https://stars.library.ucf.edu/honorstheses/1376/

Leite, R. (2023b). *The effects of Virtual Reality-Based Mindfulness Meditation on cognition* [Undergraduate Thesis]. University of Central Florida.

Letafati, M., & Otoum, S. (2023). *On the privacy and security for e-health services in the metaverse: An overview*. ScienceDirect. doi:10.1016/j.adhoc.2023.103262

Levin, J. (2023). Being in the present moment: Toward an epidemiology of mindfulness. *Mindfulness*. doi:10.100712671-023-02179-4

Li, H., & Chen, H. (2023). Research on immersive virtual reality healing design based on the Five senses Theory. In Communications in computer and information science (pp. 99–106). doi:10.1007/978-3-031-35992-7_14

Li, Y., Ma, Z., & Zhang, L. L. (2023). Research on interaction design based on artificial intelligence technology in a metaverse environment. In Lecture Notes in Computer Science (pp. 193–209). doi:10.1007/978-3-031-35699-5_15

Liang, T.-P., & Liu, Y.-H. (2018). Research landscape of business intelligence and big data analytics: A bibliometrics study. *Expert Systems with Applications*, *111*, 2–10. doi:10.1016/j.eswa.2018.05.018

Liao, Y., Huang, T., Lin, S., Wu, C., Chang, K., Hsieh, S., Lin, S., Goh, J. O. S., & Yang, C. (2023). Mediating role of resilience in the relationships of physical activity and mindful self-awareness with peace of mind among college students. *Scientific Reports*, *13*(1), 10386. doi:10.103841598-023-37416-2 PMID:37369802

Li, B., Naraine, M. L., Liang, Z., & Li, C. (2021). A magic "Bullet": Exploring sport fan usage of On-Screen, ephemeral posts during live stream sessions. *Communication & Sport*, *11*(2), 334–355. doi:10.1177/21674795211038949

Liedgren, J., Desmet, P., & Gaggioli, A. (2023). Liminal design: A conceptual framework and three-step approach for developing technology that delivers transcendence and deeper experiences. *Frontiers in Psychology*, *14*, 1043170. doi:10.3389/fpsyg.2023.1043170 PMID:36844338

Li, H.-H., Lian, J.-J., & Liao, Y.-H. (2023). *Design an Adaptive Virtual Reality Game to Promote Elderly Health*. IEEE Explore. doi:10.1109/CITS58301.2023.10188784

Li, J., Kwon, N., Pham, H., Shim, R., & Leshed, G. (2023). *Co-designing Magic Machines for Everyday Mindfulness with Practitioners*. ACM. doi:10.1145/3563657.3595976

Compilation of References

Li, K., De Oliveira Cardoso, C., Moctezuma-Ramirez, A., Elgalad, A., & Perin, E. C. (2023). (Preprint). Heart Rate Variability Measurement through a Wearable Device. *Another Breakthrough for Personal Health Monitoring*. doi:10.20944/preprints202308.0732.v1

Li, N. (2023). Application of motion tracking technology in movies, television production and photography using big data. *Soft Computing*, *27*(17), 12787–12806. doi:10.100700500-023-08963-7

Lister, P. (2023). Opening up smart learning cities - building knowledge, interactions and communities for lifelong learning and urban belonging. In Lecture Notes in Computer Science (pp. 67–85). doi:10.1007/978-3-031-34609-5_5

Liu, L., Yin, H., & Chen, Z. (2020). *Using Self-Determination Theory to Explore Enjoyment of Educational Interactive Narrative Games: A Case Study of Academical*. Research Gate.

Liu, Y., Bitter, J. L., & Spierling, U. (2023). Evaluating interaction challenges of Head-Mounted Device-Based augmented reality applications for First-Time users at museums and exhibitions. In Lecture Notes in Computer Science (pp. 150–163). doi:10.1007/978-3-031-34732-0_11

Liu, H., Liu, S., Li, X., & Bing-Quan, L. (2023). Efficacy of Baduanjin for treatment of fatigue: A systematic review and meta-analysis of randomized controlled trials. *Medicine*, *102*(32), e34707. doi:10.1097/MD.0000000000034707 PMID:37565842

Liu, Q., Luo, D., Haase, J. E., Guo, Q., Wang, X. Q., Liu, S., Xia, L., Liu, Z., Yang, J., & Yang, B. X. (2020). The experiences of health-care providers during the COVID-19 crisis in China: A qualitative study. *The Lancet. Global Health*, *8*(6), e790–e798. doi:10.1016/S2214-109X(20)30204-7 PMID:32573443

Liu, Y., Zhang, Y., Zhang, X., Han, F., & Zhao, Y. (2023). A geographical perspective on the formation of urban nightlife landscape. *Humanities & Social Sciences Communications*, *10*(1), 483. doi:10.105741599-023-01964-9

Li, X., Huang, J., Kong, Z., Sun, F., Sit, C. H. P., & Li, C. (2023). Effects of Virtual Reality-Based Exercise on Physical Fitness in People with Intellectual Disability: A Systematic Review of Randomized Controlled Trials. *Games for Health Journal*, *12*(2), 89–99. doi:10.1089/g4h.2022.0168 PMID:36716183

Li, Y., Cabano, F., & Li, P. (2023). How to attract low prosocial funders in crowdfunding? Matching among funders, project descriptions, and platform types. *Information & Management*, *103840*(7), 103840. doi:10.1016/j.im.2023.103840

Li, Y., Ch'ng, E., & Cobb, S. (2023). Factors influencing engagement in hybrid virtual and augmented reality. *ACM Transactions on Computer-Human Interaction*, *30*(4), 1–27. doi:10.1145/3589952

Loesche, J. A., Gardner, D. L., & Kalpakjian, M. L. (2021, November). Machine learning-based patient-specific prediction models for diabetic lower-extremity ulcer healing exist despite scarce reporting quality: A systematic review. *Wound Repair and Regeneration*, *29*(6), 900–911. doi:10.1111/wrr.13031

Lopes, F. (2023). *Exploring the features and benefits of Mixed Reality Toolkit 2 for developing immersive games : a reflective study*. Theseus. https://www.theseus.fi/handle/10024/803207

Lopez, J.-L. C. (2017). An IoT Approach for Wireless Sensor Networks Applied to e-Health Environmental Monitoring. *The 2017 IEEE International Conference on Internet of Things (iThings-2017)*. IEEE.

López-Ojeda, W., & Hurley, R. A. (2023). The Medical Metaverse, Part 1: Introduction, Definitions, and New Horizons for Neuropsychiatry. *The Journal of Neuropsychiatry and Clinical Neurosciences*, *35*(1), A4–A3. doi:10.1176/appi.neuropsych.20220187 PMID:36633472

Loveys, K., Sagar, M., Antoni, M., & Broadbent, E. (2023). *The impact of virtual humans on psychosomatic medicine*. Psychosomatic Medicine. doi:10.1097/PSY.0000000000001227

Lucas, I., Solé-Morata, N., Baenas, I., Rosinska, M., Fernández-Aranda, F., & Jiménez-Murcia, S. (2023). Biofeedback interventions for impulsivity-related processes in addictive disorders. *Current Addiction Reports*, *10*(3), 543–552. doi:10.100740429-023-00499-y

Lui, X. (2019). A comparison of deep learning performance against health-care professionals in detecting diseases from medical imaging: a systematic review and meta-analysis. *The Lancet, 10.* . doi:10.1016/S2589-7500(19)30123-2

Lundberg, S. M., & Lee, S. I. (2017). A unified approach to interpreting model predictions. *Advances in Neural Information Processing Systems*, 4765–4774.

Mabary, J. (2023). *Analyzing compositional strategies in video game music*. MoSpace. https://mospace.umsystem.edu/xmlui/handle/10355/96145

Mahbub, M. K., Biswas, M., Gaur, L., Alenezi, F., & Santosh, K. C. (2022). Deep features to detect pulmonary abnormalities in chest X-rays due to infectious diseases: Covid-19, pneumonia, and tuberculosis. *Information Sciences (New York)*, *592*, 389–401. doi:10.1016/j.ins.2022.01.062 PMID:36532848

Ma, J., Zhao, D., Xu, N., & Yang, J. (2023). The effectiveness of immersive virtual reality (VR) based mindfulness training on improvement mental-health in adults: A narrative systematic review. *Explore (New York, N.Y.)*, *19*(3), 310–318. doi:10.1016/j.explore.2022.08.001 PMID:36002363

Malighetti, C., Bernardelli, L., Pancini, E., Riva, G., & Villani, D. (2023). Promoting Emotional and Psychological Well-Being During COVID-19 Pandemic: A Self-Help Virtual Reality intervention for university students. *Cyberpsychology, Behavior, and Social Networking*, *26*(4), 309–317. doi:10.1089/cyber.2022.0246 PMID:36940285

Malin, Y. (2023). Others In Mind: A Systematic Review and Meta-Analysis of the Relationship between Mindfulness and Prosociality. *Mindfulness*, *14*(7), 1582–1605. doi:10.100712671-023-02150-3

Compilation of References

Manoukian, S., Stewart, S., Graves, N., Mason, H., Robertson, C., Kennedy, S., Pan, J., Kavanagh, K., Haahr, L., Adil, M., Dancer, S. J., Cook, B., & Reilly, J. (2021). Bed-days and costs associated with the inpatient burden of healthcare-associated infection in the UK. *The Journal of Hospital Infection*, *114*, 43–50. doi:10.1016/j.jhin.2020.12.027 PMID:34301395

Manto, A., & D'Oria, M. (2023). Some Ethical and Educational Perspectives on Using Artificial Intelligence in Personalized Medicine and Healthcare. In A. Cesario, M. D'Oria, C. Auffray, & G. Scambia (Eds.), *Personalised Medicine Meets Artificial Intelligence: Beyond "Hype", Towards the Metaverse* (pp. 261–269). Springer International Publishing. doi:10.1007/978-3-031-32614-1_18

Marabelli, M., & Newell, S. (2023). Responsibly strategizing with the metaverse: Business implications and DEI opportunities and challenges. *The Journal of Strategic Information Systems*, *32*(2), 101774. doi:10.1016/j.jsis.2023.101774

Mariam, G., Alemayehu, A., Tesfaye, E., Mequannt, W., Temesgen, K., Yetwale, F., & Limenih, M. A. (2017). Prevalence of Diabetic Foot Ulcer and Associated Factors among Adult Diabetic Patients Who Attend the Diabetic Follow-Up Clinic at the University of Gondar Referral Hospital, North West Ethiopia, 2016: Institutional-Based Cross-Sectional Study. *Journal of Diabetes Research*, *2017*, 1–8. doi:10.1155/2017/2879249 PMID:28791310

Maskeliunas, R., Damaševicius, R., and Segal, S. (2019). A review of internet of things technologies for ambient assisted living environments. *Future Internet, 11*(12). doi: 10.3390/fi11120259

Maskeliūnas, R., Damaševičius, R., Blažauskas, T., Canbulut, C., Adomavičienė, A., & Griškevičius, J. (2023). BioMacVR: A virtual Reality-Based system for precise human posture and motion analysis in rehabilitation exercises using depth sensors. *Electronics (Basel)*, *12*(2), 339. doi:10.3390/electronics12020339

Mathur, S., & Gaur, L. (2021). Predictability, Power and Procedures of Citation Analysis. In D. Goyal, A.K. Gupta, V. Piuri, M. Ganzha, & M. Paprzycki (Eds.), *Proceedings of the Second International Conference on Information Management and Machine Intelligence*. Springer Singapore, Singapore. 10.1007/978-981-15-9689-6_6

Matt, D.T., Arcidiacono, G., Rauch, E. (2018). Applying Lean to Healthcare Delivery Processes - a Case-based Research. *International Journal on Advanced Science, Engineering and Information Technology, 8*(123).

Maurya, A., Munoz, J. M., Gaur, L., & Singh, G. (2023). *Disruptive Technologies in International Business: Challenges and Opportunities for Emerging Markets*. Walter de Gruyter GmbH & Co KG. doi:10.1515/9783110734133

Mazlan, I., Abdullah, N., & Ahmad, N. (2023). Exploring the impact of hybrid recommender systems on personalized mental health recommendations. *International Journal of Advanced Computer Science and Applications*, *14*(6). doi:10.14569/IJACSA.2023.0140699

Mbunge, E., Muchemwa, B., & Batani, J. (2022). Are we there yet? Unbundling the potential adoption and integration of telemedicine to improve virtual healthcare services in African health systems. *Sensors International*, *3*, 100152. doi:10.1016/j.sintl.2021.100152 PMID:34901894

McCain, R. S., Diamond, A., Jones, C., & Coleman, H. G. (2018). Current practices and future prospects for the management of gallbladder polyps: A topical review. *World Journal of Gastroenterology*, *24*(26), 2844–2852. doi:10.3748/wjg.v24.i26.2844 PMID:30018479

McCaw, C. T. (2023). Contemplative practices and teacher professional becoming. *Educational Review*, 1–29. doi:10.1080/00131911.2023.2215467

McEwan, K., Krogh, K. S., Dunlop, K., Khan, M., & Krogh, A. (2023). Virtual Forest Bathing Programming as Experienced by Disabled Adults with Mobility Impairments and/or Low Energy: A Qualitative Study. *Forests*, *14*(5), 1033. doi:10.3390/f14051033

McIntyre, T., Hughes, C. D., Pauyo, T., Sullivan, S. R., Rogers, S. O. Jr, Ray-monville, M., & Meara, J. G. (2011). Emergency surgical care delivery in post-earthquake haiti: Partners in health and zanmi lasante experience. *World Journal of Surgery*, *35*(4), 745–750. doi:10.100700268-011-0961-6 PMID:21249359

McMahan, D. L. (2023). *Rethinking meditation: Buddhist Practice in the Ancient and Modern Worlds*. Academic Press.

Meena, S. D., Mithesh, G. S. S., Panyam, R., Chowdary, M. S., Sadhu, V. S., & Sheela, J. (2023). *Advancing Education through Metaverse: Components, Applications, Challenges, Case Studies and Open Issues*. IEEE Explore. doi:10.1109/ICSCSS57650.2023.10169535

Mejtoft, T., Lindahl, H., Norberg, O., Andersson, M., & Söderström, U. (2023). *Enhancing Digital Social Interaction Using Augmented Reality in Mobile Fitness Applications*. ACM. doi:10.1145/3591156.3591170

Menhas, R., Luo, Q., Saqib, Z. A., & Younas, M. (2023). The association between COVID-19 preventive strategies, virtual reality exercise, use of fitness apps, physical, and psychological health: Testing a structural equation moderation model. *Frontiers in Public Health*, *11*, 1170645. doi:10.3389/fpubh.2023.1170645 PMID:37483921

Mezei, K., & Szentgáli-Tóth, B. (2023). Some comments on the legal regulation on misinformation and cyber attacks conducted through online platforms. *Lexonomica*, *15*(1), 33–52. doi:10.18690/lexonomica.15.1.33-52.2023

Mihalj, M., Carrel, T., Gregoric, I. D., Andereggen, L., Zinn, P. O., Doll, D., Stueber, F., Gabriel, R. A., Urman, R. D., & Luedi, M. M. (2020). Telemedicine for preoperative assessment during a covid-19 pandemic: Rec-ommendations for clinical care. *Best Practice & Research. Clinical Anaesthesiology*, *34*(2), 345–351. doi:10.1016/j.bpa.2020.05.001 PMID:32711839

Miljković, I., Shlyakhetko, O., & Fedushko, S. (2023). Real estate app development based on AI/VR technologies. *Electronics (Basel)*, *12*(3), 707. doi:10.3390/electronics12030707

Miller, N., Stepanova, E. R., Desnoyers-Stewart, J., Adhikari, A., Kitson, A., Pennefather, P. P., Quesnel, D., Brauns, K., Friedl-Werner, A., Stahn, A., & Riecke, B. E. (2023). *Awedyssey: Design Tensions in Eliciting Self-transcendent Emotions in Virtual Reality to Support Mental Well-being and Connection*. ACM. doi:10.1145/3563657.3595998

Compilation of References

Miller, R. (2020). *Digital arts based research methods for teenage and young adult (TYA) cancer patients. Goldsmiths*. University of London.

Miner, H., Koenig, K., & Bozic, K. J. (2020). Value-based healthcare: Not going anywhere—why orthopaedic surgeons will continue using tele-health in a post-covid-19 world. *Clinical Orthopaedics and Related Research*, *478*(12), 2717–2719. doi:10.1097/CORR.0000000000001561 PMID:33165045

Mirlou, F., & Beker, L. (2023). Wearable Electrochemical Sensors for Healthcare Monitoring: A review of current developments and future Prospects. *IEEE Transactions on Molecular, Biological, and Multi-Scale Communications*, *1*(3), 364–373. doi:10.1109/TMBMC.2023.3304240

Mishra, N., & Bharti, T. (2023). Exploring the nexus of social support, work–life balance and life satisfaction in hybrid work scenario in learning organizations. *The Learning Organization*. doi:10.1108/TLO-08-2022-0099

Mitsea, E., Drigas, A., & Skianis, C. (2023). Brain-computer interfaces in digital mindfulness training for metacognitive, emotional and attention regulation skills: A literature review. *Research. Social Development*, *12*(3), e2512340247. doi:10.33448/rsd-v12i3.40247

Miyoung, R., Choi, Y., & Park, H. (2023). Analysis of Issues in Fitness Centers through News Articles before and after the COVID-19 Pandemic in South Korea: Applying Big Data Analysis. *Sustainability (Basel)*, *15*(3), 2660. doi:10.3390u15032660

Mogavi, R. H., Hoffman, J., Deng, C., Yihang, D., Haq, E., & Hui, P. (2023). *Envisioning an Inclusive Metaverse: Student Perspectives on Accessible and Empowering Metaverse-Enabled Learning*. doi:10.1145/3573051.3596185

Mohiuddin, S. I., Thorakkattil, S. A., Abushoumi, F., Nemr, H. S., Jabbour, R., & Al-Ghamdi, F. (2021). Implementation of pharmacist-led tele medica-tion management clinic in ambulatory care settings: A patient-centered care model in covid-19 era. *Exploratory Research in Clinical and Social Pharmacy*, *4*, 100083. doi:10.1016/j.rcsop.2021.100083 PMID:34723240

Monge, J., Ribeiro, G., Raimundo, A., Postolache, O., & Santos, J. F. D. (2023). AI-Based Smart Sensing and AR for GAIT Rehabilitation Assessment. *Information (Basel)*, *14*(7), 355. doi:10.3390/info14070355

Montalto, J. (2023). The Effects Of Mindfulness On Stress Reduction And Academic Performance In Students Studying Health Sciences. *DUNE: DigitalUNE*. https://dune.une.edu/na_capstones/51/

Moon, I., An, Y., Min, S., & Park, C. (2023). Therapeutic Effects of Metaverse Rehabilitation for Cerebral Palsy: A Randomized Controlled Trial. *International Journal of Environmental Research and Public Health*, *20*(2), 1578. doi:10.3390/ijerph20021578 PMID:36674332

Moro, C. (2023). Utilising the metaverse in anatomy and physiology. *Anatomical Sciences Education*. John Wiley & Sons. PMID:36545794

Morrell, A. L. G., Morrell-Junior, A. C., Morrell, A. G., Mendes, J. M. F., Tustumi, F., De-Oliveira-e-Silva, L. G., & Morrell, A. (2021). The history of robotic surgery and its evolution: When illusion becomes reality. *Revista do Colégio Brasileiro de Cirurgiões*, *48*, 48. doi:10.1590/0100-6991e-20202798 PMID:33470371

Morrison, A. M., & Buhalis, D. (2023). *Routledge Handbook of Trends and Issues in Global Tourism Supply and Demand*. Routledge. doi:10.4324/9781003260790

Mousazadeh, H., Ghorbani, A., Azadi, H., Almani, F. A., Ali, Z., Zhu, K., & Dávid, L. D. (2023). Developing sustainable behaviors for underground heritage tourism management: The case of Persian Qanats, a UNESCO World Heritage property. *Land (Basel)*, *12*(4), 808. doi:10.3390/land12040808

Moyer, M. A. (2023). *Engaging Technologies of the Self with Youth: A Critical Contemplative Pedagogy Action Research Project*. https://etd.ohiolink.edu/acprod/odb_etd/etd/r/1501/10?clear=10&p10_accession_num=miami1689338623782483

Mozumder, M. A. I., Sheeraz, M. M., Athar, A., Aich, S., & Kim, H.-C. (2022). Overview: Technology Roadmap of the Future Trend of Metaverse based on IoT, Blockchain, AI Technique, and Medical Domain Metaverse Activity. *2022 24th International Conference on Advanced Communication Technology (ICACT)*, (pp. 256–261). IEEE. 10.23919/ICACT53585.2022.9728808

Mozumder, M. A. I., Sheeraz, M. M., Athar, A., Aich, S., & Kim, H.-C. (2022). Overview: Technology roadmap of the future trend of metaverse based on IoT, blockchain, AI technique, and medical domain metaverse activity. In *2022 24th International Conference on Advanced Communication Technology (ICACT)*. IEEE.

Mozumder, M. I., Armand, T. P. T., Uddin, S. M. I., Athar, A., Sumon, R. I., Hussain, A., & Kim, H. C. (2023). Metaverse for Digital Anti-Aging Healthcare: An overview of potential use cases based on artificial intelligence, blockchain, IoT technologies, its challenges, and future directions. *Applied Sciences (Basel, Switzerland)*, *13*(8), 5127. doi:10.3390/app13085127

Mulders, M. (2023). Learning about Victims of Holocaust in Virtual Reality: The Main, Mediating and Moderating Effects of Technology, Instructional Method, Flow, Presence, and Prior Knowledge. *Multimodal Technologies and Interaction*, *7*(3), 28. doi:10.3390/mti7030028

Murakawa D. (2023). Decision making under virtual environment triggers more aggressive tactical solutions. *2023*. doi:10.51015/jdl.2023.3.9

Musamih, A., Yaqoob, I., Salah, K., Jayaraman, R., Al-Hammadi, Y., Omar, M., & Ellahham, S. (2022). Metaverse in healthcare:applications, challenges,and future directions. IEEE Consumer Electronics Magazine, vol. 12, no. 4, pp. 33-46, 1 July 2023, doi: 10.1109/MCE.2022.3223522..

Musamih, A., Yaqoob, I., Salah, K., Jayaraman, R., Al-Hammadi, Y., Omar, M., & Ellahham, S. (2023). Metaverse in Healthcare: Applications, Challenges, and Future Directions. *IEEE Consumer Electronics Magazine*, *12*(4), 33–46. doi:10.1109/MCE.2022.3223522

Muslihati, M. (2023). *How to prevent student mental health problems in metaverse era?* Muslihati | Jurnal Kajian Bimbingan Dan Konseling. http://journal2.um.ac.id/index.php/jkbk/article/view/37598

Musto, S. (2023). Exploring the uses of yoga nidra: An integrative review. *Nursing and Scholarship.* https://sigmapubs.onlinelibrary.wiley.com/doi/abs/10.1111/jnu.12927

Muthmainnah, Y., Al Yakin, A., & Ibna Seraj, P. M. (2023). Impact of metaverse technology on student engagement and academic performance: The Mediating role of learning motivation. *International Journal of Computations. Information and Manufacturing, 3*(1), 10–18. doi:10.54489/ijcim.v3i1.234

N, S., M, S., G, K., & R, R. (2023). *Securing the Cloud: An empirical study on best practices for ensuring data privacy and protection.* doi:10.31033/ijemr.13.2.6

Nagarajan, G. (2023, July 15). *The Role Of The Metaverse In Digital Marketing.* Universidad De Granada. https://digibug.ugr.es/handle/10481/84077

Nagelkerke, G. P., Kars, M. A., & Driessen, P. H. T. G. (2020, November). Feasibility of a mobile health tool for remotely monitoring diabetic foot ulceration. *Journal of Wound Care, 29*(11), 714–720. doi:10.12968/jowc.2020.29.11.714

Nanda, R., Nath, A., Patel, S., & Mohapatra, E. (2022, June). Machine learning algorithm to evaluate risk factors of diabetic foot ulcers and its severity. *Medical & Biological Engineering & Computing, 60*(8), 2349–2357. doi:10.100711517-022-02617-w PMID:35751828

Nath, D., Singh, N., Saini, M., Banduni, O., Kumar, N., Srivastava, M. V. P., & Mehndiratta, A. (2023). Clinical potential and neuroplastic effect of targeted virtual reality based intervention for distal upper limb in post-stroke rehabilitation: A pilot observational study. *Disability and Rehabilitation,* 1–10. doi:10.1080/09638288.2023.2228690 PMID:37383015

Naved, M., Devi, V. A., Gaur, L., & Elngar, A. A. (2023). *IoT-Enabled Convolutional Neural Networks: Techniques and Applications.* CRC Press. doi:10.1201/9781003393030

Nawaz, N. A., Abid, A., Rasheed, S., Farooq, M. S., Shahzadi, A., & Mubarik, I. (2022). Impact of telecommunication network on future of telemedicine in healthcare: A systematic literature review. *International Journal of Advanced and Applied Sciences, 9*(7), 122–138. doi:10.21833/ijaas.2022.07.013

Nee, A. Y. C., & Ong, S. K. (2023). *Springer Handbook of Augmented Reality.* Springer Nature. doi:10.1007/978-3-030-67822-7

Ning, H., Wang, H., Lin, Y., Wang, W., Dhelim, S., Farha, F., Ding, J., & Daneshmand, M. (2021). *A Survey on Metaverse: the State-of-the-art, Technologies, Applications, and Challenges.* arXiv preprint arXiv:2111.09673.

Ning, H., Wang, H., Lin, Y., Wang, W., Dhelim, S., Farha, F., Ding, J., & Daneshmand, M. (2023). A survey on the metaverse: The State-of-the-Art, technologies, applications, and challenges. *IEEE Internet of Things Journal, 1*(16), 14671–14688. doi:10.1109/JIOT.2023.3278329

Norman, K., French, A., Lake, A., Tchuisseu, Y. P., Repka, S., Vasudeva, K., Dong, C., Whitaker, R., & Bettger, J. P. (2023). Describing Perspectives of Telehealth and the Impact on Equity in Access to Health Care from Community and Provider Perspectives: A Multimethod Analysis. *Telemedicine Journal and e-Health*, tmj.2023.0036. doi:10.1089/tmj.2023.0036 PMID:37410525

O'Hagan, J., Saeghe, P., Gugenheimer, J., Medeiros, D., Marky, K., Khamis, M., & McGill, M. (2022). Privacy-Enhancing technology and everyday augmented reality. *Proceedings of the ACM on Interactive, Mobile, Wearable and Ubiquitous Technologies, 6*(4), 1–35. 10.1145/3569501

Omoregbe, N. A. I., Ndaman, I. O., Misra, S., Abayomi-Alli, O. O., & Damaševičius, R. (2020). Text messaging-based medical diagnosis using nat-ural language processing and fuzzy logic. *Journal of Healthcare Engineering*, 2020. doi: 10.1155/2020/8839524

Omranian, S., Zolnoori, M., Huang, M., Campos-Castillo, C., & McRoy, S. (2023). Predicting patient satisfaction with medications for treating opioid use Disorder: Case study Applying natural language processing to reviews of methadone and Buprenorphine/Naloxone on Health-Related Social media. *JMIR Infodemiology, 3*, e37207. doi:10.2196/37207 PMID:37113381

Oniani, S., Marques, G., Barnovi, S., Pires, I. M., & Bhoi, A. K. (2021). Artificial intelligence for internet of things and enhanced medical systems. *Bio-inspired neurocomputing*, 43-59.

Ortet, C. P., Vairinhos, M., Veloso, A. I., & Costa, L. V. (2023). Virtual Reality Hippotherapy Simulator: A model proposal for Senior citizens. In Lecture Notes in Computer Science (pp. 592–609). doi:10.1007/978-3-031-34866-2_42

Ose, S. O., Thaulow, K., Færevik, H., Hoffmann, P. L., Lestander, H., Stiles, T. C., & Lindgren, M. (2023). Development of a social skills training programme to target social isolation using virtual reality technology in primary mental health care. *Journal of Rehabilitation and Assistive Technologies Engineering, 10*. doi:10.1177/20556683231187545 PMID:37456950

Ozacar, K., Ortakci, Y., & Küçükkara, M. Y. (2023). VRArchEducation: Redesigning building survey process in architectural education using collaborative virtual reality. *Computers & Graphics, 113*, 1–9. doi:10.1016/j.cag.2023.04.008

Padilla-Castañeda, T., Téllez-Valencia, J. A., & González-González, G. A. (2019, August). A clinical decision support system for the diagnosis of diabetic foot syndrome using a Bayesian network. *BMC Medical Informatics and Decision Making, 19*(1), 167. doi:10.118612911-019-0885-5 PMID:31429747

Pak, H. S., Brown-Connolly, N. E., Bloch, C., Clarke, M., Clyburn, C., Doarn, C. R., Llewellyn, C., Merrell, R. C., Montgomery, K., Rasche, J., & Sullivan, B. (2008). Global forum on telemedicine: Connecting the world through partnerships. *Telemedicine Journal and e-Health, 14*(4), 389–395. doi:10.1089/tmj.2008.0030 PMID:18570571

Palozzi, G., Schettini, I., & Chirico, A. (2020). Enhancing the sustainable goal of access to healthcare: Findings from a literature review on telemedicine employment in rural areas. *Sustainability, 12*(8), 3318. doi:10.3390u12083318

Compilation of References

Pal, R., Adhikari, D., Heyat, M. B. B., Ullah, I., & You, Z. (2023). Yoga meets intelligent Internet of Things: Recent challenges and future directions. *Bioengineering (Basel, Switzerland)*, *10*(4), 459. doi:10.3390/bioengineering10040459 PMID:37106646

Pancini, E., Di Natale, A. F., & Villani, D. (2023). *Breathing in virtual Reality for Promoting Mental Health: A scoping review. Research Square*. Research Square. doi:10.21203/rs.3.rs-3230685/v1

Pandya, S. (2007). *Telemedicine, telehealth and e-health: An emerging role in private industry and international health policy*.

Papamichael, I., Pappas, G., Siegel, J. E., Inglezakis, V. J., Demetriou, G., Zorpas, A. A., & Hadjisavvas, C. (2023). Metaverse and circular economy. *Waste Management & Research*, *41*(9), 1393–1398. doi:10.1177/0734242X231180406 PMID:37313976

Pap, I. A., & Oniga, S. (2022). A review of converging technologies in ehealth pertaining to artificial intelligence. *International Journal of Environmental Research and Public Health*, *19*(18), 11413. doi:10.3390/ijerph191811413 PMID:36141685

Parcu, P. L., Rossi, M. A., Innocenti, N., & Carrozza, C. (2023). How real will the metaverse be? Exploring the spatial impact of virtual worlds. *European Planning Studies*, *31*(7), 1466–1488. doi:10.1080/09654313.2023.2221323

Pardini, S., Gabrielli, S., Olivetto, S., Fusina, F., Dianti, M., Forti, S., Lancini, C., & Novara, C. (2023). Personalized, naturalistic virtual reality scenarios coupled with Web-Based progressive muscle relaxation training for the general population: Protocol for a Proof-of-Principle randomized controlled trial. *JMIR Research Protocols*, *12*, e44183. doi:10.2196/44183 PMID:37067881

Park, M., Song, R., Ju, K., Shin, J. C., Seo, J., Fan, X., Gao, X., Ryu, A., & Li, Y. (2023). Effects of Tai Chi and Qigong on cognitive and physical functions in older adults: Systematic review, meta-analysis, and meta-regression of randomized clinical trials. *BMC Geriatrics*, *23*(1), 352. doi:10.118612877-023-04070-2 PMID:37280512

Parry, J., & Giesbrecht, J. (2023). Esports, real sports and the Olympic Virtual Series. *Journal of the Philosophy of Sport*, *50*(2), 1–21. doi:10.1080/00948705.2023.2216883

Pascual, K. J., Fredman, A., Naum, A., Patil, C., & Sikka, N. (2022). Should mindfulness for health care workers go virtual? A Mindfulness-Based intervention using virtual reality and heart rate variability in the emergency department. *AAOHN Journal*, *71*(4), 188–194. doi:10.1177/21650799221123258 PMID:36377263

Pastel, S., Petri, K., Chen, C. H., Cáceres, A. M. W., Stirnatis, M., Nübel, C., Schlotter, L., & Witte, K. (2022). Training in virtual reality enables learning of a complex sports movement. *Virtual Reality (Waltham Cross)*, *27*(2), 523–540. doi:10.100710055-022-00679-7

Piacevoli, Q. (2023). Metaverse and Health Care System. *PriMera Scientific Medicine and Public Health*, *2*, 06-14.

Piçarra, M., Rodrigues, A., & Guerreiro, J. (2023). *Evaluating Accessible Navigation for Blind People in Virtual Environments*. ACM. doi:10.1145/3544549.3585813

Pickhardt, P. J. (2023). *Abdominal Imaging in the Coming Decades: Better, Faster, Safer, and Cheaper?* (Vol. 307). Radiological Society of North America.

Pira, G. L., Aquilini, B., Davoli, A., Grandi, S., & Ruini, C. (2023). The Use of Virtual Reality Interventions to Promote Positive Mental Health: Systematic Literature review. *JMIR Mental Health*, *10*, e44998. doi:10.2196/44998 PMID:37410520

Pirmoazen, A. M., Khurana, A., El Kaffas, A., & Kamaya, A. (2020). Quantitative ultrasound approaches for diagnosis and monitoring hepatic steatosis in nonalcoholic fatty liver disease. *Theranostics*, *10*(9), 4277–4289. doi:10.7150/thno.40249 PMID:32226553

Pizzo, A. D. (2023). Hypercasual and Hybrid-Casual Video Gaming: A Digital Leisure perspective. *Leisure Sciences*, 1–20. doi:10.1080/01490400.2023.2211056

Placidi, G., Di Matteo, A., Lozzi, D., Polsinelli, M., & Theodoridou, E. (2023). Patient–Therapist Cooperative Hand Telerehabilitation through a Novel Framework Involving the Virtual Glove System. *Sensors (Basel)*, *23*(7), 3463. doi:10.339023073463 PMID:37050523

Ponce, P., Peffer, T., Garduno, J. I. M., Eicker, U., Molina, A., McDaniel, T., Mimo, E. D. M., Menon, R. P., Kaspar, K., & Hussain, S. (2023). Smart communities and cities as a unified concept. In Studies in big data (pp. 125–168). doi:10.1007/978-3-031-32828-2_5

Pontin, S. (2023). *AI-Based Race StrategyAssistant and Car data Monitor*. DIVA. https://www.diva-portal.org/smash/record.jsf?pid=diva2%3A1756880&dswid=-6708

Prasath, P. R., Xiong, Y., & Zhang, Q. (2023). A practical guide to planning, implementing, and evaluating the mindfulness-based well-being group for international students. *The Journal of Humanistic Counseling*, johc.12200. doi:10.1002/johc.12200

Pratviel, Y., Bouny, P., & Deschodt-Arsac, V. (2023). *Immersion in a relaxing virtual reality environment is associated with similar effects on stress and anxiety as heart rate variability biofeedback*. Research Square. doi:10.21203/rs.3.rs-3221200/v1

Priest, S. (2023). Predicting the future of experiential and adventurous learning in the metaverse. *Journal of Adventure Education and Outdoor Learning*, 1–14. doi:10.1080/14729679.2023.2220835

Protic, D., Gaur, L., Stankovic, M., & Rahman, M. A. (2022). Cybersecurity in smart cities: Detection of opposing decisions on anomalies in the computer network behavior. *Electronics MDPI*, *11*(22), 3718. doi:10.3390/electronics11223718

Purcarea, I. M. (2023). *E-Commerce Business Under Pressure To Grow*. https://ideas.repec.org/a/hmm/journl/v13y2023i2p24-30.html

Purdy, G. M., Sobierajski, F., Onazi, M. M. A., Effa, C., Venner, C. P., Tandon, P., & McNeely, M. L. (2023). Exploring participant perceptions of a virtually supported home exercise program for people with multiple myeloma using a novel eHealth application: A qualitative study. *Supportive Care in Cancer*, *31*(5), 298. doi:10.100700520-023-07762-y PMID:37097319

Compilation of References

Purwar, S. (2021, December 8). Designing User Experience for Virtual Reality (VR) applications. *Medium*. https://uxplanet.org/designing-user-experience-for-virtual-reality-vr-applications-fc8e4faadd96

Qi, J., Ma, L., Cui, Z., & Yu, Y. (2023). Computer vision-based hand gesture recognition for human-robot interaction: A review. *Complex & Intelligent Systems*. doi:10.100740747-023-01173-6

Quraishi, S. A., Berra, L., & Nozari, A. (2020). Indoor temperature and relative humidity in hospitals: Workplace considerations during the novel coronavirus pandemic. [EPub.]. *Occupational and Environmental Medicine*, 77(7), 508–512. doi:10.1136/oemed-2020-106653 PMID:32424023

Qureshi, I. (2023, July 10). *Can Music And Artificial Intelligence Influence Customer Behavior In-Store?* RC. https://rc.library.uta.edu/uta-ir/handle/10106/31524

Rachmadtullah, R., Setiawan, B., Setiawan, B., & Wicaksono, J. W. (2022). Elementary school teachers' perceptions of the potential of metaverse technology as a transformation of interactive learning media in Indonesia. *International Journal of Innovative Research and Scientific Studies*, 6(1), 128–136. doi:10.53894/ijirss.v6i1.1119

RadanlievD. P. (2023, August 1). *Accessibility and inclusiveness of new information and communication technologies for disabled users and content creators in the metaverse*. https://arxiv.org/abs/2308.01925

Rajda, J., & Paz, H. L. (2020). The future of virtual care services: A payor's perspective. *Telemedicine Journal and e-Health*, 26(3), 267–269. doi:10.1089/tmj.2019.0020 PMID:31058584

Rana, J., Gaur, L., & Santosh, K. (2022). Classifying Customers' Journey from Online Reviews of Amazon Fresh via Sentiment Analysis and Topic Modelling. *2022 3rd International Conference on Computation, Automation and Knowledge Management (ICCAKM)*, (pp. 1–6). IEEE. 10.1109/ICCAKM54721.2022.9990124

Randazzo, G., Reitano, G., Carletti, F., Iafrate, M., Betto, G., Novara, G., Moro, F. D., & Zattoni, F. (2023). Urology: A trip into metaverse. *World Journal of Urology*, 41(10), 2647–2657. doi:10.100700345-023-04560-3 PMID:37552265

Räsänen, P., Muotka, J., & Lappalainen, R. (2023). Examining coaches' asynchronous written feedback in two blended ACT-based interventions for enhancing university students' wellbeing and reducing psychological distress: A randomized study. *Journal of Contextual Behavioral Science*, 29, 98–108. doi:10.1016/j.jcbs.2023.06.006

Rasmussen, J., Moffatt, M. L., & Zhang, K. (2021, March). Standardized Assessment of diabetic foot ulcer healing in clinical trials: The SAD-FU study. *Wound Repair and Regeneration*, 29(2), 309–319. doi:10.1111/wrr.12880

Ray, P. P. (2023). ChatGPT: A comprehensive review on background, applications, key challenges, bias, ethics, limitations and future scope. *Internet of Things and Cyber-physical Systems*, 3, 121–154. doi:10.1016/j.iotcps.2023.04.003

Reardon, C. L., Hainline, B., Aron, C. M., Baron, D., Baum, A. L., Bindra, A., Budgett, R., Campriani, N., Castaldelli-Maia, J. M., Currie, A., Derevensky, J. L., Glick, I. D., Gorczynski, P., Gouttebarge, V., Grandner, M. A., Han, D. H., McDuff, D., Mountjoy, M., Polat, A., & Engebretsen, L. (2019). Mental health in elite athletes: International Olympic Committee consensus statement (2019). *British Journal of Sports Medicine*, *53*(11), 667–699. doi:10.1136/bjsports-2019-100715 PMID:31097450

Redirect notice. (n.d.). https://www.google.com/url?sa=i&url=https%3A%2F%2Fwww.shutterstock.com%2Fvideo%2Fsearch%2Fvr-meditation&psig=AOvVaw1lDxksdO4j_cUe7TWIDomo&ust=1692327355095000&source=images&cd=vfe&opi=89978449&ved=0CBIQjhxqFwoTCPDmqenY4oADFQAAAAAdAAAAABBg

Rejeb, A., Rejeb, K., & Treiblmaier, H. (2023). Mapping Metaverse research: Identifying future research areas based on bibliometric and topic modeling techniques. *Information (Basel)*, *14*(7), 356. doi:10.3390/info14070356

Ren, C. (2023). *Question the nature of reality through virtual reality Portals of Perception - ProQuest*. New York University Tandon School of Engineering.

Ren, Y., Yang, Y., Chen, J., Zhou, Y., Li, J., Xia, R., Yang, Y., Wang, Q., & Su, X. (2022). A scoping review of deep learning in cancer nursing combined with augmented reality: The era of intelligent nursing is coming. *Asia-Pacific Journal of Oncology Nursing*, *9*(12), 100135. doi:10.1016/j.apjon.2022.100135 PMID:36276884

Riches, S., Jeyarajaguru, P., Taylor, L., Fialho, C., Little, J. R., Ahmed, L., O'Brien, A., Van Driel, C., Veling, W., & Valmaggia, L. (2023). Virtual reality relaxation for people with mental health conditions: A systematic review. *Social Psychiatry and Psychiatric Epidemiology*, *58*(7), 989–1007. doi:10.100700127-022-02417-5 PMID:36658261

Riches, S., Taylor, L., Jeyarajaguru, P., Veling, W., & Valmaggia, L. (2023). Virtual reality and immersive technologies to promote workplace wellbeing: A systematic review. *Journal of Mental Health (Abingdon, England)*, 1–21. doi:10.1080/09638237.2023.2182428 PMID:36919828

Richter, S., & Richter, A. (2023). What is novel about the Metaverse? *International Journal of Information Management*, *73*, 102684. doi:10.1016/j.ijinfomgt.2023.102684

Rieger, K. L., Hack, T. F., Duff, M. A., Campbell-Enns, H., & West, C. H. (2023). Integrating mindfulness and the expressive arts for meaning making in cancer care: A grounded theory of the processes, facilitators, and challenges. *Supportive Care in Cancer*, *31*(8), 475. doi:10.100700520-023-07909-x PMID:37466723

Rob, F. M., Jaap, J., van Baal, J., & van der Heijden, F. (2020). Infrared 3D Thermography for Inflammation Detection in Diabetic Foot Disease: A Proof of Concept. *Journal of Diabetes Science and Technology*. https://journals.sagepub.com/doi/10.1177/1932296819854062

Robison, J., Walter, T., Godsey, J. A., & Robinson, J. (2023). Chairside yoga therapy alleviates symptoms in patients concurrently receiving outpatient cancer infusions: A Promising Feasibility study. *Journal of Holistic Nursing*. doi:10.1177/08980101231170482 PMID:37128683

Compilation of References

Rodriguez, S. D., Rivu, R., Mäkelä, V., & Alt, F. (2023). *Challenges in Virtual Reality Studies: Ethics and Internal and External Validity*. ACM. doi:10.1145/3582700.3582716

Rolbiecki, A. J., Govindarajan, A., & Froeliger, B. (2023). Immersive virtual reality and neurofeedback for the management of cancer symptoms during treatment. *Supportive Care in Cancer*, *31*(8), 493. doi:10.100700520-023-07957-3 PMID:37493785

Rosenberg, L. (2023). The Metaverse and Conversational AI as a Threat Vector for Targeted Influence. In *2023 IEEE 13th Annual Computing and Communication Workshop and Conference (CCWC)*. IEEE. 10.1109/ccwc57344.2023.10099167

Rospigliosi, P. (2022). Adopting the metaverse for learning environments means more use of deep learning artificial intelligence: this presents challenges and problems. *Interactive Learning Environments*. Routledge. doi:. doi:10.1080/10494820.2022.2132034

Roy, A. (2020). The fourth industrial revolution. *Journal of International Consumer Marketing*, *32*(3), 268–270. doi:10.1080/08961530.2020.1727164

Roy, B. L., Martin-Krumm, C., & Trousselard, M. (2023). Mindfulness for adaptation to analog and new technologies emergence for long-term space missions. *Frontiers in Space Technologies*, *4*. doi:10.3389/frspt.2023.1109556

Ruan, H., Pocock, I., & Ruan, H. (2023). "You just have to stick with the practice": A Long-Term weekly mindfulness group at the VA. *Group*, *47*(1–2), 91–114. doi:10.1353/grp.2023.0008

S¸ahin, E., Yavuz Veizi, B. G., and Naharci, M. I. (2021). Telemedicine inter-ventions for older adults: a systematic review. *Journal of telemedicine and telecare*. doi: 10.1177/1357633X21105834

Saadouli, H., Masmoudi, M., Jerbi, B., & Dammak, A. (2014). An optimization and simulation approach for Operating room scheduling under stochastic durations. *Proceedings - International Conference on Control, Decision and Information Technologies*. IEEE. 10.1109/CoDIT.2014.6996903

Saha, B. (n.d.). *Analysis of the adherence of MHealth applications to HIPAA Technical Safeguards*. DigitalCommons@Kennesaw State University. https://digitalcommons.kennesaw.edu/msit_etd/14/

Sahu, G., Gaur, L., & Singh, G. (2023). Investigating the impact of Personality Tendencies and Gratification Aspects on OTT Short Video Consumption: A case of YouTube Shorts. *2023 3rd International Conference on Innovative Practices in Technology and Management (ICIPTM)*, (pp. 1–6). IEEE. 10.1109/ICIPTM57143.2023.10118122

Saleh, S., Cherradi, B., Gannour, O. E., Gouiza, N., & Bouattane, O. (2023). Healthcare monitoring system for automatic database management using mo-bile application in iot environment. *Bulletin of Electrical Engineering and Informatics*, *12*(2), 1055–1068. doi:10.11591/eei.v12i2.4282

Salem, S. F., Lawry, C. A., Alanadoly, A., & Li, J. (2023). Branded experiences in the immersive spectrum: How will fashion consumers react to the Metaverse? *ResearchGate*. https://www.researchgate.net/publication/372782798_Branded_experiences_in_the_immersive_spectrum_How_will_fashion_consumers_react_to_the_Metaverse

Samant, P., & Agarwal, R. (2018, April). Machine learning techniques for medical diagnosis of diabetes using iris images. *Computer Methods and Programs in Biomedicine*, *157*, 121–128. doi:10.1016/j.cmpb.2018.01.004 PMID:29477420

Samarin, N., Kothari, S., Siyed, Z., Bjorkman, O., Yuan, R., Wijesekera, P., Alomar, N., Fischer, J., Hoofnagle, C. J., & Egelman, S. (2023). *Lessons in VCR Repair: Compliance of Android App Developers with the California Consumer Privacy Act (CCPA)*. Cornell University. doi:10.48550/arxiv.2304.00944

Sanku, B. S., Li, Y. J., & He, J. (2023). A Survey of VR-Based Neurofeedback Systems in Physiological Computing for Depression Treatment. *2023 9th International Conference on Virtual Reality (ICVR)*. 10.1109/icvr57957.2023.10169583

Şanlisoy, S., & Çiloğlu, T. (2023). A View of the Future of the Metaverse Economy on the Basis of The Global Financial System: New Opportunities and Risks. *Journal of Corporate Governance, Insurance and Risk Management*, *10*(1), 28–41. doi:10.56578/jcgirm100104

Santosh & Gaur. (2021). Artificial Intelligence and Machine Learning in Public Healthcare. SpringerLink. 10.1007-978-981-16-6768-8.

Santosh, K. C., & Gaur, L. (2021). AI in Sustainable Public Healthcare. In K. C. Santosh & L. Gaur (Eds.), *Artificial Intelligence and Machine Learning in Public Healthcare: Opportunities and Societal Impact* (pp. 33–40). doi:10.1007/978-981-16-6768-8_4

Santosh, K. C., Gaur, L., Santosh, K. C., & Gaur, L. (2021). Societal Impact:-AI in Public Health Issues. In *Artificial Intelligence and Machine Learning in Public Healthcare: Opportunities and Societal Impact* (pp. 49–54). Springer. doi:10.1007/978-981-16-6768-8_6

Santosh, K., & Gaur, L. (2021a). *Ai in precision medicine*. SpringerBriefs in Applied Sciences and Technology. doi:10.1007/978-981-16-6768-8_5

Santosh, K., & Gaur, L. (2021b). *Ai solutions to public health issues*. Springer-Briefs in Applied Sciences and Technology. doi:10.1007/978-981-16-6768-8_3

Sarasalin, P. (2023). Atmosphere of Place: A case study of a contemporary tropical home. *The International Journal of Design in Society*, *17*(1), 45–78. doi:10.18848/2325-1328/CGP/v17i01/45-78

Schäfer, A., Mathisen, A., Svendsen, K., Engberg, S., Rolighed Thomsen, T., & Kirketerp-Møller, K. (2021, February). Toward Machine-Learning-Based Decision Support in Diabetes Care: A Risk Stratification Study on Diabetic Foot Ulcer and Amputation. *Frontiers in Medicine*, *7*, 601602. doi:10.3389/fmed.2020.601602 PMID:33681236

Schlussel, H., & Frosh, P. (2023). The taste of video: Facebook videos as multi-sensory experiences. *Convergence*, *29*(4), 980–996. doi:10.1177/13548565231179958

Compilation of References

Schneider, M., Woodworth, A., Arumalla, S., Gowder, C., Hernandez, J., Kim, A., & Moorthy, B. (2023). Development of a tool for quantifying need-supportive coaching in technology-mediated exercise classes. *Psychology of Sport and Exercise*, *64*, 102321. doi:10.1016/j.psychsport.2022.102321 PMID:37665807

Schoonjans, L. J. L. M. (2021). *The dominance challenge of European ICT companies against China and the USA*. Academic Press.

Schrodt, P. A. (2019). Artificial intelligence and international relations: An overview. *Artificial Intelligence and International Politics*, 9-31.

Schwartz, K., Ganster, F. M., & Tran, U. S. (2022). Mindfulness-Based Mobile Applications and their Impact on Well-Being in Non-Clinical Populations: A Systematic Review of Randomized Controlled Trials (Preprint). *Journal of Medical Internet Research*. doi:10.2196/44638 PMID:37540550

Seetharaman, R., Avhad, S., & Rane, J. (2023). *Exploring the healing power of singing bowls: An overview of key findings and potential benefits*. Elsevier. doi:10.1016/j.explore.2023.07.007

Settimo, C., De Cola, M. C., Pironti, E., Muratore, R., Giambò, F. M., Alito, A., Tresoldi, M., La Fauci, M., De Domenico, C., Tripodi, E., Impallomeni, C., Quartarone, A., & Cucinotta, F. (2023). Virtual Reality Technology to Enhance Conventional Rehabilitation Program: Results of a Single-Blind, Randomized, Controlled Pilot Study in Patients with Global Developmental Delay. *Journal of Clinical Medicine*, *12*(15), 4962. doi:10.3390/jcm12154962 PMID:37568364

Shafiq, D. A., Jhanjhi, N. Z., & Abdullah, A. (2021). Machine Learning Approaches for Load Balancing in Cloud Computing Services. *2021 National Computing Colleges Conference (NCCC)*. 10.1109/NCCC49330.2021.9428825

Shah, A. C. & Badawy, S. M. (2021). Telemedicine in pediatrics: system-atic review of randomized controlled trials. *JMIR pediatrics and parenting, 4*(1), e22696.

Shah, I., Sial, Q., Jhanjhi, N., and Gaur, L. (2022). *The role of the IoT and digital twin in the healthcare digitalization process: IoT and digital twin in the healthcare digitalization process*. In Digital Twins and Healthcare: Trends, Techniques, and Challenges. doi: 10.4018/978-1-6684-5925-6.ch002

Shannon, L. (2023). *Interconnected realities: How the Metaverse Will Transform Our Relationship with Technology Forever*. John Wiley & Sons.

Shao, L., Tang, W., Zhang, Z., & Chen, X. (2023). Medical Metaverse: Technologies, Applications, Challenges And Future. *Journal of Mechanics in Medicine and Biology*, *23*(02), 2350028. doi:10.1142/S0219519423500288

Sharma, S., Singh, G., Gaur, L., & Afaq, A. (2022). Exploring customer adoption of autonomous shopping systems. *Telematics and Informatics*, *73*, 101861. doi:10.1016/j.tele.2022.101861

Sharmin, S. (2023, July 25). *Insights into Cognitive Engagement: Comparing the Effectiveness of Game-Based and Video-Based Learning.* https://arxiv.org/abs/2307.13637

Shen, J., Wang, J., & Zhang, J. (2023). *The Development of Digital Technology Efficiency in the Communication of Large-Scale Events.* European Union Digital Library. doi:10.4108/eai.6-1-2023.2330328

She, Y., Wang, Q., Liu, F., Lin, L., Yang, B., & Hu, B. (2023). An interaction design model for virtual reality mindfulness meditation using imagery-based transformation and positive feedback. *Computer Animation and Virtual Worlds, 34*(3-4), e2184. doi:10.1002/cav.2184

Shuai, Q., Li, Z., & Zhang, Y. (2023). E-Commerce Channels and Platforms. In Spinger Link (pp. 283–318). Springer. doi:10.1007/978-981-99-0043-5_8

Silver, F. H., Deshmukh, T., Kelkar, N., Ritter, K., Ryan, N., & Nadiminti, H. (2021). The "Virtual Biopsy" of Cancerous Lesions in 3D: Non-Invasive Differentiation between Melanoma and Other Lesions Using Vibrational Optical Coherence Tomography. *Dermatopathology (Basel, Switzerland), 8*(4), 539–551. doi:10.3390/dermatopathology8040058 PMID:34940035

Singh, S., Bhatt, P., Sharma, S. K., & Rabiu, S. (2021). Digital Transformation in Healthcare: Innovation and Technologies. In Blockchain for Healthcare Systems (pp. 61-79). CRC Press.

Singh, A., Sharma, S., Singh, A., Unanoglu, M., & Taneja, S. (2023). *Cultural marketing and metaverse for consumer engagement.* IGI Global. doi:10.4018/978-1-6684-8312-1

Singhal, V., Jain, S. P., Anand, D., Singh, A., Verma, S., Kavita, Rodrigues, J. J. P. C., Jhanjhi, N. Z., Ghosh, U., Jo, O., & Iwendi, C. (2020). Artificial Intelligence Enabled Road Vehicle-Train Collision Risk Assessment Framework for Unmanned railway level crossings. *IEEE Access : Practical Innovations, Open Solutions, 8*, 113790–113806. doi:10.1109/ACCESS.2020.3002416

Singh, K., & Saxena, G. (2023). *Religious and spiritual practices in India: A Positive Psychological Perspective.* Springer Nature. doi:10.1007/978-981-99-2397-7

Singh, M., & Kumar, A. (2023). A Critical Political Economy Perspective on Indian Television: STAR, Hotstar, and Live Sports Streaming. *TripleC, 21*(1), 18–32. doi:10.31269/triplec.v21i1.1395

Singh, R. P., Hom, G. L., Abramoff, M. D., Campbell, J. P., & Chiang, M. F. (2020). Current challenges and barriers to real-world artificial intelligence adoption for the healthcare system, provider, and the patient. *Translational Vision Science & Technology, 9*(2), 45–45. doi:10.1167/tvst.9.2.45 PMID:32879755

Siricharoen, N. (2023). Creative Brain Training Apps and Games Can Help Improve Memory, Cognitive Abilities, and Promote Good Mental Health for The Elderly. *EAI Endorsed Transactions on Context-aware Systems and Applications, 9*(1). doi:10.4108/eetcasa.v9i1.3524

Sittig, D. F., Kahol, K., & Singh, H. (2013). Sociotechnical evaluation of the safety and effectiveness of point-of-care mobile computing devices: a case study conducted in india. *Electronic Health Records: Challenges in Design and Implementation, 115.*

Compilation of References

Siwik, C., Adler, S. R., Moran, P. J., Kuyken, W., Segal, Z. V., Felder, J. N., Eisendrath, S. J., & Hecht, F. M. (2023). Preventing Depression Relapse: A Qualitative Study on the Need for Additional Structured Support Following Mindfulness-Based Cognitive Therapy. *UCSF, 12*. doi:10.1177/27536130221144247 PMID:37077178

Skalidis, I., Muller, O., & Fournier, S. (2022). CardioVerse: The cardiovascular medicine in the era of Metaverse. *Trends in Cardiovascular Medicine*. doi:10.1016/j.tcm.2022.05.004 PMID:35568263

Slater, M., Gonzalez-Liencres, C., Haggard, P., Vinkers, C., Gregory-Clarke, R., Jelley, S., Watson, Z., Breen, G., Schwarz, R., Steptoe, W., Szostak, D., Halan, S., Fox, D., & Silver, J. (2020). The ethics of realism in virtual and augmented reality. *Frontiers in Virtual Reality*, *1*, 1. doi:10.3389/frvir.2020.00001

Slivjak, E., Kirk, A., & Arch, J. J. (2023). The Psychophysiology of Self-Compassion. In Springer eBooks (pp. 291–307). Springer. doi:10.1007/978-3-031-22348-8_17

Smith, M. J., Mark, R., Nette, H., & Rhodes, R. E. (2023). Correlates and participation in community-based exercise programming for cancer patients before and during COVID-19. *Supportive Care in Cancer*, *31*(6), 319. doi:10.100700520-023-07725-3 PMID:37148447

Snodgrass, J. G. (2023). *The Avatar faculty: Ecstatic Transformations in Religion and Video Games*. Univ of California Press.

Soilemezi, D., Roberts, H., Navarta-Sánchez, M. V., Kunkel, D., Ewings, S., Reidy, C., & Portillo, M. C. (2022). Managing Parkinson's during the COVID-19 pandemic: Perspectives from people living with Parkinson's and health professionals. *Journal of Clinical Nursing*, *32*(7-8), 1421–1432. doi:10.1111/jocn.16367 PMID:35581711

Solanki, A., Jain, V., & Gaur, L. (2022). *Applications of Blockchain and Big IoT Systems: Digital Solutions for Diverse Industries*. CRC Press. doi:10.1201/9781003231332

Solas-Martínez, J. L., Suárez-Manzano, S., De La Torre-Cruz, M. J., & Ruiz-Ariza, A. (2023). Artificial Intelligence and Augmented Reality in Physical Activity: A Review of Systems and Devices. In Spinger Link (pp. 245–270). doi:10.1007/978-3-031-27166-3_14

Song, Y.-T., & Qin, J. (2022). Metaverse and Personal Healthcare. *Procedia Computer Science*, *210*, 189–197. doi:10.1016/j.procs.2022.10.136

Soni, L., & Kaur, A. (2023). *Strategies for Implementing Metaverse in Education*. IEEE Explore. doi:10.1109/ICDT57929.2023.10150886

Søvold, L. E., Naslund, J. A., Kousoulis, A. A., Saxena, S., Qoronfleh, M. W., Grobler, C., & Münter, L. (2021). Prioritizing the mental health and well-being of healthcare workers: An urgent global public health priority. *Frontiers in Public Health*, *9*, 679397. doi:10.3389/fpubh.2021.679397 PMID:34026720

Sparkes, M. (2021). What is a metaverse. *New Scientist*, *251*(3348), 18. doi:10.1016/S0262-4079(21)01450-0

Srinivasu, P. N., Ijaz, M. F., Shafi, J., Wozniak, M., & Sujatha, R. (2022). 6g driven fast computational networking framework for healthcare applications. *IEEE Access: Practical Innovations, Open Solutions*, *10*, 94235–94248. doi:10.1109/ACCESS.2022.3203061

Starekova, J., & Reeder, S. B. (2020). Liver fat quantification: Where do we stand? *Abdominal Radiology*, *45*(11), 3386–3399. doi:10.100700261-020-02783-1 PMID:33025153

Ștefan, S. C., Popa, I., & Mircioiu, C. (2023). Lessons Learned from Online Teaching and Their Implications for Students' Future Careers: Combined PLS-SEM and IPA Approach. *Electronics (Basel)*, *12*(9), 2005. doi:10.3390/electronics12092005

Steinhoff, L., & Martin, K. D. (2022). Putting Data Privacy Regulation into Action: The Differential Capabilities of Service Frontline Interfaces. *Journal of Service Research*, *26*(3), 330–350. doi:10.1177/10946705221141925

Stocker, V., Whalley, J., & Lehr, W. (2023). Beyond the pandemic: towards a digitally enabled society and economy. In Emerald Publishing Limited eBooks (pp. 245–265). doi:10.1108/978-1-80262-049-820231012

Stockly, K. J., & Wildman, W. J. (2022). Interpreting the rapidly changing landscape of spirit tech. *Religion, Brain & Behavior*, *13*(1), 109–118. doi:10.1080/2153599X.2022.2091010

Strickland, M., Wimbush, S. C., Rupich, M. W., & Long, N. J. (2019). Asymmetries in the Field and Angle Dependences of the Critical Current in HTS Tapes. *IEEE Transactions on Applied Superconductivity*, *29*(Jan), 1–4. doi:10.1109/TASC.2019.2894278

Suh, I. H., McKinney, T., & Siu, K. (2023). Current Perspective of Metaverse Application in Medical Education, Research and Patient Care. *MDPI*, *2*(2), 115–128. doi:10.3390/virtualworlds2020007

Sullivan, M., Huberty, J., Chung, Y., & Stecher, C. (2023). Mindfulness meditation app Abandonment during the COVID-19 Pandemic: An observational study. *Mindfulness*, *14*(6), 1504–1521. doi:10.100712671-023-02125-4 PMID:37362188

Sun, P. (2023). *A Guidebook for 5GTOB and 6G Vision for Deep Convergence*. Springer Nature. doi:10.1007/978-981-99-4024-0

Sun, T., Jin, T., Huang, Y., Meng, L., Yun, W., Jiang, Z., & Fu, X. (2023). Restoring Dunhuang Murals: Crafting Cultural Heritage Preservation Knowledge into Immersive Virtual Reality Experience Design. *International Journal of Human-Computer Interaction*, 1–22. doi:10.1080/10447318.2023.2232976

Surveswaran, S., & Deshpande, L. (2023). *A Glimpse into the Future*. AI in Clinical Medicine. doi:10.1002/9781119790686.ch47

SynnottC. K. (2023). Gambling companies' contracts in higher education raise concerns. *Social Science Research Network*. doi:10.2139/ssrn.4394642

Compilation of References

Tai, B., Tsou, Y., Li, S., Huang, Y., Tsai, P., & Tsai, Y. (2023). User-Driven Synthetic Dataset Generation with Quantifiable Differential Privacy. *IEEE Transactions on Services Computing*, *16*(5), 1–14. doi:10.1109/TSC.2023.3287239

Tamulis, Vasiljevas, M., Damaševičius, R., Maskeliunas, R., & Misra, S. (2022). Affective Computing for eHealth Using Low-Cost Remote Internet of Things-Based EMG Platform. *Internet of Things*. doi: 10.1007/978-3-030-81473-1_3

Tan, M. C. C., Chye, S., & Min, T. J. (2023). Teaching Social-Emotional Learning with Immersive Virtual Technology: Exploratory Considerations. In Spinger Link (pp. 169–195). doi:10.1007/978-981-99-2107-2_10

Tan, M., & Le, Q. V. (2019). *EfficientNet: Rethinking Model Scaling for Convolutional Neural Networks*. arXiv.org. https://arxiv.org/abs/1905.11946

Tan, F. F., Ram, A., Haigh, C., & Zhao, S. (2023). *Mindful Moments: Exploring On-the-go Mindfulness Practice On Smart-glasses*. ACM. doi:10.1145/3563657.3596030

Tang, P. (2016). Multimetallic catalysed radical oxidative C(sp3)–H/C(sp)–H cross-coupling between unactivated alkanes and terminal alkynes. *Nature Communications, 7*. . doi:10.1038/ncomms11676

Tan, T. F., Li, Y., Lim, J. S., Gunasekeran, D. V., Teo, Z. L., Ng, W. Y., & Ting, D. S. W. (2022). Metaverse and Virtual Health Care in Ophthalmology: Opportunities and Challenges. *Asia-Pacific Journal of Ophthalmology*, *11*(3), 237–246. doi:10.1097/APO.0000000000000537 PMID:35772084

Tayyab, M., Marjani, M., Jhanjhi, N. Z., Hashem, I. T., Usmani, R. S. A., & Qamar, F. (2023). A comprehensive review on deep learning algorithms: Security and privacy issues. *Computers & Security*, *131*, 103297. doi:10.1016/j.cose.2023.103297

Tekin, B. H., & Gutiérrez, R. U. (2023). Human-centred health-care environments: A new framework for biophilic design. *Frontiers in Medical Technology*, *5*, 1219897. doi:10.3389/fmedt.2023.1219897 PMID:37560462

Thamrongrat, P., Khundam, C., Pakdeebun, P., & Nizam, D. M. (2023). Desktop vs. Headset: A Comparative Study of User Experience and Engagement for Flexibility Exercise in. *ResearchGate*. doi:10.28991/ESJ-2023-07-04-03

Thomason, J. (2022). Metaverse, token economies, and non-communicable diseases. *Global Health Journal*, *6*(3), 164–167. doi:10.1016/j.glohj.2022.07.001

Tlili, A., Huang, R., Shehata, B., Liu, D., Zhao, J., Metwally, A. H. S., Wang, H., Denden, M., Bozkurt, A., Lee, L.-H., Beyoglu, D., Altinay, F., Sharma, R. C., Altinay, Z., Li, Z., Liu, J., Ahmad, F., Hu, Y., Salha, S., & Burgos, D. (2022). Is Metaverse in education a blessing or a curse: A combined content and bibliometric analysis. *Smart Learning Environments*, *9*(1), 24. doi:10.118640561-022-00205-x

Torky, M., Darwish, A., & Hassanien, A. E. (2023). Blockchain technology in metaverse: opportunities, applications, and open problems. In Springer eBooks (pp. 225–246). doi:10.1007/978-3-031-29132-6_13

Torrance, J., O'Hanrahan, M., Carroll, J., & Newall, P. (2022). *The structural characteristics of online sports betting: a scoping review of current product features and utility patents as indicators of potential future developments.* Taylor Francis Online. doi:10.1080/16066359.2023.2241350

Toussaint, L., Huynh, K., Kohls, N., Sirois, F. M., Alberts, H., Hirsch, J. K., Hanshans, C., Nguyen, Q., Van Der Zee-Neuen, A., & Offenbaecher, M. (2023). Expectations regarding Gastein Healing Gallery treatment and their connection to Health-Related quality of life. *International Journal of Environmental Research and Public Health*, *20*(7), 5426. doi:10.3390/ijerph20075426 PMID:37048040

Transformers in Vision Survey. (2020ACM. https://dl.acm.org/doi/abs/10.1145/3505244

Tri, H. (2019). Insecticide resistance in Aedes aegypti: An impact from human urbanization? *PlosOne, 14*(6). . doi:10.1371/journal.pone.0218079

Turdialiev, M. (2023). *Legal discussion of metaverse Law*. doi:10.59022/ijcl.36

Turoń-Skrzypińska, A., Tomska, N., Mosiejczuk, H., Rył, A., Szylińska, A., Marchelek-Myśliwiec, M., Ciechanowski, K., Nagay, R., & Rotter, I. (2023). Impact of virtual reality exercises on anxiety and depression in hemodialysis. *Nature*, *13*(1), 12435. doi:10.103841598-023-39709-y PMID:37528161

Tyagi, A., Gaur, L., Singh, G., & Kumar, A. (2022). Air Quality Index (AQI) Using Time Series Modelling During COVID Pandemic. In G. Sanyal, C.M. Travieso-González, S. Awasthi, C.M.A. Pinto, & B.R. Purushothama (Eds.), *International Conference on Artificial Intelligence and Sustainable Engineering*. Springer Singapore, Singapore. 10.1007/978-981-16-8546-0_36

Tyagi, Y., & Saxena, S. (2022). Applications of Artificial Intelligence, Metaverse and Data Science for Intelligent Healthcare. *AAYAM: AKGIM Journal of Management*, *12*(2), 141–149.

Uddin, M., Manickam, S., Ullah, H., Obaidat, M., & Dandoush, A. (2023). Unveiling the metaverse: Exploring emerging trends, multifaceted perspectives, and future challenges. *IEEE Access : Practical Innovations, Open Solutions*, *1*, 87087–87103. doi:10.1109/ACCESS.2023.3281303

Ulhaq, A., Born, J., Khan, A., Gomes, D. P. S., Chakraborty, S., & Paul, M. (2020). COVID-19 control by computer vision approaches: A survey. *IEEE Access : Practical Innovations, Open Solutions*, *8*, 179437–179456. doi:10.1109/ACCESS.2020.3027685 PMID:34812357

Ullah, H., Manickam, S., Obaidat, M., Laghari, S. A., & Uddin, M. (2023). Exploring the potential of metaverse technology in healthcare: Applications, challenges, and future directions. *IEEE Access : Practical Innovations, Open Solutions*, *11*, 69686–69707. doi:10.1109/ACCESS.2023.3286696

Compilation of References

Ullah, M., Hamayun, S., Wahab, A., Khan, S. U., Qayum, M., Ullah, A., Rehman, M. U., Mehreen, A., Awan, U. A., & Naeem, M. (2023). Smart Technologies used as Smart Tools in the Management of Cardiovascular Disease and their Future Perspective. *Current Problems in Cardiology*, *101922*(11), 101922. doi:10.1016/j.cpcardiol.2023.101922 PMID:37437703

Üstün, A., Yılmaz, R., & Yılmaz, F. G. K. (2022). Educational UTAUT-based virtual reality acceptance scale: A validity and reliability study. *Virtual Reality (Waltham Cross)*, *27*(2), 1063–1076. doi:10.100710055-022-00717-4

Vaccaro, A., Koerner, J. D., & Kim, D. H. (2016). *Recent advances in spinal surgery*. JP Medical Ltd.

Vadalà, G., De Salvatore, S., Ambrosio, L., Russo, F., Papalia, R., & Denaro, V. (2020). Robotic spine surgery and augmented reality systems: A state of the art. *Neurospine*, *17*(1), 88–100. doi:10.14245/ns.2040060.030 PMID:32252158

Van Biemen, T., Müller, D., & Mann, D. L. (2023). Virtual reality as a representative training environment for football referees. *Human Movement Science*, *89*, 103091. doi:10.1016/j.humov.2023.103091 PMID:37084551

Van Rijmenam, M. (2022). *Step into the Metaverse: How the Immersive Internet Will Unlock a Trillion-Dollar Social Economy*. John Wiley & Sons.

Van Wegen, M., Herder, J. L., Adelsberger, R., Pastore-Wapp, M., Van Wegen, E. E. H., Bohlhalter, S., Nef, T., Krack, P., & Vanbellingen, T. (2023). An overview of wearable haptic technologies and their performance in virtual object exploration. *Sensors (Basel)*, *23*(3), 1563. doi:10.339023031563 PMID:36772603

Vanagas, G., Engelbrecht, R., Damaševičius, R., Suomi, R., & Solanas, A. (2018). Ehealth solutions for the integrated healthcare. *Journal of Healthcare Engineering*, 2018. doi: 10.1155/2018/3846892 PMID:30123441

Vardasca, R., Vaz, L., Magalhaes, C., Seixas, A., & Mendes, J. (2018). Towards the Diabetic Foot Ulcers Classification with Infrared Thermal Images. *Proceedings of the 2018 International Conference on Quantitative InfraRed Thermography*. IEEE. 10.21611/qirt.2018.008

Vassallo, D., Swinfen, P., Swinfen, R., & Wootton, R. (2001). Experience with a low-cost telemedicine system in three developing countries. *Journal of Telemedicine and Telecare*, *7*(1, Suppl), 56–58. doi:10.1177/1357633X010070S123 PMID:11576493

Vaz, S. C., Oliveira, F., Herrmann, K., & Veit-Haibach, P. (2020). Nuclear medicine and molecular imaging advances in the 21st century. *The British Journal of Radiology*, *93*(1110), 20200095. doi:10.1259/bjr.20200095 PMID:32401541

Veber, M., Pesek, I., & Aberšek, B. (2023). Assessment of supporting visual learning technologies in the Immersive VET Cyber-Physical Learning Model. *Education in Science*, *13*(6), 608. doi:10.3390/educsci13060608

Velayati, F., Ayatollahi, H., Hemmat, M., & Dehghan, R. (2022). Telehealth business models and their components: Systematic review. *Journal of Medical Internet Research*, 24(3), e33128. doi:10.2196/33128 PMID:35348471

Velissaris, S. L., Davis, M., Fisher, F., Gluyas, C., & Stout, J. C. (2023). A pilot evaluation of an 8-week mindfulness-based stress reduction program for people with pre-symptomatic Huntington's disease. *Journal of Community Genetics*, 14(4), 395–405. doi:10.100712687-023-00651-1 PMID:37458974

Ventura, S., Lullini, G., & Riva, G. (2022). Cognitive Rehabilitation in the Metaverse: Insights from the Tele-Neurorehab Project. *Cyberpsychology, Behavior, and Social Networking*, 25(10), 686–687. doi:10.1089/cyber.2022.29257.ceu PMID:36264212

Venugopal, J.P., Subramanian, A.A.V. & Peatchimuthu, J. (2023). The realm of metaverse: A survey. *Computer Animation and Virtual Worlds*. John Wiley & Sons, Ltd. doi:. doi:0.1002/cav.2150

Verberk, J. D. M., Aghdassi, S. J. S., Abbas, M., Nauclér, P., Gubbels, S., Maldonado, N., Palacios-Baena, Z. R., Johansson, A. F., Gastmeier, P., Behnke, M., van Rooden, S. M., & van Mourik, M. S. M. (2022). Automated surveillance systems for healthcare-associated infections: Results from a European survey and experiences from real-life utilization. *The Journal of Hospital Infection*, 122, 35–43. doi:10.1016/j.jhin.2021.12.021 PMID:35031393

Villa-García, L., Davey, V., Pérez, L. M., Soto-Bagaria, L., Risco, E., Díaz, P., Kuluski, K., Giné-Garriga, M., Castellano-Tejedor, C., & Inzitari, M. (2023). Co-designing implementation strategies to promote remote physical activity programs in frail older community-dwellers. *Frontiers in Public Health*, 11, 1062843. doi:10.3389/fpubh.2023.1062843 PMID:36960372

Villalón, F., Moreno, M. I. B., Rivera, R. M., & Venegas, W. G. JVC, N., Soto-Mota, A., & Pemjean, A. (2023). Brief Online Mindfulness- and Compassion-Based Inter-Care Program for Students during COVID-19 Pandemic: A randomized controlled trial. *Mindfulness*. doi:10.100712671-023-02159-8

Villalonga-Gómez, C., Ortega-Fernández, E., & Borau-Boira, E. (2023). Fifteen years of metaverse in Higher Education: A systematic literature review. *IEEE Transactions on Learning Technologies*, 1–14. doi:10.1109/TLT.2023.3302382

Wagenius, M. (2021). *Complications and treatment aspects of urological stone surgery*. Lund University.

Waitt, G. R., Gordon, R., Harada, T., Gurrieri, L., Reith, G., & Ciorciari, J. (2023). Towards relational geographies of gambling harm: Orientation, affective atmosphere, and intimacy. *Progress in Human Geography*, (5), 627–644. doi:10.1177/03091325231177278

Wang, H., & Ding, S. (2017). Selection and evaluation of new reference genes for RT-qPCR analysis in Epinephelus akaara based on transcriptome data. *PlosOne*, 2. . doi:10.1371/journal.pone.0171646

Compilation of References

Wang, T. (2023, January 3). *Augmented Reality in Sports Event Videos: A Qualitative Study on Viewer experience*. Scholar Space. https://scholarspace.manoa.hawaii.edu/items/00382afd-df6e-4ece-8b84-21e7922dad76

Wang, D., Yang, Z., Zhang, P., Wang, R., Yang, B., & Ma, X. (2023). Virtual-Reality Inter-Promotion Technology for Metaverse: A survey. *IEEE Internet of Things Journal*, *1*(18), 15788–15809. doi:10.1109/JIOT.2023.3265848

Wang, G., Badal, A., Jia, X., Maltz, J. S., Mueller, K., Myers, K. J., Niu, C., Vannier, M., Yan, P., & Yu, Z. (2022). Development of metaverse for intelligent healthcare. *Nature Machine Intelligence*, 1–8. PMID:36935774

Wang, G., Badal, A., Jia, X., Maltz, J. S., Mueller, K., Myers, K. J., Niu, C., Vannier, M., Yan, P., Yu, Z., & Zeng, R. (2022). Development of metaverse for intelligent healthcare. *Nature Machine Intelligence*, *4*(11), 922–929. doi:10.103842256-022-00549-6 PMID:36935774

Wang, N., & Wen-Guang, C. (2023). The effect of playing e-sports games on young people's desire to engage in physical activity: Mediating effects of social presence perception and virtual sports experience. *PLoS One*, *18*(7), e0288608. doi:10.1371/journal.pone.0288608 PMID:37498937

Wang, Y., Su, Z., Zhang, N., Xing, R., Liu, D., Luan, T. H., & Shen, X. (2022). A survey on metaverse: Fundamentals, security, and privacy. *IEEE Communications Surveys and Tutorials*.

Wang, Y., Weng, T., Tsai, I. F., Kao, J., & Chang, Y. J. (2022). Effects of virtual reality on creativity performance and perceived immersion: A study of brain waves. *British Journal of Educational Technology*, *54*(2), 581–602. doi:10.1111/bjet.13264

Ward, P. (2018). Trust and communication in a doctor-patient relationship: A literature review. *Archives of Medicine*, *3*(3), 36.

Weber, D. J., & Rutala, W. A. (2023). Understanding and Preventing Transmission of Health-Care Associated Pathogens Due to the Contaminate Hospital Environment. *Infection Control and Hospital Epidemiology*, *34*(5), 449–452. doi:10.1086/670223 PMID:23571359

Wedig, I. J., Phillips, J. J., Kamm, K., & Elmer, S. J. (2023). Promoting Physical Activity in Rural Communities During COVID-19 with Exercise is Medicine® on Campus. *ACSM's Health & Fitness Journal*, *27*(2), 33–40. doi:10.1249/FIT.0000000000000849

Wei, W. (2023). A buzzword, a phase or the next chapter for the Internet? The status and possibilities of the metaverse for tourism. *Journal of Hospitality and Tourism Insights*. doi:. doi:10.1108/JHTI-11-2022-0568

Weinstein, R. S., Lopez, A. M., Joseph, B. A., Erps, K. A., Holcomb, M., Barker, G. P., & Krupinski, E. A. (2014). Telemedicine, telehealth, and mobile health applications that work: Opportunities and barriers. *The American Journal of Medicine*, *127*(3), 183–187. doi:10.1016/j.amjmed.2013.09.032 PMID:24384059

Weisbrod, A. V., Bohman, L., & Ramdial, K. J. (2023). From theory to practice: A novel meditation program at a global corporation. *Current Psychology (New Brunswick, N.J.)*. doi:10.100712144-023-04516-1 PMID:37359588

Wertheim, J. O., Elton, D. C., & Gibson, C. B. (2020). Self-Supervised Learning for Medical Imaging. *IEEE Transactions on Medical Imaging*, doi:10.1109/TMI.2020.3017674

Wexler, T. M., & Schellinger, J. (2022). Mindfulness-Based Stress Reduction for Nurses: An Integrative Review. *Journal of Holistic Nursing*. doi:10.1177/08980101221079472 PMID:35213264

Whiting, A., Sharma, Y., Grewal, M. K., Ghulam, Z., Sajid, W., Dewan, N., Peladeau-Pigeon, M., & Dutta, T. (2023). Virtual Accessible Bilingual conference planning: The Parks Accessibility Conference. *International Journal of Environmental Research and Public Health*, 20(3), 2302. doi:10.3390/ijerph20032302 PMID:36767670

Wieland, M., Sedlmair, M., & Machulla, T. (2023). *VR, Gaze, and Visual Impairment: An Exploratory Study of the Perception of Eye Contact across different Sensory Modalities for People with Visual Impairments in Virtual Reality*. ACM. doi:10.1145/3544549.3585726

Williams, A. M., Bhatti, U. F., Alam, H. B., & Nikolian, V. C. (2018). The role of telemedicine in postoperative care. *mHealth*, 4, 4. doi:10.21037/mhealth.2018.04.03 PMID:29963556

Williams, R. (2023). Think piece: Ethics for the virtual researcher. *Practice*, 5(1), 1–7. doi:10.1080/25783858.2023.2179893

Wong, A., Bhyat, R., Srivastava, S., Lomax, L. B., & Appireddy, R. (2021). Patient care during the COVID-19 pandemic: Use of virtual care. *Journal of Medical Internet Research*, 23(1), e20621. doi:10.2196/20621 PMID:33326410

Wong, D. H., Bolton, R. E., Sitter, K. E., & Vimalananda, V. G. (2023). Endocrinologists' experiences with telehealth: A qualitative study with impli-cations for promoting sustained use. *Endocrine Practice*, 29(2), 104–109. doi:10.1016/j.eprac.2022.11.003 PMID:36370984

Wong, I. A., Lu, M. V., Lin, S. K., & Lin, Z. (2022). The transformative virtual experience paradigm: The case of Airbnb's online experience. *International Journal of Contemporary Hospitality Management*. doi:10.1108/ijchm-12-2021-1554

Wongkitrungrueng, A., & Suprawan, L. (2023). Metaverse Meets Branding: Examining consumer responses to immersive brand experiences. *International Journal of Human-Computer Interaction*, 1–20. doi:10.1080/10447318.2023.2175162

Wootton, R. (2001). Telemedicine. British medical journal, 323(7312), 557–560.

Wu, Y. C., Maymon, C., Paden, J., & Liu, W. (2023). Launching your VR Neuroscience Laboratory. In Current topics in behavioral neurosciences. doi:10.1007/7854_2023_420

Wu, J., Tang, J., & Agyeiwaah, E. (2023). 'I had more time to listen to my inner voice': Zen meditation tourism for Generation Z. *Tourist Studies*. doi:10.1177/14687976231189833

Compilation of References

Xiang, W., Yin, J., & Lim, G. (2015). An ant colony optimization approach for solving an operating room surgery scheduling problem. *Computers & Industrial Engineering*, *85*, 335–345. doi:10.1016/j.cie.2015.04.010

Xiao, Y., & Yoogalingam, R. (2021). Reserved capacity policies for operating room scheduling. *Operations Management Research*, *14*(1-2), 107–122. doi:10.100712063-020-00172-x

Xiong, X., Wei, L., Xiao, Y., Han, Y.-C., Yang, J., Zhao, H., Yang, M., & Sun, L. (2020, October). Family history of diabetes is associated with diabetic foot complications in type 2 diabetes. *Scientific Reports*, *10*(1), 17056. doi:10.103841598-020-74071-3 PMID:33051498

Xu, Y. (2023). The evolving eSports landscape: Technology empowerment, intelligent embodiment, and digital ethics. *Sport, Ethics and Philosophy*, *17*(3), 356–368. doi:10.1080/17511321.2023.2168039

Xu, Y., Holanda, G., Souza, L. F. D. F., Silva, H., Gomes, A., Silva, I., Fer-reira, M., Jia, C., Han, T., De Albuquerque, V. H. C., & Filho, P. P. R. (2021). Deep learning-enhanced internet of medical things to analyze brain ct scans of hemorrhagic stroke patients: A new approach. *IEEE Sensors Journal*, *21*(22), 24941–24951. doi:10.1109/JSEN.2020.3032897

Yampolskiy, R. V. (2019). *Unexplainability and incomprehensibility of artificial intelligence.* arXiv preprint arXiv:1907.03869.

Yang, Y., Siau, K., Xie, W. & Sun, Y. (2022). Smart health: Intelligent healthcare systems in the metaverse, artificial intelligence, and data science era. *Journal of Organizational and End User Computing (JOEUC)*. IGI Global.

Yang, D., Zhou, J., Chen, R., Song, Y., Song, Z., Zhang, X., Wang, Q., Wang, K., Zhou, C., Sun, J., Zhang, L., Bai, L., Wang, Y., Wang, X., Lu, Y., Xin, H., Powell, C. A., Thüemmler, C., Chavannes, N. H., & Bai, C. (2022). Expert consensus on the metaverse in medicine. *Clinical EHealth*, *5*, 1–9. doi:10.1016/j.ceh.2022.02.001

Yang, Y., Siau, K., Xie, W., & Sun, Y. (2022). Smart Health: Intelligent Healthcare Systems in the Metaverse, Artificial Intelligence, and Data Science Era. *Journal of Organizational and End User Computing*, *34*(1), 1–14. doi:10.4018/JOEUC.308814

Yan, Y., Zhang, J.-W., Zang, G.-Y., & Pu, J. (2019). The primary use of artificial intelligence in cardiovascular diseases: What kind of potential role does artificial intelligence play in future medicine? *Journal of Geriatric Cardiology : JGC*, *16*(8), 585. PMID:31555325

Yap, M. H., Hachiuma, R., Alavi, A., Brüngel, R., Cassidy, B., Goyal, M., Zhu, H., Rückert, J., Olshansky, M., Huang, X., Saito, H., Hassanpour, S., Friedrich, C. M., Ascher, D. B., Song, A., Kajita, H., Gillespie, D., Reeves, N. D., Pappachan, J. M, & Frank, E. (2021, August). Deep learning in diabetic foot ulcers detection: A comprehensive evaluation. *Computers in Biology and Medicine*, *135*, 104596. doi:10.1016/j.compbiomed.2021.104596 PMID:34247133

Yaqoob, I., Salah, K., Jayaraman, R., & Omar, M. (2023). Metaverse applications in smart cities: Enabling technologies, opportunities, challenges, and future directions. *Internet of Things*, *100884*, 100884. doi:10.1016/j.iot.2023.100884

Yeung, A. W. K., Tosevska, A., Klager, E., Eibensteiner, F., Laxar, D., Stoyanov, J., Glisic, M., Zeiner, S., Kulnik, S. T., Crutzen, R., Kimberger, O., Kletecka-Pulker, M., Atanasov, A. G., & Willschke, H. (2021). Virtual and augmented reality applications in medicine: Analysis of the scientific literature. *Journal of Medical Internet Research*, *23*(2), e25499. doi:10.2196/25499 PMID:33565986

Yilmaz, M., O'Farrell, E., & Clarke, P. M. (2023). Examining the training and education potential of the metaverse: Results from an empirical study of next generation SAFe training. *Journal of Software (Malden, MA)*, *35*(9), e2531. doi:10.1002mr.2531

Yin, C., Huang, Y., Kim, D., & Kim, K. (2023). The Effect of Esports Content Attributes on Viewing Flow and Well-Being: A focus on the moderating effect of esports involvement. *Sustainability*, *15*(16), 12207. doi:10.3390u151612207

Yoo, K., Welden, R., Hewett, K., & Haenlein, M. (2023). The merchants of meta: A research agenda to understand the future of retailing in the metaverse. *Journal of Retailing*, *99*(2), 173–192. doi:10.1016/j.jretai.2023.02.002

You, Y., & Youn, C. T. (2023). Research on the happiness experience structure of elderly people in metaverse. *Han'gug Di'jain Munhwa Haghoeji*, *29*(2), 339–353. doi:10.18208/ksdc.2023.29.2.339

Yue, Y., Yi, S., Nan, X., Leo, Y.-H. L., Shigyo, K., Liwenhan, X., Wicaksana, J., & Cheng, K.-T. (2023). FoodWise: Food Waste Reduction and Behavior Change on Campus with Data Visualization and Gamification. In *Proceedings of the 6th ACM SIGCAS/SIGCHI Conference on Computing and Sustainable Societies*. ACM. 10.1145/3588001.3609364

Yunana, K., Alfa, A. A., Misra, S., Damasevicius, R., Maskeliunas, R., & Olu-ranti, J. (2021). Internet of Things: Applications, Adoptions and Components. In: Hybrid Intelligent Systems. doi: 10.1007/978-3-030-73050-5_50

Yun, S. J., Hyun, S. E., Oh, B. M., & Seo, H. G. (2023). Fully immersive virtual reality exergames with dual-task components for patients with Parkinson's disease: A feasibility study. *Journal of Neuroengineering and Rehabilitation*, *20*(1), 92. doi:10.118612984-023-01215-7 PMID:37464349

Zainab, H. E., Bawany, N. Z., Rehman, W., & Imran, J. (2023). Design and development of virtual reality exposure therapy systems: Requirements, challenges and solutions. *Multimedia Tools and Applications*. doi:10.100711042-023-15756-5

Zalan, T., & Barbesino, P. (2023). Making the metaverse real. *Digital Business*, *3*(2), 100059. doi:10.1016/j.digbus.2023.100059

Zaman, N., Gaur, L., and Humayun, M. (2022). *Approaches and applications of deep learning in virtual medical care*. IGI Global. doi: 10.4018/978-1-7998-8929-8.

Compilation of References

Zaman, N., Gaur, L., & Humayun, M. (2022). *Approaches and applications of deep learning in virtual medical care*. IGI Global. doi:10.4018/978-1-7998-8929-8

Zhang, J. (2023). *Exploring gender expression and identity in virtual reality : The interplay of avatars, role-adoption, and social interaction in VRChat*. DIVA. https://www.diva-portal.org/smash/record.jsf?pid=diva2%3A1765332&dswid=-4051

Zhang, J. (2023, June 1). *Gamification in marketing to increase customer retention*. MIT. https://dspace.mit.edu/handle/1721.1/151418

Zhang, X., Li, Y., Yang, X., Zheng, L., Long, T., &. Baker, C. (2017). A Novel Monopulse Technique for Adaptive Phased Array Radar. *PlosOne, 17.* . doi:10.3390/s17010116

Zhang, Z., Xie, X., & Geng, N. (2021). Promise surgery start times and implementation strategies. *IEEE International Conference on Automation Science and Engineering*. IEEE.

Zhang, G., Dai, Y., Wu, J., Zhu, X., & Lu, Y. (2023). Swarm Learning-based Secure and Fair Model Sharing for Metaverse Healthcare. *Mobile Networks and Applications*. doi:10.100711036-023-02236-1

Zhang, L., He, W., Cao, Z., Wang, S., Bai, H., & Billinghurst, M. (2022). HapticProxy: Providing positional vibrotactile feedback on a physical proxy for Virtual-Real interaction in augmented reality. *International Journal of Human-Computer Interaction*, 1–15. doi:10.1080/10447318.2022.2041895

Zhang, Q. (2023). Secure preschool education using machine learning and metaverse technologies. *Applied Artificial Intelligence*, *37*(1), 2222496. doi:10.1080/08839514.2023.2222496

Zhang, X., Chen, Y., Hu, L., & Wang, Y. (2022). The metaverse in education: Definition, framework, features, potential applications, challenges, and future research topics. *Frontiers in Psychology*, *13*, 6063.

Zhao, R., Zhang, Y., Zhu, Y., Lan, R., & Hua, Z. (2023). Metaverse: Security and Privacy Concerns. *Dergi Park*, *3*(2), 93–99. doi:10.57019/jmv.1286526

Zhi, L. J., Heng, T. M., & Taojun, X. (2023). Evaluating the impact of digital economy collaborations in ASEAN. In Routledge eBooks (pp. 8–27). doi:10.4324/9781003308751-2

Zhu, Q., Zhang, X., Dai, S., Satake, N., & Wang, H. (2023). ZoomBaTogether: a video conference add-on for generating interactive visual feedback for online group exercise through On-The-Fly pose tracking. *Designing Interactive Systems Conference*. 10.1145/3563703.3596653

Zikas, P., Protopsaltis, A., Lydatakis, N., Kentros, M., Geronikolakis, S., Kateros, S., Kamarianakis, M., Evangelou, G., Filippidis, A., Grigoriou, E., Angelis, D., Tamiolakis, M., Dodis, M., Kokiadis, G., Petropoulos, J., Pateraki, M., & Papagiannakis, G. (2023). MAGES 4.0: Accelerating the world's transition to VR training and democratizing the authoring of the medical metaverse. *IEEE Computer Graphics and Applications*, *43*(2), 43–56. doi:10.1109/MCG.2023.3242686

Zoe, V. R. (2023, July 17). *Development of a therapy game proof of concept using the Virtual Reality technology*. Repostori. https://repositori.uji.es/xmlui/handle/10234/203631

About the Contributors

Loveleen Gaur is currently working as an adjunct professor with Taylor University, Malaysia & University of South Pacific, Fiji and academic consultant with Australian School of Graduate Studies. Before moving to USA, she was working as Professor with Amity University, India. She has supervised several PhD scholars, Post Graduate students, mainly in Artificial Intelligence and Data Analytics for business and healthcare. Under her guidance, the AI/Data Analytics research cluster has published extensively in high impact factor journals and has established extensive research collaboration globally with several renowned professionals. She is a senior IEEE member and Series Editor with CRC and Wiley. She has high indexed publications in SCI/ABDC/WoS/Scopus and has several Patents/copyrights on her account, edited/authored many research books published by world-class publishers. She has excellent experience in supervising and co-supervising postgraduate and PhD students internationally. An ample number of Ph.D. and master's students graduated under her supervision. She is an external Ph.D./Master thesis examiner/evaluator for several universities globally. She has also served as Keynote speaker for several international conferences, presented several Webinars worldwide, chaired international conference sessions. Prof. Gaur has significantly contributed to enhancing scientific understanding by participating in many scientific conferences, symposia, and seminars, by chairing technical sessions and delivering plenary and invited talks. She has specialized in the fields of Artificial Intelligence, Machine Learning, Pattern Recognition, Internet of Things, Data Analytics and Business Intelligence. She has chaired various positions in International Conferences of repute and is a reviewer with top rated journals of IEEE, SCI and ABDC Journals. She has been honored with prestigious National and International awards. She has introduced courses related to Artificial Intelligence specialization including, Predictive Analytics, Deep and Reinforcement learning etc. She has vast experience teaching advanced-era specialized courses, including Predictive Analytics, Data Visualization, Social Network Analytics, Deep Learning, Power BI, Digital Marketing and Digital Innovation etc., besides other undergraduate and postgraduate courses, graduation projects, and thesis supervision.

About the Contributors

Noor Zaman Jhanjhi is currently working as Associate Professor, Director Center for Smart society 5.0 [CSS5], & Cluster Head for Cybersecurity, at the School of Computer Science and Engineering, Taylor's University, Malaysia. He is supervising a great number of Postgraduate students, mainly in cybersecurity for Data Science. Dr Jhanjhi serves as Associate Editor and Editorial Assistant Board for several reputable journals, received Outstanding Associate Editor Award for IEEE ACCESS for 2020, PC member for several conferences, guest editor for the reputed journals. He is awarded globally as a top 1% reviewer by Publons (WoS). His collective research Impact factor is 400 plus. He has Patents on his account, edited/authored 35 plus research books published by world-class publishers. He is an external Ph.D./Master thesis examiner/evaluator globally, completed more than 22 internationally funded research grants. Served as a keynote speaker for several conferences, presented Webinars, chaired conference sessions, provided Consultancy internationally. His research areas include Cybersecurity, IoT security, Wireless security, Data Science, Software Engineering, UAVs.

***

Abdalla Hassan Gharib earned his Ph.D. and M.Sc. in Computer Science from Universiti Malaysia Sarawak, Malaysia. Currently, he serves as a lecturer and Quality Assurance Coordinator within the Faculty of Engineering at Zanzibar University, located in Zanzibar, Tanzania. In 2022, he was honored to be appointed as a council member of the Karume Institute of Science and Technology (KIST) by the Minister of Education and Vocational Training, Zanzibar, Tanzania. With numerous research articles to his name and supervision of eight Master's degree students by the end of 2023, Dr. Abdalla Gharib has emerged as a dedicated scholar in the realm of Mobile Communication Networks. His research specialization lies in communication protocols and information dissemination within Opportunistic Networks, addressing scenarios where traditional network infrastructures may be limited or absent. Beyond his core focus, he displays versatility and a wide array of interests, encompassing Artificial Intelligence (AI), Internet of Things (IoT), Quality Assurance, Digital Transformation, Cybersecurity and Graphic Design.. Driven by a profound passion for innovation and technology, his ultimate goal is to assist organizations and communities in harnessing technology ethically for competitive advantage and sustainable societal progress.

Husin Jazri is a computer science and cybersecurity professor at the Taylor's University Malaysia. He obtained his PhD degree in Computer Science from the National Defense University of Malaysia and Master's Degree from Royal Holloway University of London and University Putra Malaysia. He has more than 30 years of

About the Contributors

blended working experience in cybersecurity serving military, government, public listed company, startup companies and universities. He is also the founder and Director of the Global Centre for Cybersafety at Taylor's University.

Samayaraj Murali Kishanlal M. received the B.E degree in Electronics and Communication Engineering from Bannari Amman Institute of Technology, Bharthiar University, India in 2002 and M.E degree in Communication system from Government College of Technology, Anna University, Chennai, India in 2004 and completed his Ph.D. (Optical Networks) in Information and Communication engineering from Anna University, Chennai, Tamil Nadu. since 2012, working as Associate Professor Tamil Nadu in the Department of Electronics and Communication Engineering at St. Joseph's group of institutions, Chennai. He had published numerous of paper publications, reviewed research paper in various domains and working in research forum of the department. His area of interest includes Optical Networks, Optical Communication, etc.

Senthil Murugan M., born in 1982, received the Doctorate of Philosophy (Ph.D.) in the field of Electronics from Satyabhama Institute of Science and Technology, Chennai in the year 2022 and Bachelor's (B.E.) degree in Electronics and communication Engineering and Master's (M.E.) degree in Applied Electronics from St. Joseph's College of Engineering, Anna University Chennai, Tamilnadu in the year 2003 and 2005. He is currently working as an Associate Professor in St. Joseph's Institute of Technology, Chennai, Tamilnadu He is interested in research on Network Security, Wireless sensor Networks, Image processing.

Karthikeyan M. V. was born in Chennai, Tamil Nadu, India, in 1982. He received the B.E degree in Electronics and Communication Engineering from Hindustan College of Engineering, Madras University, Chennai, India in 2004 and M.E degree in Communication system from Hindustan College of Engineering, Anna University, Chennai, India in 2007 and completed his Ph.D. (Body Area Security) in Information and Communication engineering from Anna University, Chennai, Tamil Nadu. since 2010, working as Associate Professor Tamil Nadu in the Department of Electronics and Communication Engineering at St. Joseph's group of institutions, Chennai. He had published numerous of paper publications, reviewed research paper in various domains and working in research forum of the department. His area of interest includes Analog Communication, Digital Communication, wireless sensor Networks and Biomedical data analysis etc.

Siva T. received the B.E degree in Electronics and Communication Engineering from Anand Institute of Higher Technology, Anna University, India in 2006 and M.E degree in Applied Electronics from St. Joseph's College of Engineering, Anna

About the Contributors

University, Chennai, India in 2009 and doing his Ph.D. (Photonics) in Information and Communication engineering from Anna University, Chennai, Tamil Nadu. since 2013, working as Assistant Professor in the Department of Electronics and Communication Engineering at St. Joseph's group of institutions, Chennai.

Tephillah S. received the B.E. degree in Electronics and Communication Engineering from GKM College of Engineering,Chennai in 2003. She received the M.E. degree in Applied Electronics from College of Engineering, Anna University, Chennai in 2006 and PhD in Security in Cognitive Radio Networks, from College of Engineering, Guindy, Anna University, Chennai. She has Sixteen years of teaching. Her research interests include Cognitive radio networks, Wireless Communication, IOT, Embedded Systems, Sensor networks.

Index

A

Air Temperature 229
Augmented Reality (AR) 2, 93, 182, 188, 190-191, 193, 290, 310

C

Challenges 5-6, 14-15, 18, 22, 27-29, 31-33, 35, 39, 43-45, 47, 56-63, 68, 70-71, 75-78, 80-81, 83-84, 89, 91, 97, 99-100, 104-105, 108, 121-123, 125, 128, 132, 134-137, 140-143, 146-148, 150, 152-153, 156, 158-159, 164, 168-170, 184, 192-194, 201-202, 262, 267-268, 270-274, 280, 283, 285, 291-292, 295, 298-303, 306, 313-315, 325-331, 333-335, 337
CO 22, 76, 78, 229, 231, 237, 243
CO2 229, 231, 237, 243
COGNITIVE RADIO NETWORKS 159, 169-170, 174, 177, 179-181

D

Deep Learning 73, 89, 91, 156, 158, 170-171, 174-175, 178-181, 203, 205-209, 213-215, 217, 219, 221-223, 225, 228, 271, 275, 280-281, 294-296, 303, 338
Diabetic Foot Ulcer Detection 203, 223
Diabetic Prediction 206
Diagnosis 2, 58, 147, 165-166, 168, 207, 219, 226, 261, 263, 279, 281-282, 287-289, 303, 309-312, 317, 321, 324, 326-327, 329, 335

Directions 30, 67, 76, 80-81, 84, 89, 91, 97, 132, 150, 219, 268, 271, 273-274, 280, 283, 288, 297, 299, 335

E

Ethical Considerations 5, 18, 28-29, 31, 46, 65, 70, 72, 79-80, 96-97, 100, 134-135, 137, 146, 193, 195, 248, 250, 256, 265, 270, 301, 330-331

H

Healthcare 1-7, 9-11, 14-15, 17-19, 23-24, 28-29, 31, 50-51, 55, 57-59, 69-70, 73, 76, 78, 81, 84, 89, 94, 102, 149, 159, 164-170, 176-177, 179, 182-189, 192-194, 196-197, 199-201, 205-206, 219-222, 226, 229, 245-265, 267-268, 270-281, 283-293, 296-301, 303-317, 320, 322, 324, 326-337
healthcare delivery 4, 19, 247, 265, 306-308, 310-312, 314-315, 326-327, 329-330

I

Interactive Workouts 24

M

MACHINE LEARNING 21, 23, 50, 54, 77, 87, 91, 141, 154, 159, 164-168, 173-174, 176-179, 181, 193-194, 196, 203, 205-207, 216, 220, 225-226, 245,

Index

268, 275, 280-282, 319, 326-327, 331

Medical Metaverse 92, 202, 277, 302

Metaverse 1-11, 13-19, 25-32, 37, 39-40, 43-45, 51-54, 56-57, 59, 61-94, 96-100, 102, 104, 106-109, 112-113, 122-124, 129-130, 133-140, 142, 144-146, 150-157, 182-189, 193-202, 232-233, 235, 237, 244-246, 248-273, 275-281, 283-293, 297-305, 310, 324, 332-333, 335

Metaverse Systems 4-7, 14-16

Mindfulness 2, 10, 12, 56-57, 93, 96-108, 110, 112-113, 115-116, 118-119, 123-124, 127-129, 132-137, 139, 141, 143-144, 147-151, 153-156, 262

O

Opportunities 2, 7, 12, 18, 22-23, 26-27, 50, 61, 65, 69, 71-72, 77, 80-81, 83, 87, 89, 91, 112, 134-136, 139, 142, 146, 177, 179, 183, 187-188, 200, 249, 255, 266, 268, 270, 272-274, 277, 286-287, 300-301, 306, 334, 337

P

Patient 2-6, 8-9, 11-14, 17, 19, 51, 55, 58-59, 73, 77, 85, 88, 150, 155, 163-165, 167-168, 176, 178, 182-183, 188-189, 191-197, 199-200, 205-206, 219-222, 230-231, 245, 249-250, 252-253, 256-265, 271, 274-282, 284-286, 289-293, 295-297, 303, 305, 307-312, 315, 317, 319-322, 324-329, 331, 334

Potential 3-6, 8-15, 17-19, 25-32, 36, 39, 43-46, 54, 57-59, 61-63, 65-72, 76, 81, 84, 86, 89, 91, 94, 96-97, 99, 102-109, 111, 113-116, 119, 121, 123, 126-128, 130-131, 133-135, 137, 140, 147, 154, 159, 168-169, 176, 183, 185-186, 189, 193-194, 198-200, 203-205, 215, 217, 219, 221-222, 224, 249, 251-254, 256-259, 263-265, 268-270, 273-276, 284-288, 296-297, 299-300, 305-306, 308-315, 326-328, 330-331

R

Real-Time Monitoring 4, 8, 17, 127, 168-169, 193, 230, 262, 311-312, 322

Rehabilitation 2, 16, 29, 50-51, 55, 69-70, 75, 80-81, 83-85, 87, 91, 119-120, 141, 182-202, 279, 285, 289, 334

S

SECRET KEY 164-168, 177-178, 180, 238

Skills 2, 4, 10, 12, 57-58, 79, 85, 127, 149, 182-183, 185, 197-199, 201, 219, 253, 278, 298

T

Technological advancements 1-2, 20, 24-25, 30, 32, 34, 54, 100, 135-137, 266, 295, 313, 330

Technologies 1-4, 18-19, 22, 24-29, 31-32, 34, 36, 39, 43, 47, 49-51, 54-55, 57, 61, 63, 65, 67, 70, 74, 76, 83-86, 89-91, 94, 96-99, 110-111, 132-133, 135-136, 139-141, 146, 150, 152-153, 155-156, 159, 170, 176-177, 181-182, 184, 186, 188-189, 193, 195, 202, 232-233, 246-247, 249, 251-252, 262, 264-265, 269, 273-274, 277, 281, 283-286, 288-294, 296, 298-299, 301-303, 306, 308, 310-312, 316, 326, 330-331, 334-336

Telemedicine 4-5, 19, 58-59, 85, 94, 182-183, 192, 220-221, 229, 249-250, 253, 270, 275-276, 281, 289, 291, 293, 296, 300, 307-338

Treatment 2, 4, 6, 9, 11, 17, 19, 55, 58-59, 79, 132, 140, 147-148, 153, 156, 161, 165, 168, 183, 185, 188, 193-195, 199-200, 205, 213, 219-221, 249, 251-252, 258-264, 275-281, 284, 286, 288-289, 291, 293, 296-297, 304, 306, 308-312, 314-317, 321-322, 324-327, 330

V

Virtual Gym 26, 29, 31, 33, 35, 43-44, 51, 55

Virtual Meditation 12, 93-94, 96-101, 105,

405

108, 110, 114-123, 125-127, 132, 134-137
Virtual Reality (VR) 2, 6, 93, 148, 152, 182, 184, 188-189, 193, 198, 257-258, 277, 309
Virtual Spaces 46, 68-70, 81, 94, 96, 98, 114-115, 135, 186
Virtual Sports 27-31, 37-39, 48, 57-58, 61-62, 64-65, 70-71, 90

W

WBAN 159-164, 169, 174, 176-179
wearable devices 8, 13, 32, 54, 81, 111, 135-136, 183, 193, 299, 311-312, 318-321, 324, 330

Recommended Reference Books

IGI Global's reference books are available in three unique pricing formats:
Print Only, E-Book Only, or Print + E-Book.
Order direct through IGI Global's Online Bookstore at www.igi-global.com or through your preferred provider.

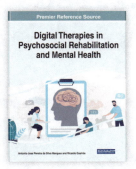

Digital Therapies in Psychosocial Rehabilitation and Mental Health

ISBN: 9781799886341
EISBN: 9781799886365
© 2022; 414 pp.
List Price: US$ 380

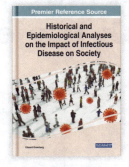

Historical and Epidemiological Analyses on the Impact of Infectious Disease on Society

ISBN: 9781799886891
EISBN: 9781799886914
© 2022; 261 pp.
List Price: US$ 325

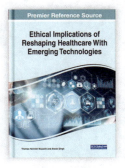

Ethical Implications of Reshaping Healthcare With Emerging Technologies

ISBN: 9781799878889
EISBN: 9781799878896
© 2022; 242 pp.
List Price: US$ 325

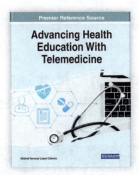

Advancing Health Education With Telemedicine

ISBN: 9781799887836
EISBN: 9781799887843
© 2022; 377 pp.
List Price: US$ 325

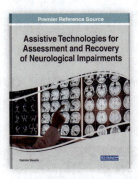

Assistive Technologies for Assessment and Recovery of Neurological Impairments

ISBN: 9781799874300
EISBN: 9781799874317
© 2022; 396 pp.
List Price: US$ 325

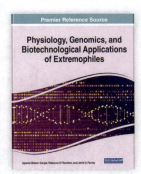

Physiology, Genomics, and Biotechnological Applications of Extremophiles

ISBN: 9781799891444
EISBN: 9781799891468
© 2022; 473 pp.
List Price: US$ 380

Do you want to stay current on the latest research trends, product announcements, news, and special offers?
Join IGI Global's mailing list to receive customized recommendations, exclusive discounts, and more.
Sign up at: www.igi-global.com/newsletters.

Publisher of Timely, Peer-Reviewed Inclusive Research Since 1988

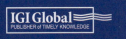

www.igi-global.com   Sign up at www.igi-global.com/newsletters   facebook.com/igiglobal   twitter.com/igiglobal

Ensure Quality Research is Introduced to the Academic Community

Become an Evaluator for IGI Global Authored Book Projects

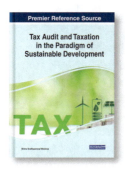 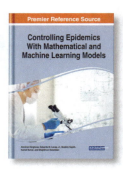 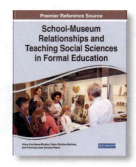 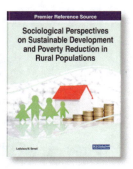

The overall success of an authored book project is dependent on quality and timely manuscript evaluations.

Applications and Inquiries may be sent to:
development@igi-global.com

Applicants must have a doctorate (or equivalent degree) as well as publishing, research, and reviewing experience. Authored Book Evaluators are appointed for one-year terms and are expected to complete at least three evaluations per term. Upon successful completion of this term, evaluators can be considered for an additional term.

If you have a colleague that may be interested in this opportunity, we encourage you to share this information with them.

Easily Identify, Acquire, and Utilize Published
Peer-Reviewed Findings in Support of Your Current Research

IGI Global OnDemand

Purchase Individual IGI Global OnDemand Book Chapters and Journal Articles

For More Information:
www.igi-global.com/e-resources/ondemand/

Browse through 150,000+ Articles and Chapters!

Find specific research related to your current studies and projects that have been contributed by international researchers from prestigious institutions, including:

 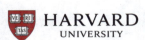 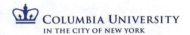 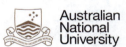

- Accurate and Advanced Search
- Affordably Acquire Research
- Instantly Access Your Content
- Benefit from the InfoSci Platform Features

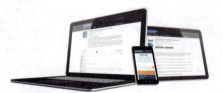

"It really provides **an excellent entry into the research literature of the field**. It presents a manageable number of **highly relevant sources** on topics of interest to a wide range of researchers. The sources are **scholarly, but also accessible** to 'practitioners'."

- Ms. Lisa Stimatz, MLS, University of North Carolina at Chapel Hill, USA

Interested in Additional Savings?

Subscribe to
IGI Global OnDemand *Plus*

Learn More

Acquire content from over 128,000+ research-focused book chapters and 33,000+ scholarly journal articles for as low as US$ 5 per article/chapter (original retail price for an article/chapter: US$ 37.50).

7,300+ E-BOOKS.
ADVANCED RESEARCH.
INCLUSIVE & AFFORDABLE.

IGI Global e-Book Collection

- **Flexible Purchasing Options** (Perpetual, Subscription, EBA, etc.)
- Multi-Year Agreements with **No Price Increases** Guaranteed
- **No Additional Charge** for Multi-User Licensing
- No Maintenance, Hosting, or Archiving Fees
- Continually Enhanced & Innovated **Accessibility Compliance Features** (WCAG)

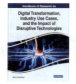

Handbook of Research on Digital Transformation, Industry Use Cases, and the Impact of Disruptive Technologies
ISBN: 9781799877127
EISBN: 9781799877141

Handbook of Research on New Investigations in Artificial Life, AI, and Machine Learning
ISBN: 9781799886860
EISBN: 9781799886877

Handbook of Research on Future of Work and Education
ISBN: 9781799882756
EISBN: 9781799882770

Research Anthology on Physical and Intellectual Disabilities in an Inclusive Society (4 Vols.)
ISBN: 9781668435427
EISBN: 9781668435434

Innovative Economic, Social, and Environmental Practices for Progressing Future Sustainability
ISBN: 9781799895909
EISBN: 9781799895923

Applied Guide for Event Study Research in Supply Chain Management
ISBN: 9781799889694
EISBN: 9781799889717

Mental Health and Wellness in Healthcare Workers
ISBN: 9781799888130
EISBN: 9781799888147

Clean Technologies and Sustainable Development in Civil Engineering
ISBN: 9781799898108
EISBN: 9781799898122

Request More Information, or Recommend the IGI Global e-Book Collection to Your Institution's Librarian

---

For More Information or to Request a Free Trial, Contact IGI Global's e-Collections Team: eresources@igi-global.com | 1-866-342-6657 ext. 100 | 717-533-8845 ext. 100

Are You Ready to Publish Your Research?

IGI Global
PUBLISHER of TIMELY KNOWLEDGE

IGI Global offers book authorship and editorship opportunities across 11 subject areas, including business, computer science, education, science and engineering, social sciences, and more!

Benefits of Publishing with IGI Global:

- Free one-on-one editorial and promotional support.
- Expedited publishing timelines that can take your book from start to finish in less than one (1) year.
- Choose from a variety of formats, including Edited and Authored References, Handbooks of Research, Encyclopedias, and Research Insights.
- Utilize IGI Global's eEditorial Discovery® submission system in support of conducting the submission and double-blind peer review process.
- IGI Global maintains a strict adherence to ethical practices due in part to our full membership with the Committee on Publication Ethics (COPE).
- Indexing potential in prestigious indices such as Scopus®, Web of Science™, PsycINFO®, and ERIC – Education Resources Information Center.
- Ability to connect your ORCID iD to your IGI Global publications.
- Earn honorariums and royalties on your full book publications as well as complimentary content and exclusive discounts.

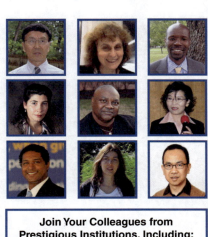

Join Your Colleagues from Prestigious Institutions, Including:

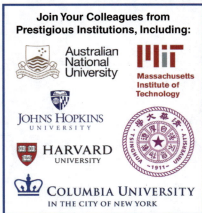

Australian National University
Massachusetts Institute of Technology
Johns Hopkins University
Harvard University
Tsinghua
Columbia University in the City of New York

Learn More at: www.igi-global.com/publish
or by Contacting the Acquisitions Department at: acquisition@igi-global.com